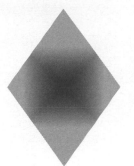

Developing Practical Nursing Skills

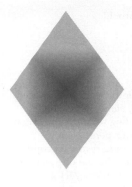

Developing Practical Nursing Skills

Edited by

Lesley Baillie

RGN, MSc(Nurs), BA(Hons), ONC, RNT

Senior Lecturer,
University of Luton

A member of the Hodder Headline Group
LONDON   NEW YORK   NEW DELHI

First published in Great Britain in 2001 by Arnold
A member of the Hodder Headline Group,
338 Euston Road, London NWI 3BH

British Library Cataloguing in Publication Data
A catalogue record for this book is available from the British Library

Library of Congress Cataloging-in-Publication Data
A catalog record for this book is available from the Library of
Congress

ISBN 0 340 76002 8

3   4   5   6   7   8   9   10

Commissioning Editor: Aileen Parlane
Production Editor: Lauren McAllister
Production Controller: Bryan Eccleshall

Typeset in 10/14 pt Palatino by
Scribe Design, Gillingham, Kent
Printed and bound in India

Contents

Contents

Contents

Preface

This book aims to provide an opportunity for nurses to develop a foundation in practical nursing skills. Whilst it has been written for student nurses who are in their common foundation programme, it will also be valuable to anybody working in a caring capacity who needs to develop skills, as well as those involved in teaching them. The idea for the book arose from the authors' experiences with students, and both lecturers' and students' concerns about developing practical skills. Interactive 'skills packages' were produced for a number of skills which enabled students to work in a self-directed manner.

As Chapter 1 emphasizes, developing clinical competence requires repeated practice with actual patients and clients. However it has been increasingly accepted that preparation for practical skills can reduce students' anxiety and improve confidence. Practitioners are more likely to be willing to demonstrate and supervize skills for students who have some prior knowledge as, with the increasing pressures within the health service, time is often limited. When students do have opportunities to practice, there is often little time to explore underpinning knowledge. This book plans to address this by including research-based rationale for skills wherever available, while also encouraging the reader to think about the 'why' of what he or she is doing, rather than just the 'how'.

The book starts by exploring the nature of practical nursing skills within the context of caring, and emphasizes how they can be carried out therapeutically. The way in which practical skills can be learnt is then examined and the role of reflection is considered. There is discussion about how learning opportunities can be maximized within the practice setting, the role of classroom learning, and the use of skills laboratories. The effect of the nurse's approach and attitude while carrying out practical nursing skills is focused on in Chapter 2, providing a foundation for the other chapters.

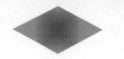

Each of the remaining chapters covers a collection of related skills. There are obvious links between the chapters and so cross-referencing occurs when relevant. Other specialized reading is referred to as appropriate. The practical nursing skills included are those which may be needed across adult, mental health, learning disability and child settings and thus how the skill can be adapted and individualized for each, is discussed. The skills chapters start with practice scenarios from the four branches of nursing, which illustrate when the skills will be needed. The content of the chapters links back to these scenarios, thus encouraging application. The reader is also asked to reflect on practice experience and to access particular equipment during placements, and within the skills laboratory. Exercises are included to help students become actively involved in the text, familiar with equipment, and to understand how and why practical skills are carried out.

Finally, a few explanatory notes. There seems to be no one acceptable term that can be used for the huge range of people whom nurses are involved with. In most mental health, community learning disability, and some adult branch settings, 'client' is the acceptable term. In residential settings, however, the term 'resident' is considered more appropriate. In many in-patient adult and child settings, particularly acute services, 'patient' is an acceptable term to be used, but in children's nursing, nurses focus on the whole family. Rather than adopt just one term within this book, a variety are used throughout. We have tried to use the most appropriate term for the content being discussed, but on occasion have stated 'patient/client'. A similar difficulty arises in relation to gender. Where what is being discussed is obviously related to a particular gender (such as female catheterization) then the obvious terms (her, she) have been used. In skills that may apply to any gender, we have arbitrarily used either, as to write 'him or her' 'she or he' throughout the text is clumsy. For simplicity, the nurse is usually referred to as 'she' throughout, but we fully recognize that it may be 'he'! We hope we have not offended anyone!

Contributors

Chapter authors

Vickie Arrowsmith (Chapters 3 and 6)
RGN, BA(Hons), PGCEA
Senior Lecturer,
University of Luton

Lesley Baillie (Chapters 1, 6, 8, 10 and 12)
RGN, MSc(Nurs), BA(Hons), ONC, RNT
Senior Lecturer,
University of Luton

Dee Burrows (Chapter 3)
BSc(Hons), RGN, RCNT, RNT, DipN(Lond), PhD
Head of Department,
Acute and Critical Care,
University of Luton

Kay Child (Chapter 4)
RGN, RCNT, BA(Hons)
Senior Lecturer,
University of Luton

Veronica Corben (Chapters 8 and 11)
RGN, MSc(Nurs), BSc(Hons), RNT, DPNP, Diploma Cancer Nursing
Principal Lecturer,
University of Luton

Sue Higham (Chapters 4, 7 and 8; reviewed and gave input into Chapters 3, 5, 6, 10 and 12)
RSCN, RGN, BSc(Hons), DPSN
Senior Lecturer,
University of Luton

Sue Maddex (Chapter 7)
RGN, BSc(Hons), Post Grad Diploma, PGCE Advanced Health Care Practice
Senior Lecturer,
University of Luton

Chrissie Major (Chapter 5)
RGN, BSc(Hons)
Senior Lecturer,
University of Luton

Nicola M. Neale (Chapter 2)
RGN, RNT, MA(Ed.), Postgrad. Diploma Cancer Care
Senior Lecturer,
University of Luton

Alex Nesbitt (Chapter 10)
RGN, BA(Hons), BSc(Hons), PGCE
Senior Lecturer,
University of Plymouth

Glynis Pellatt (Chapter 9)
RGN, MA, BA(Hons), DipN(Lond), ONC, RNT, RCNT
Senior Lecturer,
University of Luton

Joanne Sale (Chapter 2)
RMN, RGN, BSc(Hons), PGCEA, RNT
Senior Lecturer,
University of Luton

Other major contributors

Penny Goacher (Formulated biology questions)
BSc (Biology)
Senior Lecturer,
University of Luton

John O'Shaughnessy (reviewed and gave learning disability input into Chapters 4, 5, 6, 10 and 12)
RNMH, BSc(Hons), Cert.Ed.
Senior Lecturer,
University of Luton

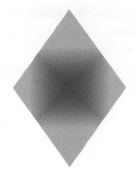

Acknowledgements

We are grateful to the many practitioners, students and colleagues in the University of Luton, who gave encouragement, inspiration and reviewed material. Many thanks also to the authors' families whose support during the writing of the chapters in the book has been much appreciated.

Special thanks to those listed below:
Alan Baillie, Staff Nurse, Acute Mental Health Admissions (under 65s)
Tracey Geddes, Senior Staff Nurse, Spinal Injuries
Paul Hannigan, Staff Nurse, Admission Ward for Elderly Mentally Ill
Hilary Hollingsworth, Senior Staff Nurse, Day Hospital
Melsina Makaza, Community Staff Nurse, Elderly Mentally Ill
Sallie McClarty and Chris Pick, Infection Control Sisters
Kirsten O'Reilly, Community Nurse for Learning Disability
Fiona Scafe, Sister, Paediatric Unit
Janine Smith, Staff Nurse, Learning Disability
Sheryl Venters, Tissue Viability Nurse
Helena Heywood, Dermatology Nurse.

Student nurses: Aoife Hughes, Joanne Roberts, Mark Prescott, Roben Gangridzo, Maxine Todd, Jennie Freeborn, Martine Stadler, Reshad Allymamod, Pauline Pennington, Louisa Grace.
Faye Riley (student nurse): illustrations: Chapters 4 and 8.

Colleagues at University of Luton:
Ann Hedges: reviewed and gave learning disability input into Chapters 8 and 9.
John Ross: reviewed and gave learning disability input into Chapter 10.
Carol Barren: reviewed and gave children's nursing input into Chapters 6, 9 and 11.
Valerie Young, who reviewed and gave helpful comments on Chapter 1.

Acknowledgements

Thanks also to Dee Burrows, who first suggested the interactive approach to learning practical nursing skills which has formed the basis for this book's approach, and carried out initial work towards seeking publication.

We would also like to thank the staff at Arnold, in particular Aileen Parlane and Lauren McAllister, for their patience and support.

Learning practical nursing skills: an introduction

Lesley Baillie

INTRODUCTION

Probably no-one would dispute that caring is an essential feature of nursing, and to demonstrate caring and caring attitudes, the nurse must be a competent practitioner (Roach 1992). The focus of this book is to assist the reader in developing the ability to carry out a range of practical skills with different client groups. Being able to perform a practical nursing skill involves not only the 'hands-on' (psychomotor) element, but needs evidence-based knowledge, effective interpersonal skills, awareness of the ethical dimension of care, creative and reflective thinking, and an appropriate professional attitude. These elements will be considered throughout the text.

To achieve the competencies required of a registered nurse does of course require more than being able to carry out a range of practical skills. However, developing ability to perform practical skills safely is necessary for all student nurses (Department of Health 1999; English National Board (ENB) 2000), and it is this specific element of nursing which is the remit of this book. There are many other texts aimed at student nurses which comprehensively cover the other necessary subjects (see later in this chapter: Recommended reading).

This chapter will be discussing the nature of practical skills in nursing, how these skills can be learnt, and how this book can help you to develop a foundation in nursing skills. There is particular emphasis on encouraging you to develop and value these practical skills as holistic, caring skills, which can also give you the opportunity to develop the therapeutic use of self. The topics covered are:

- What are practical nursing skills?
- The range of practical skills used by nurses.

- Practical skills included in this book, and use of practice scenarios
- Dimensions of practical skills:
  - The affective dimension
  - The cognitive dimension
  - The motor dimension
- Practical skills within the context of caring:
  - The experience of non-caring versus caring
  - Roach's 5Cs: a framework for caring
  - Transcultural caring
- Therapeutic nursing and practical skills
- How can you develop your practical nursing skills?
  - Stages of skill performance
  - Developing the affective, cognitive and motor elements of a skill
  - The importance of obtaining feedback
  - Learning from experience and reflection
  - The skills laboratory
  - Learning in the practice setting
- Recommended reading.

WHAT ARE PRACTICAL NURSING SKILLS?

To be a competent nurse requires mastery of a range of skills including practical, communication and management skills. These are often integrated within the nursing role, because carrying out practical nursing skills effectively will also require skills in, for example, communication, teamwork and delegation. What, however, are practical nursing skills? Bjork (1999a) defines practical nursing skills as 'hands-on actions that promote the patients' physical comfort, hygiene and safe medical treatment (which are) . . . commonly referred to as procedures or psychomotor skills'. This definition appears to imply a purely physical perspective. However there is no doubt that practical skills will often enhance social and psychological comfort and well-being too; oral hygiene is a good example of this. Bradshaw (1994) notes that physical, social, psychological, and spiritual care is actually an integrated whole and cannot be separated. Thus while a practical nursing skill may appear to be a physical procedure, it will not result only in a physical effect.

Romyn (1999) argues that deciding what constitutes a practical nursing skill is problematic, as many skills, which are carried out by nurses, are not solely their domain, for example, injections can be given by doctors too. In this book it is assumed that practical nursing skills are skills which involve 'hands-on' care by nurses with clients, although some of these skills may also be performed by other professionals. There are a vast range of practical skills which nurses use, and they must adapt these skills in different situations with differing client groups.

THE RANGE OF PRACTICAL SKILLS USED BY NURSES

Traditionally there has been a hierarchy of skills within nursing with experienced nurses undertaking more technical, medical skills such as those to do with medication, and junior staff carrying out what was sometimes referred to as 'basic nursing care', that is, assisting the client with activities of daily living such as hygiene and elimination. This system has been considered biomedical and task-focused (McMahon 1998) rather than being client-focused with the nurse delivering all the care required by that particular client. The term 'basic' has often been used in a derisory fashion, the implication being that these skills are not as important as more technical ones. Yet to help an elderly person regain the ability to wash and dress, or to help a person with confusion to maintain continence, might be a much more complex skill than many which are apparently more technical and medically orientated, such as removal of clips from a wound. Bjork (1999b), in a longitudinal in-depth study of practical skill development, analyzed the skill of mobilizing a post operative patient, and highlighted the complexity of this apparently 'simple' skill. She noted the effect of numerous individual factors, such as the patient's ability to respond to instructions and general physical and mental well-being, which affected how the skill was carried out.

The notion of delivering individualized care for clients, operationalized through the nursing process (assessing, planning, implementing and evaluating care), and based on the framework of a nursing (rather than medical) model, has become widely accepted within nursing. How nursing models are developed and chosen by practitioners is discussed by Johns (1994), and an overview of nursing models can be found in Schober (1998). However, with the role expansion of registered nurses (with many taking on skills previously carried out by doctors, such as intravenous cannulation), and the increasing use of health-care assistants whose training is competency based, to deny that a skills hierarchy does not exist is probably unrealistic. However it is hoped that practical skills can still be client centred and delivered within the context of a caring philosophy, with value attached to fundamental as well as technical care.

PRACTICAL SKILLS INCLUDED IN THIS BOOK, AND USE OF PRACTICE SCENARIOS

While developing our new pre-registration curriculum at University of Luton, we extensively surveyed practitioners from all branches and settings (hospital/residential and community), to investigate what skills would be considered essential or desirable in a newly registered nurse within that setting. From this data we were able to identify what we termed 'core skills', which were skills considered essential or desirable, across a range of settings: adult, child, learning disability and mental health. This book, as a foundation text, includes the core skills which students should expect to develop a foundation in by the end of the common foundation programme (CFP). Note that although ability to perform basic life support is an expected skill of all registered nurses, this skill requires training with thorough classroom practice and is covered in depth in the current first aid manual (Webb *et al.* 1997). For these reasons basic life support is not covered within this text.

Each chapter begins with a scenario from adult, child, learning disability and mental health-care settings, and the chapter will link the content back to these patients/clients, thus encouraging theory–practice links. This use of practice-based scenarios as a basis for study, will be a familiar approach for many students, with the increasing use of problem/enquiry/evidence based curricula; these have been recently endorsed by the ENB (2000). It has been aimed to include a selection of scenarios, from a variety of settings, but it is not intended that all possible situations are represented. All scenarios are based on real situations but identifying details have been changed or omitted, with pseudonyms allocated at random.

PRACTICAL SKILLS: MOTOR, COGNITIVE AND AFFECTIVE DIMENSIONS

Activity | Everyone will have had an injection at some stage, and indeed you may have had recent immunizations to enter the nursing programme. You probably took it for granted that the skill would be performed competently, but try to identify the different elements that this skill would have entailed.

You probably considered that there are technical aspects such as drawing up the correct drug accurately using sterile equipment, but may also have identified that the skill would have required underlying knowledge of the drug's actions and potential side effects, and that the nurse would have used a calm and friendly approach to relax you and relieve anxiety. This example illustrates that effective practical nursing skills will require a skilled motor performance (the 'doing' element), a sound knowledge base (based on best evidence), and an appropriate attitude towards the client. Bjork (1999a) reviews the concept of nursing practical skills and concludes that they were for many years commonly considered to comprise the art of nursing. However, she identifies that more recently these skills have been termed motor or psychomotor skills, and it has been the technical, motor element that has been emphasized.

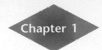

Oermann (1990) also suggests that the motor (doing) element of a practical (psychomotor) skill is often emphasized to the exclusion of the cognitive and affective component. She highlights the importance of the cognitive base (the scientific principles underlying the performance of the skill) and the affective domain, which reflects the nurse's values and concern for the client while the skill is being performed. It can be argued that in order to provide high quality care, the nurse must be competent to apply theory and skill in each clinical situation, which includes knowledge, and mastery in each of the psychomotor, cognitive and affective domains (Fitzpatrick *et al.* 1992). These three aspects will now be discussed.

The affective dimension

The affective domain of a practical skill includes the nurse's attitude and approach to the client as well as the ethical dimension. Bush and Barr's (1997) study of critical care nurses' experiences of caring identified the affective process as including sensitivity, empathy, concern and interest. One participant is quoted as saying: 'instead of just saying, "I'm taking your blood pressure, your temperature" you really care about what the patient is going through – how they must feel – you kind of put yourself in their position, and how you'd want to be taken care of yourself instead of just a mechanical (action) . . .'. Bjork (1999a) argues that it is the intentional element of practical nursing skills which sets them apart from other skills. She suggests that caring intentions are necessary in practical nursing actions because 'they can transform the acts of handling and helping into tolerable or even meaningful experiences for the patient'. She goes on to suggest that within the application of a practical skill, the nurse can use the situation to convey respect for and interest in the patient, conveying the message that 'it is not just a body that is being handled'. While carrying out a practical skill, such as bathing, a nurse can take the opportunity to foster confidence and develop a trusting relationship, as being involved in such activities offers the nurse the opportunity of becoming closer to the patient or client (Wharton and Pearson 1988). Bjork (1999a) highlights the importance of being aware of the meaning of the practical skill for the individual, and how it fits into the person's overall experience. For example, a wound dressing may exemplify the change in body image following invasive surgery, and bathing someone may highlight their loss of independence due to physical or mental health problems.

Each time you carry out a practical skill with a patient/client, you will be conveying a message about your state of being (Paterson and Zderad 1988); for example are you anxious, in a hurry, distracted or uninterested? The nurse's approach to clients during practical nursing skills application is considered in Chapter 2.

The cognitive dimension

This reflects the 'thinking' element behind the skill, including the application of research to practice and problem solving, and is what makes the nurse a 'knowledgeable doer'. Being able to adapt a skill in the practice setting requires a sound underlying knowledge of why it is being performed and the rationale for each stage. For example, understanding the principles behind the administration of oxygen therapy will enable the nurse to choose a method of administration which is acceptable to a client in a specific clinical situation. There is increasing emphasis on 'evidence-based care' throughout health care with the aim that all health-care professionals should be applying best evidence to their practice. Nurses need to choose best options when implementing care, and be reflective decision makers (Watkins 1997). In many cases this knowledge will be derived from empirical evidence–research, but it may also be based on the nurse's experience, and knowledge gained through reflection on practice. In Benner's (1984) work she identifies that practice is always more complex and presents many more realities than theory ever can, and she highlights the value of theory derived from practice (see later section: 'Learning from experience and reflection').

Various theorists have tried to explain the nature of knowledge within nursing. One of the first of these theorists was Carper (1978), who identified four 'ways of knowing': empirics (scientific knowledge); aesthetics (the art of nursing); personal (knowledge of self); and ethical. Empirical knowledge is that based on tested theory, such as research conducted to trial the effect of a specific wound dressing on wound healing. Aesthetic knowledge would be based on the nurse's intuitive grasp of the whole unique situation, for example, the meaning of the patient's wound to him and the ability to skilfully individualize care. The nurse's personal knowledge would involve the nurse knowing herself, and the effect she is having on the interaction with the patient who is having the wound dressing. Ethical knowing will focus on moral decision making and values, for example, the ethical response if the patient refused to have the dressing done or if the nurse feels that the care being delivered is inadequate. Bearing in mind the position of a registered nurse as an accountable practitioner, it is important to be able to explain the knowledge base for practical skills. Manley (1997) examines a range of theory relating to the foundation of nursing knowledge and its philosophical underpinnings.

The difference between practical and theoretical knowledge is discussed by Benner (1984). She cites philosophers such as Kuhn (1970) and Polanyi (1958) who have observed that 'knowing-how' (for example, how to take a temperature) is different from 'knowing-that', (for example, what a normal temperature recording is and what might cause a low or high reading).

Benner (1984) goes on to explore how expert nurses develop knowledge from their practice, learning to recognize, for example, subtle changes in clients' conditions.

Not all nursing skills will have a firm evidence base on which to implement practice, but in many areas such research based knowledge is obtainable (Chapman 1997). Clients should be able to assume that practical skills carried out by nurses will be based on sound evidence if it is available, rather than on ritual or unsubstantiated knowledge. There have been a number of centres set up with a specific remit for the generation and use of research-based knowledge in the NHS: the Centre for Reviews and Dissemination, the Cochrane Database, the National Clinical Audit Information and Dissemination Centre, the UK Outcome Clearing House and The Centre for Evidence-Based Medicine. Most recently the National Institute for Clinical Excellence (NICE) has been established, to develop standards for health-care practice based on best evidence.

The motor dimension

Mastering the motor dimension of a skill is important in achieving a good outcome as lack of a skilled motor performance could jeopardise both safety and comfort. Knowing how to do a practical skill can be termed 'know-how' type of knowledge – practical expertise and skill, which is really acquired through practice and experience (Manley 1997). The characteristics of a skilled motor performance have been identified by Quinn (1995) and are shown in Table 1.1, applied to the administration of an injection. Nursing skills are performed in a changing clinical environment, with people who will respond and react in different ways, so the nurse will need to adapt the skill accordingly. This need for adaptability in practical nursing skills means that they can never be wholly automatic in nature.

Three types of motor skills have been identified (Oermann 1990). Fine motor skills are precision orientated tasks, for example drawing up and giving an injection. Manual skills are repetitive and often include eye–arm action, such as washing someone, and gross manual skills involve the whole body such as when assisting a person to walk. Quinn (1995) also explains that a motor skill may be continuous, requiring continuous adjustment and repetition (e.g. removing sutures), while a discrete skill is a one off movement (e.g. giving an injection). A further classification of a motor skill is 'closed loop' versus 'open loop'. A closed loop skill could be performed with the eyes closed as it needs no external stimuli, while an open loop skill needs reaction and feedback at each stage, such as when a wound dressing is being performed. As practical nursing skills involve people, they will be open loop in every situation.

Table 1.1 Characteristics of a skilled motor performance, illustrated by injection administration

Criteria	Explanation	Illustration
Accuracy	Performed with precision.	The injection is drawn up accurately maintaining asepsis and the needle is inserted into the correct body area.
Speed	Movements swift and confident.	The injection is performed without hesitation and once injected, the needle is withdrawn quickly.
Efficiency	Movements economical, leaving spare capacity available.	The nurse gathers equipment at the start and positions herself and equipment to avoid awkward movement.
Timing	Accurate timing and correct sequential order.	The steps in preparing the injection and administration are in the correct order, and the time given to each stage is appropriate.
Consistency	Results are consistent.	The injection is performed in this manner on each occasion.
Anticipation	Can anticipate events quickly and respond accordingly.	The nurse anticipates that the client may become tense or move suddenly, and is able to respond effectively by steadying the injection and using appropriate communication.
Adaptability	Can adapt the skill to current circumstances.	Adapts injection administration taking into account factors such as age, level of anxiety and physical build of the client.
Perception	Can obtain maximum information from a minimum of cues.	Quickly takes in factors which could affect the skill. For example perceives the client's reluctance to have an injection from minimal observation and questioning.

PRACTICAL SKILLS WITHIN THE CONTEXT OF CARING

You were probably asked to state reasons for wanting to study nursing in your application, and almost certainly cited a desire to care, amongst them. That caring is inherent within nursing is a theme to be found in many nurse theorists' work. Watson (1979) has stated that 'the practice of caring is central to nursing' (p. 9). Benner and Wrubel (1989) consider that the 'nature of the caring relationship is central to most nursing interventions' (p. 5). They identify that the same act done in a non-caring way, as opposed to a caring way, will have very different consequences, thus 'nursing can never be reduced to mere technique' (p. 4). Caring is identified by Roach (1992) as both a natural concomitant of being a human and as the core of nursing. McMahon (1998) considers that in Britain, it is widely accepted that the concept of care is the nurse's domain. Bjork (1999b) presents a model of practical skill performance, which includes aspects such as sequence and fluency, but also includes caring comportment. This, she views, as being how the nurse creates a respectful, accepting, and encouraging atmosphere, which includes concern for the whole person.

The experience of non-caring versus caring

The detrimental effects of skills being implemented without a caring context are identified in a study by Halldorsdottir (1991). The in-depth interviews which she conducted with former patients highlighted the vulnerability of patients who found uncaring encounters with nurses to be discouraging and distressing. Patients described being initially puzzled and disbelieving, followed by feelings of anger and resentment, and then despair and helplessness. She found that dependent people being uncared for developed feelings of a sense of loss, and of being betrayed by those counted on for caring. Non-caring nurses were described as being 'cold human beings, like computers'. Box 1.1 illustrates the effect on an individual of feeling uncared for. Halldorsdottir describes this feeling as dehumanization, with the person feeling that he has no value as a person and is 'an object': 'I was . . . a piece of dust on the floor'. The uncaring nurse, Halldorsdottir found, did carry out the routine tasks (as the nurse in Box 1.1 did leave a vomit bowl for Jane), but was perceived as not 'caring about the patient as a person'.

> Jane, aged 14 years, was in hospital following orthopaedic surgery. During the night she felt very nauseated and then started to vomit. She was unable to reach her call bell. Eventually a nearby patient called a nurse. The nurse told her off for not pressing her call bell, left a bowl on her table and walked away. Jane described feeling 'upset, unwanted and a waste of space'.

Box 1.1 Illustrative example of feeling uncared for

With application of this research to practical skills, to carry out observation of blood pressure in a technically competent manner would not, in itself, be perceived as caring. It is the nurse's approach to the client that makes the person feel cared for and of value. Fernandez's (1997) reflective account details how while carrying out 'routine' observations of blood pressure and pulse on a patient, she built rapport, trust and mutual respect, which led to the patient talking about his personal life crisis. Woodward's (1997) analysis of the literature on professional caring identifies these two elements as instrumental caring (the technique comprising skills and knowledge) and expressive caring (the emotional element which includes respect for the individual). It is expressive caring which, she suggests, transforms nursing actions into caring. Halldorsdottir (1991) identifies a 'life-sustaining mode of being with a patient' which includes 'compassionate competence, genuine concern for the patient as a person, undivided attention when the nurse is with the patient, and cheerfulness'. This approach is described as 'professional caring'. Participants in the research felt relief when they felt cared for, and believed that this diminished anxiety and gave them time to concentrate on getting better.

Roach (1992) has made a study of caring in relation to nursing and developed a framework: the five Cs. These are compassion, competence, confidence, conscience and commitment.

Roach's 5Cs: a framework for caring

Compassion is defined by Roach (1992) as 'a way of living born out of an awareness of one's relationship to all living creatures; engendering a response of participation in the experience of another; a sensitivity to the pain and brokenness of the other; a quality of presence which allows one to share with and make room for the other' (p. 58). Roach argues that compassion is needed more than ever to humanize the ever increasing cold and impersonal technology used within health care. Box 1.2 illustrates this with a nurse's act of compassion which occurred in the highly technical environment of the intensive therapy unit.

James was in the final stages of heart and lung failure and his nurse, about to go home after a 12-hour shift and knowing that she would not see him again, asked him if there was anything she could get him before she left. He replied 'Oh a port and brandy please!' Phone calls around the hospital were unsuccessful in locating any and the nurse went off shift. She returned half an hour later with a small glass of port and brandy brought from home. As James was unable to swallow she dipped sponge mouth sticks into the drink and put them in his mouth for him to suck. James grinned and said it was 'wonderful'. This act of compassion brought tenderness to this patient's final hours and made an immeasurable difference to his relatives' feelings about his death.

Box 1.2 Compassion: an illustrative example from an intensive therapy unit

To ensure safe and effective care, practical skills must be carried out competently. Roach (1992) defines competence as having the 'knowledge, judgement, skills, energy, experience and motivation required to respond adequately to the demands of one's professional responsibilities' (p. 61). Roach goes on to state that 'while competence without compassion can be brutal and inhumane, compassion without competence may be no more than a meaningless, if not harmful, intrusion into the life of a person or persons needing help'. Wallis's (1998) in-depth study of patients' experiences of being cared for in a coronary care unit, found that patients viewed competence as essential in a caring nurse, e.g. 'You have got to have a competent nurse to start with'. It seemed that technical competence was reassuring to patients, and that this competence then allowed the nurse to 'transcend' the technology and become close to the patient. Competence also requires that healthy and safety is maintained, and this must be for the nurse as well as for the client.

Confidence is defined by Roach as 'the quality which fosters trusting relationships' (p. 62). Roach discusses the importance of not deceiving clients and states that 'caring confidence fosters trust without dependency; communicates truth without violence; and creates a relationship of respect without paternalism or without engendering a response borne out of professional caring' (p. 63). Consider a situation whereby a person who has had a hip fracture due to a fall is regaining mobility and independence. The client may lack confidence and be afraid of falling again, but the nurse's approach will enable a trusting relationship to be built. The nurse can help the client to set and reach realistic goals in mobilization, giving the client praise for achievements, and helping her to believe in her abilities.

Conscience is, according to Roach (1992), a 'state of moral awareness' (p. 63) and this will be exuded throughout the nurse's approach when undertaking practical skills. Roach considers that conscience grows out of experience, 'out of a process of valuing self and others' (p. 64). The nurse can demonstrate whether she values the person, and respects his right to dignified and humane care. She will also speak out if she feels that the client's care is compromised in any way.

Commitment is defined by Roach (1992) as 'a complex affective response characterized by a convergence between one's desires and one's obligations, and by a deliberate choice to act in accordance with them' (p. 65). This very much conjures up a picture of duty; the nurse may sometimes not want to carry out a certain practical skill, but commitment means that if it is necessary then she will do so. The situation discussed in Box 1.2 which exemplified compassion, also demonstrated commitment from the nurse to James, in her decision to bring in the drink from home despite just finishing a 12-hour shift.

Roach's five Cs act as a useful framework when considering how a practical skill can be carried out in a caring manner.

Activity

Think about the skill of feeding someone in a caring manner using the framework of the five Cs. Can you think of relevant points in relation to compassion, competence, confidence, conscience and commitment?

11

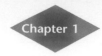

A few points in relation to each of the five Cs are discussed below, but you may well have thought of other issues. A compassionate approach to feeding someone entails being understanding and empathetic in manner, showing insight into the individual's experience of being fed, and using effective communication to convey this. This would include sitting at the person's level and not appearing rushed. Competence means that the nurse has knowledge about what nutrients the person needs, and can help the person to make informed menu choices. The competent nurse is aware of any potential problems such as swallowing difficulties, and ensures that the person is positioned so as to minimize problems. The nurse has the knowledge and skill to deal with choking if it occurs and if the person's nutritional input is being monitored, ensures that the meal is recorded accurately. The nurse also has knowledge about any special utensils deemed necessary. Confidence means that the nurse is honest in her dealings with the client, and realistic about his ability to regain independence in feeding. Realistic goals are set and the nurse encourages the client to work towards them. Conscience promotes awareness of moral dimensions, such as the approach to take if the person refuses food. Commitment on the nurse's part ensures that she is there to feed the client on time so that the food does not become cold, and that if the meal is unsuitable for the client, she makes the effort to contact the kitchens and ensure that a more acceptable meal is provided.

Transcultural caring

We live in a multicultural society, and practical nursing skills must be carried out with sensitivity and in a culturally appropriate manner for each individual and family. The American nurse and anthropologist, Madeleine Leininger, has studied transcultural caring over many years, and has identified how acts of caring, such as comforting and physical care, and the meaning attached to them, can vary between cultures (Leininger 1981). Leininger suggests that culture and caring cannot be separated within nursing actions and decision making. An overview of her theory can be found in Reynolds and Leininger (1993). Papadopoulos *et al.* (1998) have developed a model for the development of transcultural skills, consisting of four linked elements: cultural awareness, knowledge, sensitivity and competence.

- Cultural awareness includes examining and questioning one's personal value system (see Chapter 2: section on self-awareness), thus leading, the authors suggest, to the exploration of different views.
- Cultural knowledge may be drawn from sources such as sociology and research, and from experience of people. Where appropriate to specific practical skills, cultural variations (particularly related to religious beliefs)

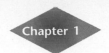

will be considered in this book. However there will often be individual and regional variations, and it is important to avoid stereotyping and making ethnocentric judgements; these are barriers to cultural sensitivity.

■ Cultural sensitivity, the third dimension of Papadoulos *et al.*'s model, can be achieved by nurses working with clients as partners, offering choices in care. Very important here are communication skills, respect and empathy (see Chapter 2: approach to clients and patients).

■ Cultural competence is achieved when practice is both antidiscriminatory and anti-oppressive. Papadopoulos *et al.* (1998)'s chapter includes a number of useful exercises aimed at promoting the development of transcultural caring skills.

THERAPEUTIC NURSING AND PRACTICAL SKILLS

The term therapeutic nursing can be defined as nursing which 'deliberately leads to beneficial outcomes for the patient' (McMahon, 1998, p. 7). At first glance it might seem obvious that this is what nursing seeks to attain, and if you look back to the discussion of feeding above, the care described should certainly have a positive effect on the client. However, read through Box 1.3, which illustrates how care relating to nutrition can be non-therapeutic. A recent headline in the Nursing Times ('This week' 2000) stated: 'Nurses "failed to feed us", patients say'. The article detailed that a Community Health Council had reported that nurses 'placed food out of patients' reach and failed to help them eat'. Thus unfortunate examples such as these illustrate that nursing does not always have a therapeutic effect on an individual. Indeed it might be said that some patients get better despite their nursing care, not because of it (McMahon 1998).

> Ellen had metastatic cancer at its last stages, was severely visually impaired and was being nursed in a side room. A plate of food was left in front of her wordlessly. When the nurse returned to collect the plate some while later, she remarked 'Oh you weren't hungry today then?' Ellen had not even known that the food was there. She could not see it, and would have been unable to reach it or feed herself anyway. She told the nurse that she had not known the food was there as she could not see. The nurse said 'Oh', picked up the tray and walked out.

Box 1.3 Non-therapeutic nursing: an illustrative example

McMahon (1998) identifies a number of activities in nursing (*see* Box 1.4) which can be considered therapeutic. Note that complementary health practices include such activities as massage, aromatherapy and reflexology. These require qualifications which are not usually included as part of pre-registration education, as the courses are quite extensive. NHS Trusts will usually have protocols for implementing complementary health practices. It is likely that they will only be performed by registered nurses holding the appropriate qualifications.

- Developing
  - partnership
  - intimacy
  - reciprocity in the nurse-patient relationship
- Caring and comforting
- Using evidence-based physical interventions
- Teaching
- Manipulating the environment
- Adopting complementary health practices.

Box 1.4 Therapeutic activities in nursing (McMahon 1998)

McMahon's (1998) framework will now be discussed, again in relation to feeding. Feeding a client is an ideal time to develop the nurse–patient relationship as it involves being physically close to the person, and giving one-to-one care. The nurse can use effective communication skills through-out the process to value the person. The very act of feeding should be comforting and make the person feel cared for as long as it is done consid-erately, without being rushed, and with the nurse aiming to meet individ-ual preferences. An evidence-based physical intervention could be the use of a nutritional assessment scale, and the whole process of feeding is a good opportunity for education. Examples include teaching the person to feed himself with special utensils, explaining about nutritional food choices, or the best position for eating to avoid choking. The nurse can promote a conducive environment for eating, by trying to ensure that it is comfortable and relaxed, and if the client wishes, encouraging meals to be social occasions.

Work by Ersser (1998) identified three core categories which he found reflected views about nurses' therapeutic actions. These were presentation of the nurse, such as non-verbal communication and greeting the patient, relat-ing to patients as when developing rapport, and specific actions of the nurse which are largely instrumental or procedural such as doing a wound dress-ing. When carrying out any practical nursing skill you need to consider how your actions can be therapeutic. For example, what will engender bathing a person a therapeutic action as opposed to simply attending to hygiene needs?

Reflecting on your practice can help you to identify how you could provide a more positive outcome for the client (see later section: 'Learning from experience and reflection').

HOW CAN YOU DEVELOP YOUR PRACTICAL NURSING SKILLS?

Activity

To understand how nurses acquire practical skills, reflect back on a practical skill which you have learnt previously, for example learning to drive. How did you learn this skill?

You may recall that you had to build up the skill in step by step stages, learning each sub-skill at a time. You could probably focus only on the skill, and found that it was difficult to do anything else (e.g. have a conversation) at the same time. Benner (1984) has identified that when learning any new skill, the performance will initially be 'halting and rigid' (p. 37) and that one must pay careful attention to the explicit rules relating to the skill.

It is important to realize that as a student you are not expected to be an expert in your practical skills! Benner's (1984) research adapted a skill acquisition model by Dreyfus and Dreyfus (1980) to describe different levels of performance in nurses. She conducted paired interviews with beginners and experienced nurses as well as doing participant observation with nurses at various levels of experience. The five stages of performance identified are outlined below.

Stages of skill performance

Stage 1: Novice

The novice nurse will have no experience on which to draw (new students but also experienced nurses moving to an unfamiliar area of practice). Benner describes the novice as being 'rule governed' in behaviour. By this she means that the novice will need explicit guidelines about what to do and in which sequence. However, these guidelines will need adapting to the actual situation, and the novice nurse will need help and guidance to do this.

Stage 2: Advanced beginner

At this stage the nurse can use previous experience and apply it in practice but will continue to need adequate support, particularly with aspects which are situational, such as prioritizing. She will have difficulty in seeing a situation as a whole and will focus on the specific skill to be carried out, regardless of additional situational factors.

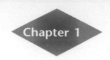

Stage 3: Competent

The competent nurse will be able to carry out conscious and deliberate planning, and prioritize and manage her work. However she lacks the flexibility and speed of the proficient nurse.

Stage 4: Proficient

The nurse can perceive situations holistically, recognize important and less important elements, and make decisions quickly. Benner found proficiency in nurses who have worked in an area for some time.

Stage 5: Expert

The expert nurse has a deep understanding and an intuitive grasp of situations, gained from substantial experience in the practice setting. You may observe this level in some practitioners with whom you work. In her book Benner gives many examples of expert nurses' care for clients. Such nurses may be excellent and inspirational role models but it is important not to feel inadequate or overawed by such expertise.

Developing the affective, cognitive and motor elements of a skill

A detailed review of theories about learning psychomotor skills can be found in Knight (1998).

Woodward's (1997) analysis indicates that developing the affective domain of a skill requires practice and perseverance, just as will the motor element. Roach (1992) has suggested that while nursing students may start their course with rudimentary expressive caring skills, these may sometimes go unrecognized and unvalued, and may be eroded rather than developed further. This book will include exercises throughout which focus on the affective dimension, asking you to think about, for example, how a patient might be feeling in a particular situation. Chapter 2 concentrates on the affective dimension of practical skills, and will help you to understand the concept of self-awareness, and how your values might affect how you carry out your care. Developing the cognitive domain of a skill will involve you in undertaking activities to acquire and understand the underpinning knowledge and rationale. Throughout this book research findings which underpin nursing practice will be discussed, but there will also be activities encouraging you to access other sources of knowledge, such as reflection on experience. It is hoped to encourage you to develop an enquiring and problem solving approach to your nursing practice.

To learn the motor dimension of a psychomotor skill requires practice; the opportunity to try out and repeat performance (Oermann 1990). It is only with practice that movement becomes refined and a smooth co-ordinated performance can be developed. The amount of practice needed will vary according to motivation to learn the skill, previous related skills learning, familiarity with equipment, level of anxiety, and the physical resources and co-ordination of the learner (Oermann 1990). Practice needs vary but more complex skills need more practice. Motivation affects mastery as many skills may be initially difficult, but a highly motivated student will persevere. If you have had previous experience of a related skill, some component parts of the skill will be familiar, so then your practice can focus on parts of the skill not already learned. Familiarity with equipment will also ease the learning of a new skill. The stages which a learner will move through, when acquiring a new skill, are identified in Box 1.5.

- **Perception**: at this stage the learner has watched the skill and can perceive what it is going to entail.
- **Set**: physically and psychologically, the learner is ready to attempt the skill.
- **Guided response**: the skill is performed under guidance.
- **Mechanism**: becomes habitual.
- **Complex overt response**: a typical skilled performance.
- **Adaptation**: the skill can be adapted to each individual situation.
- **Origination**: creation of original movement patterns. The skill can be carried out creatively.

Box 1.5 The stages which a learner will move through when learning a new skill (Simpson 1972, cited by Quinn 1995)

Understanding the different stages which you are likely to go through when learning a new skill can help you to be systematic and realistic in your approach. You will understand, for example, that you will initially need guidance and that being adaptable and creative is unlikely to be possible until you have mastered the routine stages of the skill. You may find that the person who has reached stage seven, origination, may carry out the skill in such a fluent manner that he will find it difficult to break the skill down into sub-skills at all. It may also mean that you see the skill carried out in different ways by different nurses with different clients, due to the adaptations which they have made. Students can sometimes be very concerned about learning the skill the 'right' way. An understanding of the cognitive and affective dimensions can enable adaptations to be made which enhance rather than

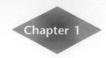

compromise practice. When you are learning a new skill Quinn (1995) has identified some key points which a facilitator can do to help (see Box 1.6).

- Provide an atmosphere conducive to learning
- Carry out a skills analysis
- Determine sequence
- Assess student's prior knowledge
- Teach sequence
- Teach skill by either whole learning or part learning
- Allocate sufficient time to practise
- Provide feedback
- Prompt student to self-evaluate
- Encourage transfer of skills.

Box 1.6 How a facilitator can help a student learn a practical skill (Quinn 1995)

You yourself can be active about promoting these conditions. For example, the time to ask a nurse to supervise you drawing up an injection is probably not in the middle of an emergency situation, as the stress and anxiety in the environment are unlikely to be conducive to learning. Thus when asking to be supervised carrying out a skill for the first time, pick the right moment! You can yourself be forthcoming about your prior knowledge, saying explicitly that you have, for example, observed a number of injections, and now feel ready to be supervised administering one.

De Tornyay and Thompson (1987) highlight some other issues too. They identify that learners need to handle equipment as this diffuses anxiety, therefore always take opportunities to become familiar with equipment that you are likely to use. This book will help by explaining what type of equipment is used for the skills discussed, and will include illustrations. There is also advice about where you might be able to access equipment with which to become familiar. De Tornyay and Thompson (1987) highlight that adult learners can be self-conscious when trying out new skills. You will need to be supervised when practising a new skill, but you may wish to ensure that there won't be too big an audience if you feel that you will be self-conscious! A warm and accepting learning environment will help to reduce excess anxiety which might adversely affect your performance. While it is suggested that a supervisor should avoid the temptation to 'take over', if client safety is compromised then the supervising practitioner would need to do so. De Tornyay and Thompson (1987) also suggest that when learning a new skill feedback is crucial – to reinforce correct behaviour and eliminate error.

The importance of obtaining feedback

Gaining feedback when you are developing skills will be important for your learning. From whom can you gain feedback? Obviously the nurse supervising you can give you feedback. It is best if the comments are as specific as possible rather than a general comment such as 'very good', or 'you need to be quicker'. It will be helpful to your supervisor if you yourself identify any aspects in particular that you want feedback on. For example, you might state that when performing the skill last time, the supervisor had said that you needed to give a clearer explanation to the client, and ask that she gives you feedback on this aspect in particular. The client may also be able to give you feedback. He may make spontaneous comments, such as that he feels 'much more comfortable now', but you can also seek feedback specifically, e.g. by asking how he feels at different stages of the skill. Hopefully if you are approachable in the way you seek feedback, the client will give an honest response. However, your observation of the client during the skill will also give you feedback, e.g. you can observe for facial expressions which might indicate fear or discomfort.

These sources of feedback outlined so far are what would be termed 'extrinsic feedback'. This combined with intrinsic feedback should give you a balanced view of your performance. Intrinsic feedback involves you reflecting on your performance, and asking yourself what were the strengths and weaknesses and how you could improve your performance next time. Some universities have equipment to video performance of skills. Watching this objectively and identifying your strengths and areas for improvement will help you to develop your skills performance.

Learning from experience and reflection

Becoming skilled at learning from experience is essential if you are going to benefit fully from your practice placements. We have already established that to develop competency, practice is necessary. But is it inevitable that experience will lead to learning, and improved performance? Bjork's (1999b) study followed the progress of four newly qualified nurses' practical skill development. Her focus was on the skill of mobilizing a post-operative patient. In fact their skills performance did not necessarily improve over time. Some aspects in some nurses improved while other aspects deteriorated. Bjork's findings led her to question how it could be that nurses with 8 to 14 months experience '. . . do not give the patient sufficient physical support during ambulation, or that basic attention to the patient's clothing and comfort is missing?' She also found that nurses became quicker and seemingly efficient, but learnt to cut corners in a way which was culturally acceptable, such as not washing

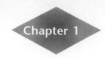

hands. Andrews *et al.* (1998) suggest that continued repetition of skills may lead to merely habitual behaviour, rather than conscious analysis of actions.

Bjork (1999b) theorizes a number of possible reasons why these nurses' performance did not necessarily improve with experience. She questions whether their knowledge base was adequate, believing that some skills are inadequately described in nursing text books. She identifies therefore that nurses cannot use in practice knowledge which they do not have but equally, they may not use in practice the knowledge which they do have. However she also identifies lack of reflection on experience as a possible cause. She suggests that nurses are often intent on long-term outcomes and that opportunity to reflect and learn from practice is delayed or embedded in a broader context. The results of our actions in every day life are often clear and direct therefore making an obvious connection between our action and its result. For example, if you leave a cake in the oven too long it will burn, so you might take more care next time. The result of a nurse's failure to wash her hands after dealing with a patient is unlikely to be immediately obvious.

Dewey, an educational theorist, has argued that we do not 'learn by doing' but by 'doing and realizing what came of what we did' (Dewey, 1929, p. 367). Dewey's theories were developed further by Kolb and Fry (1975), and then more fully by Kolb (1984). The theory of how we learn from experience is often referred to as experiential learning. The Kolb experiential learning cycle (*see* Fig. 1.1) separates action from reflection, the theory being that learning takes place during reflection once action has taken place. The cycle starts at the point of experience, continues with reflective observation, onto abstract conceptualization, where new ideas are developed, and then to active experimentation – where the new knowledge arising from the experience is applied to practice.

It has been proposed by Honey (1982) that students will tend to have a preferred learning style, and may be stronger in one component of the learning cycle than the others. Four learning styles have been identified: activists,

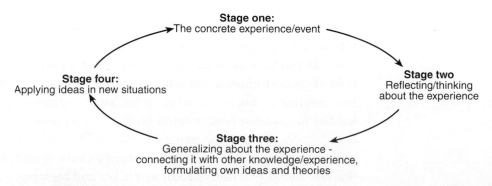

Figure 1.1 Kolb's (1984) learning cycle

who are open to new experiences; reflectors who are cautious and like to observe; theorists who are logical and rational; and pragmatists, who like to experiment and try out new ideas. Identifying your preferred learning style can give you useful insights. It can also help you to focus on developing your skills in the other learning styles thus enabling you to learn from experience more effectively.

Reflection enables you to consider what you did and why, and provides opportunities to develop knowledge from experience and link theory and practice. Johns (1994) defines reflective practice as involving 'the practitioner paying attention to "significant" aspects of experience in order to make sense of it within the context of their intention' (p. 7). Andrews *et al.* (1998) emphasize that reflection is not just recalling events but is a purposeful activity, which requires the nurse to want to change behaviour. Knowledge gained as a result of reflection on practice has been termed 'practical knowledge' (Schon 1987). It has been asserted that reflection can enable the uncovering of knowledge embedded in practice (Lawler 1991). Furthermore, Johns (1994) considers that reflection can enable the practitioner to become aware of conflicts between aims of care and the reality of practice, and these insights can enable the nurse to become more effective.

How guided reflection can help nurses to learn from their experience and 'assert and realize caring as an everyday reality' is explored in Johns (1996). Schon (1983) has suggested that there is also such a thing as reflection-in-action. In relation to practical skills this would mean that rather than dealing with the client's incontinence and reflecting on your care afterwards, gaining new insights for application on the next occasion, you would be reflecting and acquiring knowledge while you are carrying out the care. Reflection-on-action is usually a conscious act but reflection-in-action may not be, making it difficult to articulate knowledge gained in this way. An analysis of both experiential learning and reflection is discussed in some detail by Powell (1998), who suggests that it is unrealistic for nurses to use reflection on every occasion; rather reflective techniques can be applied to specific situations.

To think over or mull over an event is commonplace, but without an analytical and purposeful approach it may not lead to new ways of thinking or behaving (Andrews *et al.* 1998). To help you to develop your reflective skills you will probably be encouraged to keep a reflective journal, recording and reflecting on significant events which you experience in your nursing practice. This activity can assist you in developing evaluative and decision-making skills, and help you to link theory and practice (Howard 1999). It is essential, however, that you do not identify patients or clients (either by name or by using other identifying material) in your reflective writing, to maintain confidentiality (UKCC 1992). You are also likely to take part in reflective activities within the classroom setting where you will be encouraged to reflect on a specific incident from practice. You will probably be recommended a reflective model, which can help you to be structured about your reflection.

The skills laboratory

As it is recognized that students need opportunities to rehearse skills in a safe environment and handle equipment, most universities will have skills laboratories or centres (formerly called practical rooms). These will vary in complexity, but will usually contain equipment for practising technical procedures. Some skills, such as blood pressure recording, can be practised safely on your peers, but there may be models for simulation of other practices. Some skills laboratories organize volunteer 'patients' for students' practice (Smith 1995). Universities will have different systems for learning in the skills laboratory, which you will need to become familiar with. There may be compulsory sessions, optional workshops, and formal or informal sessions. Exercises within the chapters of this book will often suggest that you access equipment to practise with. You will need to find out about your local policies/procedures for use of equipment in the skills laboratory.

At one stage in nurse education, learning skills in the classroom setting went out of favour (Knight and Mowforth 1998). Some educationalists felt that skills could only be learnt in the practice setting with actual patients/clients, and that skills learnt in the classroom could not in any case be readily transferred to the practice setting (Neary 1997). However, without any classroom-based practical skills learning, students have often reported feeling unprepared and lacking in confidence (Neary 1997). Practice staff do not always have the time to teach skills 'from scratch', and can be reluctant to involve students in practical skills which they have not been 'taught'. When skills are taught in the practice setting, the focus is usually on the physical procedure and manual dexterity, while the cognitive and affective dimensions are omitted. This is probably due, again, to time constraints on practitioners. Students have also reported anxiety about practising skills in the clinical setting without previous experience (Neary 1997). McAdams *et al.* (1989) in a survey of 59 students, found that students believed classroom-based skills learning reduced anxiety, increased feelings of mastery, enhanced patient safety and provided hands-on, pre-clinical experience. Some would consider that it is only fair to patients/clients that students should have had some prior preparation before practising on such vulnerable people. Clinical practice on patients must certainly be carried out safely (McAdams *et al.* 1989).

Some researchers have attempted evaluation of whether practice in skills laboratories actually does enhance performance in the clinical setting (Erickson Megel *et al.* 1987; McAdams *et al.* 1989; Hallal and Welch 1984; Love *et al.* 1989; Gomez and Gomez 1987) with varied results. Knight's (1998) critical review of some of these studies casts doubt on some of their conclusions. Gomez and Gomez (1987) explain the difference between 'open' and 'closed' psychomotor skills. A closed psychomotor skill within nursing would be making an unoccupied bed. This skill will not be greatly affected by situational variables and is therefore easier to transfer from the classroom to the clinical setting. Skills performed in dynamic environments such as taking a patient's blood pressure, are called 'open' psychomotor skills as there could be many different factors which will vary how this skill has to be performed. For example, noise within a ward setting, relatives looking on, and a patient who has difficulty in fully straightening his arm, are all unpredictable variables, which would not be present if the student was practising the skill in the classroom setting. Thus practising the skill of taking a blood pressure in the classroom, while beneficial in leading to familiarity with equipment and the sequence of steps in the procedure, has recognized limitations. To actually become competent and confident in this skill requires repeated practice in the clinical setting.

Knight's (1998) extensive review of the literature on learning psychomotor skills in nursing supports the use of a controlled and safe environment to facilitate initial skills practice. She identifies that learning a skill requires a structured and systematic approach, which enables practice in a safe environment. Overall, most educationalists would support the view that students should have classroom preparation for practical skills, and these facilities are now generally available. The use of skills laboratories has also recently been endorsed by the ENB (2000), as a means to enable students to become safe and effective in practice. Their use in no way replaces the need for practice of skills within clinical placements. However, the classroom provides a more controlled environment for familiarization with practical skills than the clinical setting, and if students are familiar with some skills and equipment they can focus on learning aspects which cannot be simulated in the classroom (Hallal and Welch 1984). Some skills laboratories include video equipment so that students can analyse their performance afterwards (Smith 1995; Knight and Mowforth 1998). Increasingly students are also being tested in the classroom, often through a system termed 'objective structured clinical examination' (OSCE). Patient scenarios are used, and the components of competence are assessed objectively against pre-set criteria, which have been determined in advance from course content and objectives (Harden 1988).

Learning in the practice setting

Clinical placement experience has been stated to be 'central to the development of nursing practice skills' (Nolan 1998). Indeed, actual practice with clients in the clinical environment is essential to enable competence to be developed. It is important, however, not to see clients as just people to be practised on, therefore objectifying them (Roach 1992). Roach (1992) suggests that instead, students should see themselves as being 'in a helping therapeutic relationship with clients who freely collaborate in the educational enterprise' (p. 120). Practical skills development and practice should therefore take place within the context of the relationship between you and the client, as part of his holistic care. I was once told of a student who refused to help a patient to wash, as she said she already knew how to do that! Obviously you should take every opportunity to develop new skills, but not within a task orientated framework which is dehumanizing and objectifies the client. Learning practical skills should thus occur within the total care required for the individual.

In Nolan's (1998) qualitative study about learning in clinical placements, she cites a student starting a new placement as saying: 'You are so scared and wondering, Oh God, I want to do this right'. When starting a new clinical placement you may well feel anxious or even fearful and it is important to be aware that you are not alone in these feelings. Starting a new clinical placement has been likened to starting a new job! Each placement will have its own culture, and you will need to familiarize yourself with the environment, staff and routines (Nolan 1998). Until you 'settle in' to the placement and start to feel part of the team, effective learning can be difficult. Some placements send you information prior to your placement to help you feel welcome and reduce anxiety, and often a pre-placement visit is encouraged.

When students enter a new practice placement they can also sometimes feel overwhelmed by the extent of learning opportunities. To help you to focus on the specific opportunities available in your placement, the ENB (1998) suggests that each placement area identifies what opportunities are available, and these will of course include practical skills.

In any practice setting you will have an assigned assessor, whose remit will include supporting you in:

1. Identifying your learning needs.
2. Addressing these learning needs through enabling you to practise, and giving feedback.
3. Assessing your performance at the end of the placement.

Your role should be an active one throughout this process.

Identifying your learning needs

When, with support from your assessor, you identify your learning needs you should take into account:

- The learning outcomes for your stage of the course.
- Your prior learning, from previous practice placements, and any relevant experience prior to entering nurse education.
- Any learning needs which were identified from your previous practice placement.
- The specific learning opportunities specified by the placement.

Your assessor will discuss these learning needs with you, and can advise you of the learning opportunities in the placement which can help to meet these learning needs but it will be up to you to be honest, about your strengths and areas for improvement. Your learning needs are likely to include practical skills but will include a range of other needs too.

Addressing learning needs

Unfortunately some studies have found that students do not always learn whilst in clinical placements as effectively as they could do (Ashworth and Morrison 1989; Melia 1987). The earlier section 'Learning from experience and reflection' can give you some insight into how you can most benefit from your clinical experience. Further suggestions are given below.

You should work with your assessor for a minimum of 2 days per week (ENB 1998) and you will need to be active in seeking out your learning opportunities. Being aware of how practical skills are learnt will help you to make the best use of opportunities available, ensuring that you observe a skill first, and ask for supervised practice until you feel confident to practise the skill independently. While some skills will need minimal practice, others are much more complex and will need repeated practice. It is very important not to attempt a skill unsupervised unless you are confident of your ability. You will be given formative feedback during the placement to guide your learning. As discussed before, the practical skills which you develop should be considered within the holistic care of the patient, and not as isolated tasks which you have learnt to perform.

Being proactive about learning in the practice setting can be helped if you are aware of different learning methods which you might employ. There is much that you can learn from observing others in the practice setting but you will need to identify who is a 'good' professional role model and who is a 'poor' one. In some practice settings there may be formal teaching sessions organized. This might be particularly appropriate when there are several students in a placement area, and where workload is predictable and so a specific time can be set aside for a teaching session. Formal teaching sessions enable you to prepare, by pre-reading for example. Informal teaching occurs more spontaneously 'on the spot'. Such sessions can be particularly meaningful as they are likely to be directly linked with the clinical practice occurring at that time. This type of learning is called 'action learning' (Howard 1999). Sometimes a critical incident can be used as a basis for reflection in the practice setting. This might be a situation that has occurred which was difficult or challenging, such as where a relative has complained about lack of care by the staff. Critical incident analysis can aid reflection and learning from such a situation.

An example of how you might employ different learning methods in the practice setting is now given. When taking part in drug administration, you can actively observe the qualified nurse, asking questions as necessary, either at the time (if appropriate) or making a note of questions for later, or specific drugs which you wish to find out about. The nurse you are with may also ask you questions in order to check your understanding and encourage you to think about what is happening. You may be able to take part in practical elements such as dispensing of tablets or preparing a nebulizer. If a difficult situation occurs, for example a patient refuses his tablets, you could use this incident to reflect afterwards and develop knowledge from this experience. You could consider, for example, whether a different approach to the patient would have made any difference, or whether an adequate explanation about the tablets was given. You could also follow up later by looking up drugs which you encountered and were not familiar with.

Assessment

All universities are required to have in place continuous assessment schemes (ENB 1998), so your final (summative) assessment should be based on your performance throughout your placement. You will be expected to self-evaluate which many students find difficult, especially at first. However, learning to self evaluate is an important professional skill – *see* Chapter 2 (Self-awareness).

Recommended reading

As stated earlier, the remit of this book is to help you to develop a foundation in practical nursing skills. For guidance about reading material for other aspects you should refer to your university's recommended reading list for your course. Books containing chapters on all the main topic areas which student nurses are required to study, include those by Hinchliff *et al.* (1998) and Perry and Jolley (1997).

Many practical nursing skills require an underlying biological knowledge base. For example when taking and recording blood pressure, it is necessary to understand what blood pressure is and how it is maintained.

A foundation in biology is not, however, within the scope of this book and it is assumed that students will gain their biological knowledge from one or more of those texts available, many of which are aimed specifically at student nurses. When working through each chapter of this book, it would be sensible to have an understanding of the related biology, so each chapter includes questions on the related biology. You are advised to use your recommended text to check your biological knowledge, by finding out the answers to the questions posed. Studying the relevant biology and then working through the relevant skills chapter, can help to bring the biology alive, making it more comprehensible and memorable, as you can see its immediate relevance and applicability to nursing practice.

CHAPTER SUMMARY

- Competence in a range of practical nursing skills is required of all registered nurses.
- There is a vast range of practical skills. This book addresses core skills but not those which are branch specific.
- Practical nursing skills include motor, affective and cognitive dimensions. To become competent requires all three dimensions to be developed.
- Practical nursing skills should be carried out therapeutically and within the context of caring.
- To develop competence requires practice and experience, which should include gaining feedback, and reflection, thus maximizing learning from experience.
- There are stages in developing skills which have been identified as ranging from novice to expert.
- Classroom preparation in a skills laboratory or equivalent, can familiarize with equipment and the sequential steps of a skill. The cognitive and affective domain can also be introduced.
- Carrying out practical skills in the dynamic and variable environment of the clinical setting will be affected by many factors.
- Repeated practice in the clinical setting will be needed in order to become competent and confident in a skill.

REFERENCES

Andrews, M.; Gidman, J. and Humphreys, A. 1998. Reflection: does it enhance professional nursing practice? *British Journal of Nursing* **7**, 413–17.

Ashworth, P. and Morrison, P. 1989. Some ambiguities of the student's role in undergraduate nurse training. *Journal of Advanced Nursing* **14**, 1009–15.

Benner, P. 1984. *From Novice to Expert*. Massachusetts: Addison-Wesley Publishing.

Benner, P. and Wrubel, J. 1989. *The Primacy of Caring*. Massachusetts: Addison-Wesley Publishing.

Bjork, I.T. 1999a. What constitutes a nursing practical skill? *Western Journal of Nursing Research* **21** (1), 51–70.

Bjork, I.T. 1999b. Practical skill development in new nurses. *Nursing Inquiry* **6**, 34–47.

Bradshaw, A. 1994: *Lighting the Lamp: The Spiritual Dimension of Nursing Care*. Harrow: Scutari Press.

Bush, H.A. and Barr, W.J. 1997. Critical Care Nurses' lived experiences of caring. *Heart and Lung* **26**, 387–98.

Carper, B.A. 1978. Fundamental patterns of knowing in nursing. *Advances in Nursing Science* 1, 13–23.

Chapman, E.J. 1997. Research – what it is and what it is not. In: Perry, A. and Jolley, M. (ed.) *Nursing: A Knowledge Base for Practice*, 2nd edn. London: Arnold, 33–54.

Department of Health. 1999. *Making a Difference: Strengthening the Nursing, Midwifery and Health Visiting Contribution to Nealth and Nealth Care*. London: DOH.

de Tornyay R. and Thompson, M.A. 1987. *Strategies for Teaching Nursing*, 3rd edn. New York: Delmar Publishing.

Dewey, J. 1929. *Experience and Nature*. New York: Grove Press.

English National Board. 1998. *Standards for Approval of Higher Education Institutions and Programmes*. London: ENB.

English National Board. 2000. *Education in Focus: Strengthening Pre-registration Nursing and Midwifery Education*. London: ENB.

Erickson Megel, M., Wilken, M.K. and Volcek, M.K. 1987. Nursing students' performance: administering injections in laboratory and clinical area. *Journal of Nursing Education* **26**, 288–93.

Ersser, S. 1998. The presentation of the nurse: a neglected dimension of therapeutic nurse-patient interaction? In: McMahon, R. and Pearson, A. (eds.) *Nursing as Therapy*, 2nd edn. Cheltenham: Stanley Thornes (Publishers), 36–63.

Fernandez, E. 1997. Just 'doing the observations': reflective practice in nursing. *British Journal of Nursing* **6**, 939–943.

Fitzpatrick, J.M., While, A.E. and Roberts, J.D. 1992. The role of the nurse in high-quality patient care: a review of the literature. *Journal of Advanced Nursing* **17**, 1210–19.

Gomez, G.E. and Gomez, E.A. 1987. Learning of psychomotor skills: laboratory versus patient care setting. *Journal of Nursing Education* **26**, 20–24.

Hallal, J.C. and Welch, M.D. 1984. Using the competency laboratory to learn psychomotor skills. *Nurse Educator* **9**, 34–8.

Halldorsdottir, S. 1991. Five basic modes of being with another. In: Gaut, D.A. and Leininger, M.M. (eds.) *Caring: The Compassionate Healer*. New York: National League for Nursing Press, 37–49.

Harden, R.M. 1988. What is OSCE? *Medical Teacher* **10**, 19–22.

Hinchliff, S., Norman, S. and Schober, J. (eds.) 1998. *Nursing Practice and Health Care: A Foundation Text*, 3rd edn. London: Arnold.

Howard, A. 1999. Strategies for meeting learning needs. In: Hinchliff, S. (ed) *The Practitioner as Teacher*, 2nd edn. Edinburgh: Ballière Tindall, 107–21.

Honey, P. 1982. *The Manual of Learning Styles*. Maidenhead: Honey and Munford.

Johns, C. 1994. A philosophical basis for nursing practice. In: Johns, C. (ed.) *The Burford NDU Model: Caring in Practice*. Oxford: Blackwell Science, 3–19.

Johns, C. 1996. Visualising and realising caring in practice through guided reflection. *Journal of Advanced Nursing* **24**, 1135–13.

Knight, C. 1998. Evaluating a skills centre: the acquisition of psychomotor skills in nursing – a review of the literature. *Nurse Education Today* **18**, 441–47.

Knight, C.M. and Mowforth, G.M. 1998. Skills centre: why we did it, how we did it. *Nurse Education Today* **18**, 389–93.

Kolb, D.A. 1984. *Experiential Learning*. London: Prentice Hall.

Kolb, D.A. and Fry, R. 1975. Towards an applied theory of experiential learning. In: Cooper, C.L. (ed.) *Theories of Group Processes*. London: John Wiley.

Lawler, J. 1991. *Behind the Screens: Nursing Somology and the Problem of the Body*. London: Churchill Livingstone.

Leininger, M. 1981. Transcultural nursing: its progress and its future. *Nursing and Health Care* **2**, 365–71.

Love, B., McAdams, C., Patton, D.M. *et al.* 1989. Teaching psychomotor skills in nursing: a randomised control trial. *Journal of Advanced Nursing* **14**, 970–75.

Manley, K. 1997. Knowledge for nursing practice. In: Perry, A. and Jolley, M. (ed) *Nursing: A Knowledge Base for Practice*, 2nd edn. London: Arnold, 301–33.

McAdams, C., Rankin, E., Love, B. and Patton, D. 1989. Psychomotor skills laboratories as self-directed learning: a study of nursing students' perceptions. *Journal of Advanced Nursing* **14**, 788–96.

McMahon, R. 1998. Therapeutic nursing: theory, issues and practice. In: McMahon, R. and Pearson, A. (eds.) *Nursing as Therapy*, 2nd edn. Cheltenham: Stanley Thornes (Publishers), 1–20.

Melia, K. 1987. *Learning and Working: The Occupational Socialisation of Nursing*. London: Tavistock Publications.

Neary, M. 1997. Project 2000 students' survival kit: a return to the practical room (nursing skills laboratory). *Nurse Education Today* **17**, 46–52.

Nolan, C.A. 1998. Learning on clinical placement: the experience of six Australian student nurses. *Nurse Education Today* **18** 622–29.

Oermann, M.H. 1990. Psychomotor skill development. *The Journal of Continuing Education in Nursing* **21**, 202–4.

Papadopoulus, I., Tilki, M. and Taylor, G. 1998. Developing trans-cultural skills. In: Papadopoulus, I., Tilki, M. and Taylor, G. (eds.) *Trans-Cultural Care: A Guide for Health Care Professionals*. Dinton, Salisbury: Quay Books, Mark Allen Publishing, 175–211.

Paterson, J. and Zderad, L. 1988. *Humanistic Nursing*. New York: League for Nursing.

Perry, A. and Jolley, M. (ed.) 1997: *Nursing: A Knowledge Base for Practice*, 2nd edn. London: Arnold.

Powell, J. 1998. Reflection and the evaluation of experience: prerequisites for therapeutic practice. In: McMahon, R. and Pearson, A. (eds.) *Nursing as Therapy*, 2nd edn. Cheltenham: Stanley Thornes (Publishers), 21–36.

Quinn, F. 1995. *The Principles and Practice of Nurse Education*. 3rd edn. Cheltenham: Stanley Thorns (Publishers).

Reynolds, C.L. and Leininger, M. 1993. *Madeleine Leininger: Cultural Care Diversity and Universality Theory*. Newbury Park: Sage Publications.

Roach, M.S. 1992. *The Human Act of Caring: A Blueprint for the Health Professions*, revised edn. Ottawa: Canadian Hospital Association Press.

Romyn, D.M. 1999. Commentary. *Western Journal of Nursing Research* **21**, 64–70.

Schober, J. 1998. Nursing: issues for effective practice. In: Hinchliff, S., Norman, S. and Schober, J. (eds) *Nursing Practice and Health Care: A Foundation Text*, 3rd edn. London: Arnold, 251–73.

Schon, D. 1983. *The Reflective Practitioner*. London: Temple Smith.

Schon, D. 1987. *Educating the Reflective Practitioner*. San Fransisco: Jossey-Bass.

Smith, K. 1995. All taped. *Nursing Times*, **91** (1), 16.

'This Week' 2000. Nurses 'failed to feed us,' patients say. *Nursing Times*. **96**(1), 9.

United Kingdom Central Council 1992. *Code for Professional Conduct*. London: UKCC.

Wallis, M.C. 1998. Responding to suffering: the experience of professional nurse caring in the coronary care unit. *International Journal for Human Caring* **2** (2), 35–44.

Watkins, M. 1997. Nursing knowledge in nursing practice. In: Perry, A. and Jolley, M. (ed.) *Nursing: a Knowledge Base for Practice*, 2nd edn. London: Arnold, 1–31.

Watson, J. 1979. *Nursing: The Philosophy and Science of Caring*. Boston: Little Brown.

Webb, M., Bond, M. and Beale, P. 1997. *First Aid Manual: The Authorized Manual of St John Ambulance, St Andrews Ambulance Association and the Red Cross*, 7th edn. London: Dorling Kindersley.

Wharton, A. and Pearson, A. 1988. Nursing and intimate physical care – the key to therapeutic nursing. In: Pearson, A. (ed.) *Primary Nursing: Nursing in the Burford and Oxford Nursing development Units*. London: Chapman and Hall, 117–24.

Woodward, V.M. 1997. Professional caring: a contradiction in terms? *Journal of Advanced Nursing* **26**, 999–1004.

Chapter

2

The nurse's approach: self-awareness and communication

Nicola M. Neale and Joanne Sale

> Other people's behaviour doesn't happen in a vacuum. When they relate to us, they are relating to *us*, to the people we are. Their behaviour towards us is a response, in no small measure, to our behaviour towards them . . .
>
> (Fontana 1990, cited in Niven and Robinson 1994, p. 11)

As Fontana suggests, any interaction is a two-way process and therefore it is important that nurses are aware that their approach to clients/patients in any setting will affect the outcome. Childs (1995), when discussing quality in relation to the Patient's Charter, suggests that treatments should be given with respect rather than seen solely as a task to be performed. This book is addressing practical skills required by nurses and this chapter focuses on the nurse/patient interactions whilst carrying out these skills.

Included in this chapter are:
- Developing self awareness.
- Communication skills in a range of care settings with a variety of clients.

The above sections will incorporate ethical considerations when caring for individuals and their families.

> **Recommended reading**
>
> The following books are particularly helpful when developing knowledge and understanding related to this chapter:
>
> - Gross, R. 1996. Psychology: *The Science of Mind and Behaviour*, 3rd edn. London: Hodder and Stoughton.
> - Hargie, O., Saunders, C. and Dickson, D. 1994. *Social Skills in Interpersonal Communication*, 3rd edn. London: Routledge.
> - Williams, D. 1996. *Communication Skills in Practice: A Practical Guide for Health Professionals*. London: Jessica Kingsley.

PRACTICE SCENARIOS

The following scenarios, taken from later chapters in this book, will be referred to during the text.

■ **Adult**

Mr Ronald Atkinson is a 70-year-old man who is taken to the Accident and Emergency Unit by ambulance following a suspected **cerebrovascular accident (CVA)**. He had been found on the floor at home. On his arrival, you take over his care. During his assessment you are required to measure and record his temperature, pulse and blood pressure and a set of neurological observations. His family are present. You will meet Mr Atkinson again in Chapter 7, Monitoring vital signs.

■ **Child**

Kevin O'Riordan, aged 14 years, has undergone an emergency appendicetomy for a perforated appendix, leading to **peritonitis**. He has an abdominal wound, is receiving intravenous fluids, and is nil by mouth. He seems quiet and uncommunicative. Kevin has two younger sisters. His parents spend part of each day at the hospital with him. You will meet Kevin again in Chapter 5, Meeting hygiene needs.

■ **Learning disability**

Clara Wright is a 43-year-old woman with a learning disability who lives in a small staffed unit. She has epilepsy and, this morning, had a prolonged fit for which a rectal muscle relaxant (diazepam) was administered. She is now very drowsy and unresponsive and you have been advised that her respirations need to be monitored carefully. You will meet Clara Wright again in Chapter 8, Assessing and managing respiratory needs.

Cerebrovascular accident (CVA):
Cerebral damage caused either by decreased blood flow or haemorrhage. Effects vary but often causes paralysis down one side of the body (hemiplegia), and speech, swallowing and elimination difficulties. Commonly called a 'stroke'.

Peritonitis:
Inflammation of the peritoneum, the membrane lining the abdominal cavity. Results in pain, tenderness and fever.

■ **Mental health**

Mrs Vera Wilson aged 80 years has been readmitted to the ward for the elderly mentally ill after a marked deterioration in her mental state. Her mood is low and she appears confused, disorientated, agitated and restless. She also seems frightened. You will meet Mrs Wilson again in Chapter 6, Meeting elimination needs.

DEVELOPING SELF-AWARENESS

Definition: Self-awareness is the evolving and expanding sense of noticing and taking account of a wide range of aspects of self (Burnard 1994).

Learning outcomes

By the end of this section you will be able to:

1. Reflect upon the importance of self and self-awareness in a caring context.
2. Understand the terms self-concept and body image and recognize their relevance to nursing practice.
3. Show insight into the relevance of understanding aspects of personality.
4. Discuss attitudes, values and beliefs and their impact in the care environment.

Learning outcome 1:
Reflect upon the importance of self and self-awareness in a caring context

■ **Activity**

• Describe yourself. Spend five minutes writing down the aspects of yourself that you would like a stranger to know.
• Highlight what you see as your strengths and weaknesses.

Check out what you have written with a friend:

■ Does their view match yours?
■ Were there things that you did not know about yourself?
■ What do any differences tell you about yourself? (The authors accept no responsibility for the break-up of friendships!)

Figure 2.1 displays the Johari window, which was used by the authors, Luft and Ingram (1955), to help individuals to identify aspects of self. This model suggests that through self-disclosure, i.e. telling others about yourself and seeking feedback from others, e.g. the exercise that you have just completed, there will be an effect on your awareness of self. This occurs because there is

	You know	You don't know
Others know	Public area	Blind area
Others don't know	Hidden area	Unknown area

Figure 2.1 The Johari window (Luft and Ingram 1955)

an increase in the size of the public area in relation to the other three – so you will acquire a greater understanding of your own strengths and weaknesses.

Activity

How may this understanding of these aspects of self, affect you as a care-giver when carrying out practical skills?

You may have considered several different aspects. **For example**: If you have had an argument at home, you may understand why you feel impatient with a client who appears to lack motivation to assist with hygiene needs. As a result of this awareness you could adapt your behaviour accordingly.

It is important that health-care professionals develop an appreciation of how and why they behave in certain ways in certain circumstances and as suggested by Irving and Hazlett (1999, p. 270), 'self-awareness is a important precursor of effective communication'. Therefore the crucial point about self-awareness is how it helps us to recognize how our behaviour affects others.

Activity

Think of a recent situation where you think that your behaviour had an impact on the outcome of a particular incident.

Learning outcome 2:
Understand the terms self-concept and body image and recognize their relevance to nursing practice

Self-concept can be defined as the information and beliefs that individuals have about their own nature, qualities, and behaviour (Rogers 1961). Body image is the individual's interpretation of their 'bodily self' and includes aspects such as their physical characteristics – tall, short, fat, thin, brown-eyed, blond-haired (Gross 1996). It is generally accepted that there are three components to the self-concept: self-image, self-esteem and ideal-self (Gross 1996).

Self-image

Self-image is the way in which we would describe ourselves. Kuhn and McPartland (1954) (cited by Gross 1996) suggest that this can be found by asking a person to answer the question 'who am I' twenty times. The answer might include social roles, personality traits and physical characteristics (as in body image).

Look back to your strengths and weaknesses, identified earlier. Do any of these match up with the above three categories? Adams and Bromley (1998) suggest three additional categories: sexuality, spirituality and lifestyle. You may find that some of your responses fit into these more readily.

However, how many of your strengths and weaknesses relate to physical characteristics? Price (1990) identifies three aspects of body image:

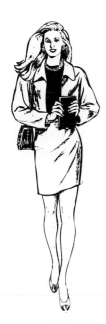

- Body reality is the way we are.
- Body ideal is how we would like to look. Sometimes this is guided by society's views and is a dynamic process. Thus in Figure 2.2 we (the authors) have interpreted society's view of the ideal female as being tall and slim, with long, blonde hair. (Unfortunately neither author conforms to this ideal!)
- Body presentation is how we present ourselves, so **we** need to go out and buy long, blonde wigs and platform shoes, if we want to live up to our perceptions of body ideal.

Another aspect of body presentation is how we behave. It is likely that you would not only choose different clothes to wear to a party than for a job interview, but that you would also probably act differently. Niebuhr (1963) suggests that self-conduct is a fundamental aspect of accountability and for nurses, professional behaviour is important in order to remain a registered nurse. In relation to the above discussion about body presentation, nurses are expected to have a certain standard of dress when on duty and to conform to a certain standard of behaviour. Reflect on what effect you think that having dirty nails when carrying out the monitoring of vital signs would have. It is unlikely to demonstrate a 'professional' manner, and might well affect the client's confidence in the nurse and the interaction which follows.

Figure 2.2 The ideal woman in society's eyes?

For each of the scenarios, how might the person's perceptions of their self-image be influenced by what they are experiencing?

You might have identified that Kevin, as an adolescent, is already in a period of transition and has to cope with new social and emotional roles. However, in addition, he is now coping with emergency surgery, leading to an abdominal scar, and time off school, which may be a source of anxiety to him. All these factors may have an effect on his self-image. As discussed earlier, body image is a dynamic process and Kevin is particularly vulnerable because adolescence is already a period of major changes. Mr Atkinson may have been very independent prior to admission, but now, due to his CVA, he could be reliant upon health-care professionals for his essential needs. For Clara Wright, having epilepsy, may be influential on her view of 'self' and this may have been reinforced by society's perceptions of 'being an epileptic'. Mrs Wilson's mental health status may have affected her sense of self, and depression, confusion and disorientation may all contribute to a distorted view of self.

Self-esteem

Self-esteem is the extent to which we value and approve of ourselves, relating to how much we like the person we are. These judgements can be global or specific (Gross 1996). For example, we might like ourselves on the whole, but might not like a particular aspect, say the size of our nose, or our tendency to be short-tempered. Self-esteem and self-image are connected; if your self-image is positive, then it is likely that you will also have good self-esteem and vice versa.

The ideal self

The ideal self is the person we would like to be. Although this is similar to Price's concepts discussed earlier, it is not just about physical characteristics, but also considers wider issues such as personality and relationships. We might want to change some aspects of ourselves or we might wish we were a different person altogether, perhaps kinder, less judgmental or more intelligent. Rogers (1961) suggests that the greater the gap between our self-image and our ideal-self, the lower our self-esteem.

■ *Activity*   Think about how illness might effect someone's ideal-self and/or self-esteem.

Some of the things that you might have thought of are: disfigurement; loss of hair due to treatment; loss or gaining of weight (as a result of treatment or the illness process); loss of self-worth (e.g. Mrs Wilson's depressed mood might affect her ideal-self and her self-esteem), and loss of function (e.g. Mr Atkinson, due to his CVA).

It is likely that all of the individuals in the scenarios will have changes to their self-concept and body image to a greater or lesser extent as a result of their illness experiences. Thus the approach of the nurse whilst carrying out care can do much to either reinforce these views, or to improve self-esteem or self-worth.

Learning outcome 3:
Show insight into the relevance of understanding aspects of personality

Definition

Personality is 'those relatively stable and enduring aspects of individuals which distinguish them from other people, making them unique, but which at the same time allow people to be compared with each other' Gross (1996, p. 744). This is just one of many attempts to define personality.

> **Activity**
>
> Go back to your list of strengths and weaknesses. Which of these would you describe as being relatively stable and secure aspects of your personality?

Eysenck (1965, cited in Gross 1996), proposed that there were two principal dimensions of personality, these being introversion/extroversion and neuroticism/stability. Each individual lies within one of the four quadrants. Considering the diagram in Figure 2.3, where do you think you would lie?

An introverted nurse may find communicating with clients or colleagues in a group setting more stressful than an extrovert one. However on a one-to-one basis, there may be little difference.

The personality of the client is important too, as this will affect any interaction. Eysenck (1965, cited in Ryckman 1989) found that extroverts were more tolerant to pain stimuli; however, Adams and Bromley (1998) suggest that evidence from practice is contrary to this, and that extroverts are prone to displaying their emotions and pain behaviour. The behaviour that you observe may give only a small indication as to the person's personality, but

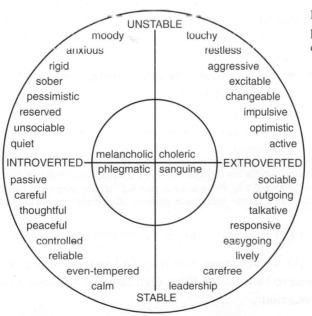

Figure 2.3 Dimensions of personality (Eysenck 1965, cited in Gross 1996)

it would be an important glimpse. For example in the scenario, Kevin is quiet and uncommunicative. What conclusions would you draw from this? You might decide that Kevin is an introverted, shy boy, or that he is a thoughtful, polite boy. Conversely you might think that Kevin is unusual for a boy of his age and therefore you might put his behaviour down to his physical condition. All of these would say something about his personality, as you see it.

Learning outcome 4:
Discuss attitudes, values and beliefs and their impact on the care environment.

Definitions

Value
The judgement that a person places on the desirability, worth or utility of obtaining some outcome (Adams and Bromley 1998).

Belief
The opinions held about something – the information, knowledge or thoughts about a particular thing (Stahlberg and Frey 1994, cited in Adams and Bromley 1998).

Our values and beliefs feed into our attitudes and these are of interest because they can, and do, affect how we behave with others.

Attitude
These are our 'likes and dislikes' (Bem 1970).

For example – what is your opinion about smokers receiving health care? You may value life, but believe in the right to freedom of choice, therefore your attitude towards smokers receiving care may be ambivalent.

Hoveland and Rosenberg (1960, cited in Gross 1996) suggest that there are three components to attitudes. The affective component is how the individual feels about a person, object etc. The cognitive component concerns those thoughts and perceptions that the individual holds toward the person, object etc. Finally the behavioural component reflects how we act toward the person, object etc.

Activity

Consider the following: be as honest with yourself as possible. Would you feel any differently about Mr Atkinson if his collapse had been as a result of alcohol abuse, rather than a CVA? How would you feel if you were told in handover that Kevin O'Riordhan's father had been verbally aggressive towards staff?

The sort of responses you may have thought of might include:

■ With Mr Atkinson, you may feel less keen to care for him because you believe his collapse is his own fault, or you may even openly criticize his behaviour.

■ With Kevin's father you may be wary of him and also avoid anything but basic contact with Kevin when his father is present. You may believe that he presents a danger to you.

Morrison and Burnard (1997) suggest that those in caring roles are constantly making decisions about whether or not individuals are deserving of care and cite Rajecki (1982) who suggests that attitudes play a crucial part in influencing caring behaviours.

Activity   Are there other illnesses or health problems where health professionals may decide that the individual or their lifestyle is responsible for this?

Some examples we have thought of are:

■ A person who is HIV positive as a result of unsafe sex or as a result of an infected blood transfusion.
■ A child with a chest infection from a travelling family as opposed to one from the local boarding school.
■ A person who has mistakenly taken an overdose of drugs in comparison to someone who has deliberately taken an overdose.

The examples above are linked to social class and diagnosis, however in reality there are many subtle, social factors that influence our judgements in client-centred relationships (Johnson and Webb 1995). You may have thought of other examples; however, the main consideration is to be aware of how our values, beliefs and attitudes are paramount in affecting how we behave.

Activity   In your practice placements listen to how nurses and other health-care professionals talk to each other about clients and their families.

Are value judgements being made and are these affecting care relationships? If so – how? We will come back to some of these issues in the section about stereotyping and labelling.

Summary
■ Developing self-awareness will improve the nurse's approach to patients/clients.
■ Aspects of self awareness include: self, self-concept, and body image.
■ Personality and attitudes are also influential, in affecting the nurse's approach and interactions with patients/clients.

COMMUNICATION SKILLS IN A RANGE OF CARE SETTINGS WITH A VARIETY OF CLIENTS

Learning outcomes

By the end of this section you will be able to:

1. Discuss interpersonal perception and the relevance to communication.
2. Understand the terms stereotyping and labelling.
3. Discuss relevant aspects of communicating with the individual who is anxious, angry, or confused.

Learning outcome 1:
Discuss interpersonal perception and the relevance to communication

Definitions

Interpersonal perception
Interpersonal perception is 'all about how we decide what other people are like and the meanings we give to their actions' (Hinton 1993, p. ix).

Communication
Communication is 'the process involving the transmission of information from sender to receiver' (Forgas 1985, cited in Long 1999, p. 10).

Interpersonal skills
Interpersonal skills are 'a set of goal-directed, interrelated, situationally appropriate social behaviours (that can be learned and are under the control of the individual)' (Hargie 1986, p. 12).

How nurses perceive others is fundamental to skilful interactions, however often our perceptions are influenced by our own thoughts, feelings and attitudes. Wilmot (1995) (cited in Hargie and Tourish 1997) suggests that 'our perception of the other, whilst seeming certain, is grounded in permanent uncertainty'. This misperception can lead to errors in communication, for example we might assume that Kevin's father's anger is directed at health-care professionals due to his dissatisfaction with Kevin's care. However there may be many other reasons for his behaviour. Hargie *et al.* (1994) suggest that where negative emotions are directed towards the carer, they can interfere with effective listening.

Activity	Make a list of the factors that might affect your perceptions of behaviour in a social setting. You might like to observe people in a variety of different social settings and try to analyze what you saw and heard, and how the setting influenced the behaviours.

You may have found it difficult to differentiate between what you actually observed and how you interpreted these observations. Kagan *et al.* (1986)

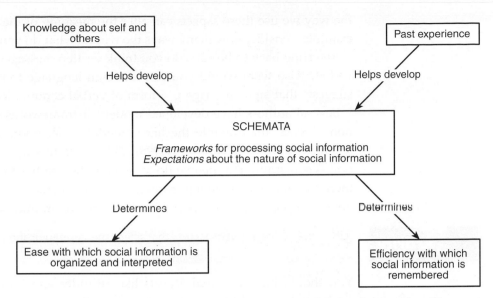

Figure 2.4 The development and function of schemata in social perception (Kagan *et al.* 1986, p. 69)

suggest that as we grow up we develop schemata that help us to organize, interpret and remember social information. Schemata are cognitive or mental frameworks and these are formed from knowledge of ourselves, others and our general life experiences (*see* Fig. 2.4).

Communication is a two way process, whereby one individual sends a message and another person receives it.

Activity | Write down as many different ways that you can think of to send a message.

You may have thought of talking to someone either face to face or on the telephone, by writing a note or sending an e-mail. Did you also think about how we send messages by gestures, facial expressions etc.? Petrie (1997) suggests that there are two forms of interpersonal communication, these being verbal and non-verbal (*see* Box 2.1).

Aspects of our conversations, such as tone of voice, express our emotions and communicate information about our interpersonal attitudes. Sometimes

---

Verbal: The words we use and how we use them e.g. pitch, tone, volume, accent, pauses and speed.
Non-verbal: Proximity, touch, eye-contact and eye-gaze, facial expression, gesture, body movements and posture.

Box 2.1 Forms of communication: verbal and non-verbal (Petrie 1997)

the way we use these aspects can alter the meaning of the words we use. For example, consider how many ways the words 'what do you want' can be said?

Referring back to Box 2.1, do you think written messages are verbal or non-verbal? Also what would you consider sign language to be? Williams (1996) suggests that sign language is a form of verbal communication.

Several authors have developed models or frameworks of the communication process, for example the linear model of Shannon and Weaver (1949) (cited in Adams and Bromley 1998). This tends to suggest that communication is something that people do to one another, rather than a process where there is continual receiving, responding and interacting. Many frameworks now incorporate wider aspects in relation to communication.

■ *Activity*	List some of the relevant factors that affect the communication process.

You should have included aspects like attitudes and intrapersonal issues as we have discussed these earlier. However, did you consider the environment or context, culture, age or gender? For example, when helping Kevin with hygiene needs, we may want to consider the effects of his age on the interpersonal relationship and how comfortable he may feel if talking to a young female nurse. There are alternative frameworks of communication that explore other factors that are important to developing our understanding, and you might like to explore some of these.

Long (1999) suggests that interpersonal skills form the tools necessary for effective communication.

■ *Activity*	Try to identify at least five interpersonal skills. It may help to think about a recent experience in practice when you were performing a practical skill. For example when helping an agitated client to use the toilet (perhaps like Mrs Wilson), or when recording blood pressure (for example Mr Atkinson).

There are many skills which you may have identified. Hargie *et al*. (1994) propose the following:

■ Being able to initiate an interaction successfully
■ Listening
■ Non-verbal communication
■ Giving clear explanations
■ Questioning appropriately
■ Praising others and accepting praise
■ The ability to reflect others' thoughts and feelings
■ Being assertive
■ Effective group-work
■ Being able to finish interactions appropriately.

We will explore the first five areas in more detail in the following sections.

Initiating a successful interaction

■ **Activity** Imagine you are meeting the people from the scenarios at the beginning of the chapter. Write down how you think you would introduce yourself to each of them.

You may introduce yourself giving your first name, for example 'Hello, I'm Jane' or 'I'm Jane Smith' or perhaps you may say 'Hello I'm Student Nurse Smith'. You need to be aware that if you offer your first name you may make it difficult for the client not to also give you his. Some clients may prefer to be called by their formal titles, for example Mr Atkinson or Mrs Wilson. Usually if the person wants you to call him by his first name, he will give you permission some time in the relationship. The use of a formal title is a sign of respect whilst the use of first names implies intimacy or familiarity. Think back to the first time you met the practitioner in charge of a recent placement – how did you address her? It is likely that you adopted a formal approach until told otherwise.

With children or younger people it may be more appropriate to use their first names as a way of putting them at ease. However it is still important to find out their preferred manner of address. For example with Kevin he may like to be called 'Kev' or perhaps a nickname. Look back to the exercise above – how would you address Clara Wright? Would you call her Miss Wright or just Clara? It is particularly important for clients who have a learning disability to be addressed in an appropriate way. You would need to find out what she usually likes to be called, from Clara herself or perhaps from family, friends or from the record in the nursing notes. It is a very important aspect of beginning a relationship with a client that you respect their wishes regarding their chosen names.

There are also cultural aspects that may need to be considered so it is important that what may seem to be a trivial aspect of the relationship is given due attention. For example it may be very disrespectful for a nurse to call a Sikh gentleman by his first name. Cultural norms determine all aspects of the communication process, not only the verbal component as discussed above but also the non-verbal, for example touch, interpersonal distance, use of gestures, eye contact and facial expressions (Burgoon 1994).

■ **Activity** Imagine that you have been asked to measure Mr Atkinson's blood pressure. You are meeting him for the first time – how would you establish rapport?

Knapp and Vangelisti, (1992, cited in Hargie and Tourish 1997) suggest that relationships develop in a number of stages and the first of these is initiating. In this stage, they propose that opening introductions and reactions often involve a degree of small talk. You might, for example, note that Mr Atkinson comes from a local village with which you are familiar, and comment: 'I see you come from Whitchurch. That's a lovely village – have you lived there long?' Note that this conversation should put Mr Atkinson at ease, thus enabling your assessment of him to be more accurate, and also helping you to assess his level of consciousness (*see* Chapter 7: Monitoring vital signs).

Listening and non-verbal communication

There are many different definitions of listening emphasizing the aural (hearing), oral (spoken) and environmental aspects. However Smith (1986) underlines the importance of recognizing listening as an active process that requires concentration and effort to enable the development of the appropriate skills.

Activity

Reflect on the last occasion you were:
- speaking to a friend in a social setting
- speaking to a colleague at work
- speaking to a client.

What can you recall about
- Verbal ways that you showed that you were listening
- Body positions: yours and their's
- Eye contact and facial expression
- Other non-verbal skills.

What can you remember about the content?

Weaver (1972, cited in Bostrom 1997) suggests that our attitudes and culture determine the selection, perception and retention of any received message – do you consider these aspects are relevant to your examples? Was it easier to remember what you discussed with your friend rather than a colleague? This exercise may demonstrate to you how important attention and memory are within the listening process.

Egan (1990) uses the acronym SOLER to help us to remember how to use our body position to help us to focus on the skill of listening.

- **S**it squarely in relation to the client
- Maintain an **O**pen position
- **L**ean slightly towards the client
- Maintain reasonable **E**ye contact
- **R**elax.

Were these aspects of body language apparent in your examples? You may also have reflected on your or others' use of space, silence, touch and gestures, such as nodding the head in agreement or the use of facial expression to show interest or understanding. You may also be aware of how you or others used verbal signals to indicate that you were listening, for example the use of 'umm, aah, uh-huh, oh, I see'. There is always a danger that when we are supposed to be actively listening, we can slip into automatic pilot and are not really fully responsive to the message. Kagan *et al.* (1986) refer to this as minimal listening.

When we are with clients it may be particularly useful to develop the skill of 'reflecting'. Kagan *et al.* (1986) suggest that reflecting is the ability of being able to demonstrate to the speaker that we have **heard and understood** both the emotional and factual content of the message. This means that we must also be alert to any non-verbal messages, for example, Kevin, when asked, may say that he is OK. However you may determine from his non-verbal cues that he is very anxious. In order to recognize this incongruence between the verbal and non-verbal message, the development of sensitive observational skills and an empathetic approach is required. Empathy entails thoughts and emotions related to understanding the client's position, and may be portrayed non-verbally and through the nurse's words and actions (Baillie 1996). The skills of empathy thus include appropriate use of touch, eye contact and use of voice. Vocal features may encompass not only the words we use but as importantly, the tone and manner – perhaps through the use of a calm and soothing voice.

Another skill of listening that relates to verbal aspects is called 'paraphrasing'. This is the ability to put what an individual has said into different words without losing the original meaning. For example when suggesting to Kevin that he might like to have a wash and clean his teeth, he may say:

'No thank you. I'm not bothered about having a wash today. I'm not dirty anyway'.

How would you respond to Kevin using paraphrasing? Another issue that this scenario highlights is that of Kevin's right to refuse care. Consider why Kevin might be refusing care. There may be many reasons – for example:

- He may be shy.
- He may prefer another nurse or his parents to help him but feel that he cannot tell you.
- He may be afraid that washing will cause him pain or make his wound bleed.
- He may simply just not want a wash today.

The Code of Professional Conduct (UKCC 1992) states in clause one that the nurse will 'act always in such a manner as to promote and safeguard the interests and well-being of patients/clients'. In relation to the above example, Kevin would not suffer undue physical harm in if he went without a wash. He will be able to get up to the bathroom and attend to his own hygiene needs before very long. It would, however, be in his best interests to allow his wound dressing to be checked for oozing, and without mouthwashes, his

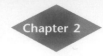

mouth would become dry and unpleasant. It might be that with support from his parents, he will be more confident to accept care. Mr Atkinson is likely to be dependent longer, and skin care will be a necessary part of his management. If he were to refuse care the nurse would need to have an understanding of *why* he was refusing care as there may be an underlying psychological need that requires addressing.

Clear explanations

Perhaps what Mr Atkinson would need in this situation is clear explanations, e.g. as to why his skin needs to be observed and cared for. One of the key elements of the new NHS Charter (Department of Health 1998) is the aspect of effective communication, and it suggests that individuals should receive comprehensive information about all aspects of their care. In providing explanations, nurses should take into account language (e.g. if the person does not speak English), age, child development, and, particularly with clients with learning disability, methods of communication which might include non-verbal and use of signing. Issues relating to providing sufficient and understandable information so that informed consent can be obtained from children and parents are explored by Colson (2000), who recommends that play activities can help with the child's understanding. An important part of giving information is paying attention to the words that we use and as nurses we need to develop an understanding of the power of language. Crawford (1999) suggests that language shapes relationships and Fairclough (1989) investigated how language can be used to dominate others.

One response to Kevin could have been:

'Come on, don't be a baby – you're old enough to be sensible – what would your mother say?' It would be easy to take a dominant stance and make it difficult for Kevin to assert himself. The way that nurses talk to clients can be beneficial and supportive or it can be detrimental by being patronizing or debilitating. Imagine that Mrs Wilson needed to wear an incontinence pad, and the nurse said: 'Come on Granny – let's put your nappy on'. How do you think she may feel? How would you feel if someone spoke to your mother or grandmother in this way? Crawford (1999, p. 49) emphasizes the unacceptability of 'secondary baby talk' and the harmful effects it may have on the nurse–client relationship. The way that we use language is also an important aspect of labelling which will be discussed later.

Questioning appropriately

There are many different types of questions that have been identified.

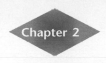

Activity   Can you list some different types of questions and give an example for each?

Niven and Robinson(1994) suggest the following types of questions:

- **Closed questions**, e.g. Do you want a cup of tea? Have you got pain? These questions are useful for gaining factual information, but they do not allow further exploration or elaboration. Often this type of question may be used in the initial assessment of a patient and can lead on to the second major type of question.

- **Open questions**, e.g. How is your diet? How would you describe your pain? These kind of questions allow a fuller response and enable people to reply in their own manner. Sometimes open questions can precipitate a long and not necessarily relevant response and it may be appropriate to use a closed question to refocus the conversation. Thus both closed and open questions are extremely valuable when interviewing clients.

- **Probing questions**, e.g. 'You say that the pain is worse in the mornings. Tell me when else it is particularly bad?' The use of probes or prompts can assist clients in talking about their thoughts and feelings and enable them to address their concerns.

- **Leading questions**, e.g. 'you don't look as if you are in pain – are you?' These kind of questions are better avoided as they can pressure the client to respond in a particular way. However, nurses are often unaware of using them.

- **Affective questions**. These are specifically used to address the emotions of the client and will indicate our concern. For example Kevin, who is quiet and uncommunicative, may need to be asked how he feels about being in hospital. In order to ask this kind of question we need to have established a good rapport and should ensure that we can give time to the client for his response. We should also know our own limitations in terms of helping responses.

Learning outcome 2:
Understand the terms stereotyping and labelling

Stereotyping is the assigning of individuals to categories as a result of assumptions that have been made (Tourish 1999). Labelling is a form of stereotyping where we categorize people by, for example, aspects such as their behaviour, their dress or their age. As previously discussed, when we were considering attitudes, the judgements we make of others may affect the care we give. Sometimes we make these judgements as a result of our personal bias, and as a result we fail to see the individual as a unique human being. This can lead to the nurse being prejudiced in the care that is given. Prejudice means to 'pre-judge'.

Activity

You are to admit a new patient. The only information you have is the patient's name, Albert Higginbottom, and limited background information, i.e. that he is aged 58 years, lives in a hostel, has fallen whilst under the influence of alcohol and has a fractured right femur. Describe how you might imagine Albert to be, e.g. his personality and his physical characteristics.

You may have decided that Albert has an alcohol problem, is scruffy, has no supporting relatives, and is possibly uncooperative. You would thus already be starting to form judgements about the patient and this might affect how you approach him. On the other hand, you might have decided to keep a completely open mind!

There are two manifestations of prejudice – direct and indirect (Pettigrew and Meertens 1995). Direct or open prejudice is just that: it is blatant and obvious. An example of this might be a patient refusing to be looked after by a nurse who is black. Whereas indirect or closed prejudice is more subtle, for example a nurse avoiding a patient that she does not approve of.

Activity

Consider the practice scenarios. How might both direct and indirect prejudice manifest itself?

You may have felt that Kevin would be seen as a young boy and therefore he may not be involved in decisions about his hygiene needs. Mr Atkinson, on the other hand, may be seen as a old man who would not understand the implications of possible treatment choices, and could therefore be excluded from the process. Clara may be judged as a result of her unresponsiveness, and as a result, care staff may not tell her what they are doing when performing practical skills. Vera may be avoided by staff as a result of her agitation and confusion and as a result may be incontinent.

We make these attempts at ordering the world around us in an effort to understand what is happening, but as we've already seen, at times this leads us to erroneous perceptions. This can then affect the care that is delivered, usually negatively though sometimes in a positive way. Included in this is how we communicate with our patients/clients as this can reflect our underlying prejudices.

Labelling of patients was initially thought to be fairly fixed in nature, so that once labelled, this would remain with the patient/client (Stockwell 1972). However Johnson and Webb (1995) found that labels were flexible and transient, and could change with time and experience. Therefore when approaching people to undertake a practical skill you need to aware of whether your behaviour is affected by any labels or stereotypical views held about the person.

Learning outcome 3:
Discuss relevant aspects of communicating with the individual who is anxious, angry or confused

The anxious person

Many people are anxious when admitted to hospital or faced with a new situation or uncertainty about the future. Anxiety is defined as 'a palpable but transitory emotional state or condition characterized by feelings of tension and apprehension and heightened autonomic nervous system arousal' (Speilberger *et al.* 1968, cited in Adams and Bromley, 1998, p. 15).

Anxiety is one of our basic emotions and can range from mild to very severe. It can serve as a warning and a certain amount can help us to cope with any threatening situations, but if it becomes excessive this may become detrimental to the patient and can interfere with their normal functioning. Sometimes anxiety is referred to as either 'state' or 'trait'. State anxiety means that it is the state the person is in that causes the state of anxiety. Trait anxiety refers to the fact that some people are naturally more anxious than others. For example Kevin may be anxious because of his hospitalization, or he may be a naturally anxious adolescent.

Activity	(a) What are the cues that may lead you to think a person is anxious?
	(b) What aspects of their situation may give rise to anxiety for Clara Wright or Mrs Wilson?

For activity (a) you may have considered: facial expression; restlessness; wringing hands; and profuse sweating, which are some indicators that an individual is anxious. You will find out more about the effects of anxiety upon the vital signs when reading Chapter 7 (Monitoring vital signs).

For activity (b), anxiety about illness and the implications for the future, are often linked to fearfulness and/or uncertainty about the future. Recipients of health care may have:

■ Fear of needles and pain
■ Fear of finding out something is wrong – pulse, blood pressure
■ Fear of being harmed – for example, use of the hoist or falling when being helped
■ Fear of the unknown environment.

It is important that we make no assumptions about what may be causing an individual's anxiety. Careful assessment and development of a trusting relationship will enable the nurse to more accurately identify the cause for their anxiety.

Once the nurse has recognized that the person is experiencing anxiety, there are some steps that can be taken to help to reduce the symptoms. Anxiety management techniques include the following:

■ Explanation of the process of anxiety and the symptoms experienced
■ Breathing control
■ Relaxation therapy
■ Challenging of cognition (thoughts)
■ Assertiveness training.

If anxiety is not addressed then it can impact on the individual's physical and emotional well-being. Adams and Bromley (1998) suggested the following are some examples of outcomes of unmanaged anxiety: angina; migraine; aggravation of skin disorders; disturbance in bowel movement; unstable diabetes; vulnerability to infections, and cognitive impairment, including poor concentration, memory and motivation. The factors relating to impairment of thinking may be particularly important to be aware of if you need to teach a patient a practical skill. Anxiety can also act as a barrier to communication

Activity — Identify other factors that may act as barriers to your communication and relationship with clients?

It is sometimes helpful to think about barriers in terms of physical, psychological and social.

Physical barriers
These may be:

■ Visual impairment
■ Auditory impairment
■ Pain
■ How the surrounding environment is organized (a desk between two participants, one person sitting whilst the other is standing, or a loud television in the background).

Psychological barriers
These may relate to aspects that we have discussed earlier:

■ Personality – if someone is very shy
■ Attitudes, beliefs and labelling – either the care-giver's or the client's
■ Emotional state of either party (e.g. anxiety).

Social barriers
These may include aspects such as:

■ Culture (this could include the culture of the ward for example whether there is team nursing or a named nurse approach)

■ Religious beliefs
■ Social status.

This list is not exhaustive and the distinction between the physical, psychological and social are not always clear-cut. However we need to be aware of these barriers and the effect that they may exert.

The angry person

Anger is a natural human emotion, associated with displeasure; it is often passionately felt and can be expressed in a number of ways, if expressed at all (Adams and Bromley 1998). Nurses are sometimes confronted with people who are displaying strong emotions such as anger and aggression. It is very important for nurses to employ good interpersonal skills at these times. This can help to minimize the psychological impact of the emotions.

Activity	How would you recognize that a client was becoming angry?

You may be able to divide your answers into the following categories; verbal and non verbal. Examples of verbal indications may be a raised voice, fast speech or the use of obscenities. Non-verbal indications include changes in body language – the patient may display exaggerated movements, clenched fists, pace back and forth, throw or kick objects. There may be changes in facial expression, e.g. frowning, eye contact may be negligible or it might be extended – glaring. These are just some of the indications that an individual is becoming angry. It is important that the nurse having recognized these, acts to disperse the anger. This is done by:

■ Listening actively to what the person has to say, thus showing a non-judgemental stance. However it is also important that eye contact is not held for too long, as this may be seen as threatening (Williams 1996).
■ Acknowledge the anger. This demonstrates empathy with what the client is feeling (Williams 1996).
■ Encourage the client to identify the cause of the anger – this is done through skilful questioning.
■ Where possible empower the person to resolve any causes.

Thus the aim is the peaceful resolution of the situation. However, if the nurse confronts anger with anger, through direct confrontation, defensiveness or questioning of the client's feelings, then this will probably lead to an escalation in anger, maybe to aggression. You may find it useful to reflect upon the scenarios and try to identify possible causes of anger.

The confused person

Confusion is defined as 'any condition in which there is a loss of orientation or difficulty ... with memory, attention span or other cognitive function' (Adams and Bromley 1998, p. 179).

Activity   Mrs Wilson is confused. Identify what could be the possible causes of this.

Confusion may be a relatively permanent feature of her condition, e.g. related to dementia. However, again we must avoid making assumptions as it may be due to number of factors for example malnutrition, dehydration, constipation or an acute infection.

Activity   You think that Mrs Wilson needs to use the toilet as she is becoming more agitated. Suggest some principles in helping her in this confused state.

Principles to consider include:

- Orientation to time and place, for example 'Mrs Wilson, I'm student nurse Smith and I'm here to help you to the toilet'.
- Use of appropriate and understandable language.
- A calm and clear voice.
- A calm manner for example avoiding sudden or exaggerated movements.
- The use of active listening skills.

Sometimes despite all attempts to help the person, their confusion may make it difficult for them to make their needs known and for us to identify the appropriate interventions. In these situations the safety of the person will be paramount, and continued observation and assessment will be crucial.

Summary

- Communication takes many forms and has verbal and non-verbal components.
- Nurses need to be able to use a range of interpersonal skills effectively. In relation to practical nursing skills, initiating interaction, listening, non-verbal communication, questioning and giving explanations are all of particular importance.
- Stereotyping of people can detract from an individual approach to care.
- There are many situations where communication is challenging and requires the nurse to be skilled and empathetic. Examples include when caring for people who are anxious, angry or confused.

CHAPTER SUMMARY

In the chapters following, specific practical nursing skills will be focused on; the importance of the approach of the nurse whilst carrying out these skills cannot be over-emphasized. In conclusion, this chapter has aimed to provide some insights into the importance of the nurse – client relationship. It has included a discussion about the impact of self within this relationship, and how this will inevitably affect communication and thus the care of people. It has also highlighted some principles of communication and their applications in a variety of care settings with a range of different clients, linked to the scenarios. As suggested by Niven and Robinson (1994) one of the most crucial features of communicating with others is that we understand *ourselves* and those with whom we are communicating.

REFERENCES

Adams, B. and Bromley, B. 1998. *Psychology for Health Care: Key Terms and Concepts*. London: Macmillan Press.

Baillie, L. 1996. A phenomenological study of the nature of empathy. *Journal of Advanced Nursing* **24**, 1300–8.

Bem, D.J. 1970. *Beliefs, Attitudes and Human Affairs*. Belmont, California: Brooks/Cole Publishing.

Bostrom, R.N. 1997. The process of listening. In: Hargie, O. (ed.) *Handbook of Communication Skills*, 2nd edn. New York: Routledge, 236–58.

Burgoon, J. 1994. Nonverbal signals. In: Knapp, M. and Miller, G. (eds.) *Handbook of Interpersonal Communication*, California: Sage, 344–93.

Burnard, P. 1994. *Counselling Skills for Health Professionals*, 2nd edn, London: Chapman and Hall.

Childs, A. 1995. A nurse's view. In: Tschudin, V. (ed.) *Ethics: The Patients' Charter*, London: Scutari Press, 1–34.

Colson, J. 2000. Concepts. In: Huband, S. and Trigg, E. (eds.) *Practices in Children's Nursing: Guidelines for Hospital and Community*, Edinburgh: Churchill Livingstone, 1–12.

Crawford, P. 1999. Nursing language: uses and abuses. *Nursing Times* **95** (6), 48–49.

Department of Health 1998. *The NHS Charter*. London: Department of Health.

Egan, G. 1990. *The Skilled Helper: A Systematic Approach to Effective Helping*, 4th edn. California:Brooks/Cole.

Fairclough, N. 1989. *Language and Power* London: Longman.

Gross, R. 1996. *Psychology: The Science of Mind and Behaviour*, 3rd edn. London: Hodder and Stoughton.

Hargie, O. 1986. Communication as a skilled behaviour. In: Hargie, O. (ed.) *A Handbook of Communication Skills*, London: Routledge, 7–21.

Hargie, O., Saunders, C. and Dickson, D. 1994. *Social Skills in Interpersonal Communication*, 3rd edn. London: Routledge.

Hargie C. T. and Tourish D. 1997. Relational communication. In: Hargie, O. (ed.) *A Handbook of Communication Skills*, 2nd edn. London: Routledge, 358–82.

Hinton, P. 1993. *The Psychology of Interpersonal Perception*. London: Routledge.

Irving, P. and Hazlett, D. 1999. Communicating with challenging clients. In: Long, A. (ed.) *Interaction for Practice in Community Nursing*. Basingstoke: Macmillan Press, 260–85.

Johnson M. and Webb C. 1995. Rediscovering unpopular patients: concept of social judgement, *Journal of Advanced Nursing*, **21**, 466–75.

Kagan, C, Evans, J and Kay, B. 1986. *A Manual of Interpersonal Skills for Nurses, an Experiential Approach*. London: Harper and Row.

Long, A. 1999. Introduction. In: Long, A. (ed.) *Interaction for Practice in Community Nursing*. London: Macmillan Press, 1–23.

Luft, J. and Ingram H.1955. *The Johari Window: A Graphic Model of Interpersonal Relations*. Los Angeles, CA: University of Los Angeles Press.

Morrison, P. and Burnard, P. 1997. *Caring and Communicating: The Interpersonal Relationship in Nursing*, 2nd edn. Basingstoke: Macmillan Press.

Niebuhr, H.R. 1963. *The Responsible Self*. New York: Harper and Row.

Niven, N. and Robinson, J. 1994: *The Psychology of Nursing Care*. London: Macmillan Press.

Petrie, P. 1997. *Communicating with Children and Adults: Interpersonal Skills for Early Years and Playwork*, 2nd edn. London: Arnold.

Pettigrew, T. and Meertens, R. 1995. Subtle and blatant prejudice in Western Europe. *European Journal of Social Psychology* **25**, 55–75.

Price, B. 1990. *Body Image: Nursing Concepts and Care*. London: Prentice Hall.

Rogers, C.R.1961. *On Becoming a Person*. Boston: Houghton Mifflin.

Ryckman, R.M. 1989. *Theories of Personality* 4th edn. Pacific Grove, CA: Brookes/Cole.

Smith V. 1986. Listening. In: Hargie, O. (ed.) *A Handbook of Communication Skills*. London: Routledge, 246–65.

Stockwell F. 1972. *The Unpopular Patient*. London: Royal College of Nursing.

Tourish, D. 1999. Communicating beyond individual bias. In: Long, A. (ed.) *Interaction for Practice in Community Nursing*, London: Macmillan Press, 190–216.

United Kingdom Central Council 1992: *Code of Professional Conduct* London: UKCC.

Williams, D. 1996. *Communication Skills in Practice: A Practical Guide for Health Professionals*. London: Jessica Kingsley.

Preventing cross-infection

Vickie Arrowsmith and Dee Burrows

Many micro-organisms exist but not all cause infection in individuals. Those that cause disease are called pathogens. When pathogens are acquired from another person, or from the environment, they are described as **exogenous**. The transmission of pathogens, between people and across environments, is termed **cross-infection**. When micro-organisms, colonizing one site on the host, enter another site on the same person and cause further infection, this is called self-infection or **endogenous infection**.

The prevention of cross-infection means breaking the 'chain of infection'. The chain consists of the source of infection, or reservoir, the route of transmission, the portal of entry and the incubation period leading to the infection. The power of this chain can be affected by the need for a minimum infectious dose and/or the aggression of the microbe, together with the competence of the victim's immune system (Meers *et al.* 1995). Preventing cross-infection is essential within the everyday activities of almost all nurses. There is an ethical and legal duty to protect patients against infection (Fletcher and Buka 1999). This is relevant within any setting, but within hospital and residential situations, the risk of cross-infection is considerably greater.

Hospital acquired infection, sometimes referred to as **nosocomial** infection, is a large problem with recent national prevalence surveys indicating rates of around 9% (Emmerson *et al.* 1996). Rapid improvements in medical technology and the consequent changes in the way care is delivered have increased the risk of infection and the subsequent personal and financial costs. In addition, as pointed out by Perry (1998), infection control can no longer be considered just a hospital issue. The increasingly rapid trend of early discharge of patients from hospital settings means that hospital acquired infection will often first become evident in the community. Furthermore, nursing homes are carrying out more invasive and technical care. Without taking adequate care, nurses may unwittingly transmit micro-organisms from one person to another, and cross-infection can also occur directly between individuals. Some people may be extra vulnerable to infection as their immune systems are compromised. Resistant micro-organisms are also posing an increasing problem.

This introduction gives some of the reasons why skills in preventing cross-infection are necessary.

Included in this chapter are:
- Universal precautions
- Hand washing
- Use of gloves and aprons
- Non-touch technique
- Specimen collection
- Source isolation
- Sharps disposal
- Waste disposal.

Recommended biology reading:

These questions will help you to focus on the biology underpinning the skills required to prevent cross-infection. Use your recommended textbook to find out:

- What are micro-organisms? Where are they found? Are all micro-organisms harmful?
- Identify some of the beneficial roles of micro-organisms.
- How do micro-organisms enter the body?
- What is meant by the terms: commensal, symbiont, pathogen, normal flora?
- What mechanisms does the body employ to defend itself from infection? (Think about non-specific defences e.g. secretions, reflexes, barriers etc. as well as specific mechanisms). Review the structure of the skin.
- What is infection?
- How does the body fight infections?
- What are the clinical signs of infection?
- What causes infections?
- How can these infective agents be prevented from being transferred between people?
- Which people may be more vulnerable to infections?
- Why are they more vulnerable and how could they be protected?

- Which cells are involved in the specific immune response? Where are they found?
- What is the difference between humoral and cell-mediated immunity?
- What are antibodies? How do they help protect us from infection?
- How do we achieve an immunological memory?
- What factors can affect an individual's immune system?

PRACTICE SCENARIOS

As discussed above, prevention of cross-infection must be part of the nurse's role in almost all practice settings. The following scenarios will be referred to during the text when discussing the practical skills which are covered in this chapter.

MRSA
Methicillin resistant *Staphylococcus aureus* is a highly resistant micro-organism, which is discussed in detail in the section on source isolation.

Bronchiolitis
An acute viral infection of the respiratory tract, causing inflammation and obstruction of the bronchioles. Respiratory syncytial virus (RSV) causes 50–90% of cases and is easily spread. It is very common, infecting 69% of all children in the first years of life (Pursell and Gould 1997).

■ **Adult**
Mrs Ethel Wrights is an 85-year-old lady who was admitted from a nursing home to hospital after feeling dizzy, and falling heavily onto the left side of her body. She sustained lacerations to her left knee and elbow, which need dressing. Her notes indicate that she is an MRSA carrier and swabs have been taken to confirm her current status.

■ **Child**
Tiffany Wells is 7 weeks old and is in hospital with bronchiolitis. She is receiving oxygen therapy via a headbox (*see* Chapter 8, Oxygen therapy), and is having feeds of her mother's expressed breast milk via a nasogastric tube (*see* Chapter 4, Supporting the breast-feeding mother; enteral feeding). Her condition is being monitored closely, and she is stable at present. Tiffany has two older brothers aged 5 and 3 years. Her mother is resident in the cubicle with her.

■ **Learning disability**
Mary Paine, who is 20 years old, has Downs syndrome and lives in a small staffed residence. Over the last 24 hours she has developed diarrhoea and vomiting. A stool specimen needs to be collected.

■ **Mental health**
Tony Morello is a 34-year-old man with a history of schizophrenic type illness. He does not like leaving the house during daylight hours. Tony receives anti-psychotic medication in the form of zuclopenthixol decanoate 200 mg every 3 weeks by intramuscular injection. The community psychiatric nurse gives the injection at Tony's home, whilst at the same time assessing his condition.

UNIVERSAL PRECAUTIONS

Activity   Consider the admission to the Accident and Emergency Department of any new patient. How do you think staff would know what infection control procedures to use, bearing in mind that they may know nothing of the person's history at all?

You may be aware that 'universal precautions' are recommended for *every* patient, which thus eliminates any random inappropriate practice (Howells-Johnson 1997). It is, for example, impossible to identify all those who are seropositive to human immunodeficiency virus (HIV) or hepatitis B. Thus every patient should be considered as a potential hazard and appropriate barrier methods used to prevent contamination by blood/body fluids (Royal College of Nursing 1997). Universal precautions not only protect health-care staff from infection with blood-borne viruses, but also prevent transmission of organisms between patients (McDougall 1999). Table 3.1 summarizes the routes of transmission of micro-organisms.

Table 3.1 Routes of transmission (adapted from Parker 1999)

Route	*Explanation*	*Example*
Direct or indirect contact	Transfer from body surface to body surface between an infected or colonized person and a susceptible host, or via an intermediate object.	**Direct**: Patient to patient e.g. through touch, or staff to patient when carrying out patient care activities e.g. moving and handling. **Indirect**: Patient touched by a nurse's unwashed hands or gloves that have not been changed, after contact with a patient who is infected/colonized.
Inanimate objects and equipment	Susceptible host is infected by an object which is contaminated with micro-organisms.	Beds, curtains, toys, bedpans, tables can all be contaminated and spread infection, sometimes via the hands of staff.
Droplet	Micro-organisms transmitted through the air within droplets, mainly saliva.	Coughing, sneezing, talking and singing can transmit microorganisms. Can also occur during procedures e.g. bronchoscopy or suctioning.
Airborne	Micro-organisms carried in droplet nuclei (small particle residue), or by dust particles (made of e.g. dead skin scales, clothing fibres).	Carried by air currents in the environment and breathed in by a susceptible host, or they settle on horizontal surfaces. Some bacteria form spores and survive for months in such conditions.
Ingestion	Ingested into the body with food or water causing gastrointestinal infections and excreted in faeces. Known as the faecal–oral route.	Food may be contaminated when hands that have been in contact with faeces transfer the organisms onto food that someone then eats.
Vector	Transmission via insects or rodents.	Cockroaches, rats, mice and ants can cause contamination of food. Mosquitoes spread malaria and yellow fever; ticks spread Lyme disease and typhus

Historically, the 'traditional' approach tried to identify which patients were infected and with what, so that particular approaches could be adopted for specific infections. If the same precautions are taken for all people (universal precautions), the process is simplified. Similarly, if the same precautions are taken for all body fluids, there is no need to identify different levels of protection for different diseases. For example, salmonella is transmitted by contact with faeces, but if the correct precautions are routinely adhered to when dealing with faeces, then additional precautions are not necessary for infected patients. The recommended policy for universal precautions (Royal College of Nursing 1997) can be found in Box 3.1. Subsequent sections in this chapter will look at many of these elements in more detail.

- **Hand washing**: essential, before and after all patient contact and after skin contamination with body fluid.
- **Gloves and aprons**: when direct contact with blood/body fluid is anticipated.
- **Eye protection**: if there is a danger of flying, contaminated debris or blood splashes.
- **Irrigation**: if conjunctiva or mucous membranes are splashed with body fluids, irrigate with plenty of saline.
- **Cuts/abrasions**: should be covered with waterproof dressings.
- **Sharps disposal**: extreme care when using and disposing of sharps. No resheathing of needles, or over-filling of sharps boxes.
- **Instructions for action in the event of blood spillage**: put on gloves and apron, cover the spillage with paper towels, treat with 10,000 ppm sodium hypochlorite or household bleach 1 to 10 dilution, leave for a few minutes, and then clean up and dispose as clinical waste.
- **Contaminated waste**: disposed of in yellow clinical sacks.

Box 3.1 Universal precautions (Royal College of Nursing 1997)

HAND WASHING

Definition

Hand washing can be defined as the careful and systematic cleaning and drying of the hands in order to remove soiling and transient bacteria to prevent cross-infection.

Learning outcomes

By the end of this section you will be able to:

1. State the purpose and importance of hand washing for the care and safety of both patients and nurses.
2. Assess when hand washing is needed.
3. Carry out hand washing effectively.
4. Understand the factors that influence effective hand washing practice.

Learning outcome 1:
State the purpose and importance of hand washing for the care and safety of both patients and nurses

Hungarian obstetrician Ignaz Semmelweis (1815–1865), succeeded in reducing the death rate of his patients from around 1 in 8, to 1 in 79, by the simple action of persuading his colleagues and medical students to wash their hands in a solution of chlorinated lime. However, he failed as a communicator, alienated his colleagues and had to leave his post (Meers *et al.* 1995). Happily, since that time it has become widely recognized that the hands of those employed in health-care settings are an important route for the transmission of infection (Gould 1997; Kerr 1998). However, Ayliffe *et al.* (1999) state that there is little statistical evidence, from controlled trials, to support this statement. Nonetheless, they concede that it is rational to consider that the hands of staff represent one of the main routes by which infection is spread. Consequently, it has long been recognized that hand washing is the most important and basic technique for preventing the transmission of pathogens (Sedgwick 1984).

Activity

Using the scenarios at the beginning of the chapter, discuss with a colleague the factors which may make each of the individuals susceptible to cross-infection, self-infection and infection from the environment.

You may have identified the following:
Mrs Wrights is elderly and unwell. Such patients' defence mechanisms are impaired, so their infections tend to be more severe and those due to hospital strains may be more difficult to treat (Meers *et al.* 1995). If Mrs Wrights was to have a device *in situ*, such as an intravenous infusion or urinary catheter, the device may allow bacteria to enter the body directly. This may increase susceptibility to infection.

Tiffany is very young. Her immune system is not yet fully developed and she has not yet received any vaccinations. This is why it is common practice for very young infants to be nursed in single cubicles when admitted to hospital.

Mary and Tony, along with the general population, require a basic knowledge of hygiene and infection control, including hand washing, in order to reduce their susceptibility. A structured behavioural programme may be necessary in order to teach Mary effective handwashing. According to developmental level this may require the use of backward chaining techniques. This involves teaching the final stage of the skill first, and then working consecutively backwards. Encouragement and reinforcement by the nurse are very important. These techniques for teaching self-help skills such as hand washing, are covered in detail by Carr and Wilson (1987).

Thus individuals vary widely in their ability to resist infection. Age, general health, state of nutrition, previous exposure to infection and vaccinations all affect levels of risk (Wilson 1995). Infants and small children are susceptible as their immune systems are not yet fully developed, and their immunity could be lowered further by treatments such as cytotoxic drugs or steroids (Simpson 1998). You may have thought of other reasons for susceptibility to infection.

In a series of classic studies, Price (1938) discovered two populations of bacteria present on hands: resident organisms and transient organisms. **Resident organisms**, sometimes called normal flora, lie deep in the stratum corneum of the skin and are difficult to remove. Because they are so difficult to remove they are less likely to be implicated in cross-infection. **Transient flora** are acquired from the environment and are carried temporarily on the hands. These organisms may be transferred between nurse and client, resulting in cross-infection as the nurse moves from one person to another, or handles different sites on the same person. The aim of hand washing is to remove transient bacteria to below the level likely to cause infection.

Activity   Try to think of some of the ways in which you might pick up transient organisms on your hands whilst in a practice scenario.

You might have thought of:

1. Following the care of an incontinent person.
2. When emptying urine bags and bedpans.
3. When handling the bed linen of an infected or incontinent person.
4. When bed bathing and handling wash bowls.
5. When touching furniture.
6. During bed making.
7. When taking a patient's pulse or temperature.

Ayliffe *et al*. (1999) state that studies in their laboratories, using finger impressions, indicate that significant contamination can follow activities 1, 2, 3, 4 and less so 5, 6 and 7.

Transferring bacteria from your hands, to a patient, can lead to infection in the patient. In the second national prevalence survey of infections in hospital, the prevalence of hospital acquired infection (HAI) was found to range from 2–29%, with an average of 9% (Emmerson *et al*. 1996). The most common infection sites identified were the urinary tract (23.2%); lower respiratory tract (22.9%); surgical wounds (10.7%); and the skin (9.6%). In special care baby units the HAI rate is estimated as 14.2% (5.2% septicaemia), and in children's wards, the rate is 5.6% (Simpson 1998). Effective hand washing can reduce the incidence of HAI in all settings.

HAIs are very costly. They cause patient distress and anxiety and increase the length of hospital stay. There is also the additional cost of specific treatments, such as antibiotics and disinfectants, and the cost of materials ranging from protective clothing to dressings. Nursing and other professional care costs are also increased. Delay in returning to work has negative financial implications for both the patient and the state. Finally, there is the cost related to the delayed admission for other people needing hospital treatment.

Learning outcome 2:
Assess when hand washing is needed

■ **Activity** | With a colleague, make a list of the times when you think it is important to wash your hands.

Your answers could include:
Generally:

- Before and after direct contact with patients/clients, especially those who are immuno-supressed.

More specifically:

- Before aseptic procedures.
- Before and after handling invasive devices.
- Before and after handling food.
- After removing gloves.
- When hands become visibly soiled.
- After using the toilet.
- When leaving the clinical area.

Importantly, pathogens are likely to be acquired on the hands in greatest number when handling moist, heavily contaminated substances, such as body fluids and hand washing should be carried out at this time. Ayliffe *et al*. (1999) suggest the following useful practical guideline when assessing when to hand wash:

Imagine that the next thing you are going to do is to eat a sandwich. Would you wash your hands first?

Learning outcome 3:
Carry out hand washing effectively

Lowbury (1991) describes three levels of hand washing:

■ **Social hand washing**: this uses non-medicated soap or detergent and water and is effective under most circumstances. 99% of transient organisms are removed in this way (Ayliffe *et al.*1999), by the mechanical action.

Disinfection
Is the process of removing or destroying most, but not all, viable micro-organisms.

■ **Hygienic hand disinfection**: hands are washed for 15–30 seconds and an antiseptic detergent may be used and/or an alcohol solution. This removes or destroys most/all transient micro-organisms and conveys a residual effect. This procedure would be used during an outbreak situation, before aseptic/invasive procedures and following contact with blood and body fluids.

■ **Surgical scrub**: this removes or destroys transient micro-organisms, reduces resident organisms and confers a prolonged effect. The nails are scraped or brushed and the hands and forearms are washed with an antiseptic for a minimum of 2 minutes. This technique is used before invasive procedures, especially surgery.

The most common antiseptic handwashes are chlorhexidine, iodine, and alcoholic hand rubs. Hand rubs, which contain 70% isopropanol alcohol, rapidly destroy micro-organisms and can be used as an alternative to hand washing on visibly clean hands. Their value, particularly when workload is high, has been clearly demonstrated (Gould and Chamberlaine 1995). They are also useful in settings, such as the community, where hand washing facilities may not be readily available (Kerr 1998).

■ ***Activity*** | For each of the scenarios, identify when you would socially hand wash and when you may need to hygienically hand disinfect.

Now check your answers:

Mrs Wrights
Hygienic hand disinfection would be employed before and after direct patient contact and especially when aseptically replacing her dressings.

Tiffany
Hygienic hand washing would be needed before and after direct contact, any invasive procedures, and when dealing with body fluids. Social hand washing is indicated before and after giving feeds.

Mary

Mary would be encouraged to socially hand wash after visiting the toilet. The nurse should hygienically hand wash following contact with body fluids. Under other circumstances, such as when serving food, social hand washing would be appropriate.

Tony

Before and after giving his intramuscular injection and for social interactions, social hand washing would be appropriate. Depending upon the availability of hand washing facilities, alcohol hand rubs may be a useful alternative.

■   **Activity**

Find out if you can access pink dye hand washing solution. This may be available in the skills laboratory or via the infection control nurse. Wash your hands with this solution and then take note of those areas that you have not covered with the dye.

Figure 3.1 shows a diagram of the areas most frequently missed. How does this compare with your hand washing result?

Thoroughness in applying the hand washing solution may be more important than the time spent on hand washing or the agent used (Ayliffe *et al.* 1999). Figure 3.2 outlines a seven-step guide to effective hand washing.

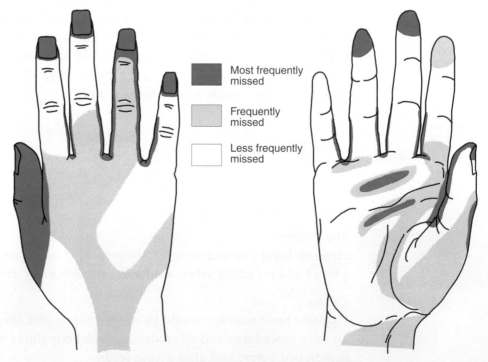

Most frequently missed

Frequently missed

Less frequently missed

Figure 3.1 Areas most frequently missed when hand washing

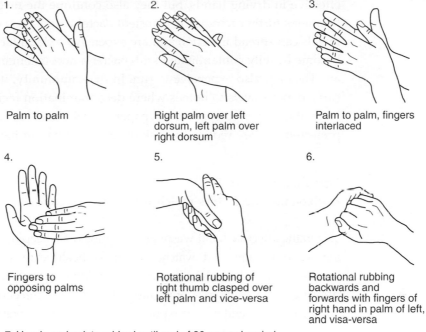

1. Palm to palm

2. Right palm over left dorsum, left palm over right dorsum

3. Palm to palm, fingers interlaced

4. Fingers to opposing palms

5. Rotational rubbing of right thumb clasped over left palm and vice-versa

6. Rotational rubbing backwards and forwards with fingers of right hand in palm of left, and visa-versa

7. Hands and wrists rubbed until end of 30-second period

Figure 3.2 A seven step guide to hand washing

> ■ *Activity*
> With the diagram in front of you, practise the seven steps. If pink dye is available, re-wash your hands using the guide and note any improvement.

The amount of time you wash your hands for is important, as the mechanical action helps to remove bacteria. Bowell (1992) recommends that thorough hand washing takes 30 seconds. However, Ayliffe *et al.* (1999) state that the average time spent hand washing is 10–20 seconds. How long did you spend washing your hands?

Drying hands

The thoroughness with which you dry your hands also influences the effectiveness of the whole hand washing procedure.

> ■ *Activity*
> Which of the following do you think is the most effective hand-drying medium?
> • Paper towels
> • Linen towels
> • Hot-air dryers

The results of a study by Gould (1994a), indicated that the right answer is **paper towels**, for the following reasons. Not only are these inexpensive and effective in drying hands, but they also continue the mechanical action which promotes further removal of transient bacteria and loose dead skin cells. Linen towels can spread infection and are expensive to launder. Hot-air hand dryers become heavily contaminated with bacteria and recontaminate hands and the air. They are also expensive to run. In the community, it may be necessary to carry paper towels to homes where decontamination facilities are inadequate. Note that when disposing of paper towels, foot operated pedal bins are preferred as they reduce the risk of recontaminating hands after washing.

Learning outcome 4:
Understand the factors which influence effective hand washing practice

Generally, effective hand washing is promoted by keeping nails short and avoiding wearing rings and watches. In most health-care settings, the only hand jewellery allowed is a wedding ring. Covering cuts and abrasions with occlusive dressings reduces the risk of acquiring blood-borne infections such as hepatitis B and C, and HIV, and may also prevent superficial infections from bacteria or fungi.

Activity   What other factors can you think of which may influence effective hand washing? In particular think about when you would need to hand wash in either the community or hospital setting. Referring to the scenarios will help you.

By referring to the scenarios you will probably have noted how frequently nurses would need to wash their hands. Frequent hand washing can cause damage to skin, especially if antiseptic solutions are used, or if hands are not dried properly. Cracked skin may harbour more bacteria and increase the risk of cross-infection.

   Gould (1994b) suggests five ways to reduce the likelihood of skin soreness:

1.   Wet skin before applying soap and antiseptic. This ensures that solutions are diluted and therefore less harsh to the skin.
2.   Rinse thoroughly to remove any traces of the solutions.
3.   Dry thoroughly.
4.   Use your own hand cream at the end of each shift. A shared hand cream is a potential source of infection.
5.   Protect any skin breaks with a waterproof dressing.

   Other reasons you may have thought of which could deter nurses from washing their hands include:

■   Inadequate and inconveniently placed hand washing facilities (Gould 1995). Kesavan *et al.* (1998) suggest that the most common problem in ward settings is the lack of suitable cleansing agents, particularly antiseptic solutions. Furthermore, taps and dispensers should be elbow operated and good facilities should exist for dispensing and disposing of paper towels.

■ Lack of education concerning the importance of hand washing.
■ Lack of emphasis on hand washing by peers and managers.
■ The use of gloves incorrectly seen as obviating the need for hand washing.

Summary

■ Effective hand washing is an essential tool in the prevention of cross-infection.
■ There are different levels of hand washing and nurses need to be aware of which are appropriate in different situations.
■ Hand washing must be performed thoroughly and for an adequate length of time. Hands must be dried carefully with paper towels.
■ There are a number of barriers to effective hand washing, but these must be overcome to prevent cross-infection.

USE OF GLOVES AND APRONS

Introduction

Gloves are worn for two main reasons:

■ To protect the patient from organisms present on the carer's hands.
■ To protect the wearer from contamination with patient's blood or other body fluids.

Similarly, aprons are worn to both protect the clothes of the carer and reduce the probability of transmission of hospital acquired infection.

Learning outcomes

On completion of this section you will be able to:

1. Identify the procedures for which sterile gloves are recommended.
2. Discuss the procedures for which non-sterile gloves are recommended.
3. Consider procedures for which gloves are not usually necessary.
4. Show awareness of the materials commonly used in the manufacture of disposable gloves, their relative values and costs.
5. Discuss when plastic aprons should be worn, stating the rationale.

Learning outcome 1:

Identify the procedures for which sterile gloves are recommended

Activity   Referring to each scenario at the beginning of the chapter, write down those clinical procedures and situations for which you believe sterile gloves should be worn.

You may have identified the following:

Mrs Wrights:

A non-touch technique (see later section) will be necessary to dress Mrs Wrights' wounds. It would be difficult to use forceps effectively on Mrs Wrights' jagged wounds, so sterile gloves will therefore need to be worn when her lacerations need cleansing and dressing.

Tiffany, Mary and Tony
None.

As you should have concluded from the above exercise, sterile gloves are only necessary for invasive procedures and for direct contact with non-intact skin (O'Toole 1997). Neither Tiffany, Mary or Tony are undergoing any invasive procedures.

Learning outcome 2:

Discuss the procedures for which non-sterile gloves are recommended

Activity   Look again at the scenarios and list those clinical procedures and situations when nurses should use non-sterile gloves.

Your list might include:

Mrs Wrights

As she is an MRSA carrier, gloves should be used when touching her. Additionally, gloves must be worn when there is potential contact with faeces, urine or any other body fluid (O'Toole 1997). The domestic cleaner should be instructed to wear gloves when cleaning the room and to discard them before leaving.

Tiffany

As Tiffany is vulnerable to infection from others and is also a potential source of infection to others, and non-sterile gloves should be worn for any contact with body fluids, especially respiratory secretions.

Mary

Contact with faeces, urine and vomit would necessitate the use of non-sterile gloves. Non-sterile gloves must therefore be worn when collecting the stool specimen.

Tony

None. Unless there is potential for contact with blood, the use of non-sterile gloves for injection would not be required.

In addition to the points above, it is worth noting that local policy concerning the handling and preparation of specific drugs, such as antibiotics and cytotoxic materials, may necessitate the use of gloves in order to protect the nurse. You should therefore check your local drug policy.

Learning outcome 3:
Consider clinical procedures for which gloves are not usually necessary

Activity

With reference to the scenarios, make a list of the procedures and situations for which gloves are usually unnecessary. Think particularly of all the individuals who may come into contact with the patient/client and try to decide if they need to wear gloves.

You may have identified the following:

Mrs Wrights

As stated above there are many occasions when gloves should be worn when attending to Mrs Wrights. However, the risk to visitors is minimal as most do not have contact with body fluids and do not therefore need to wear gloves. Nevertheless, they should be instructed to wash their hands before leaving the room. If Mrs Wrights has to be transported to another department, then the porter need not wear gloves, but should be advised to wash his hands after the journey to prevent cross-infection.

Tiffany

Gloves will not normally be necessary when caring for Tiffany, but all those in contact with her must wash their hands to prevent cross infection. In particular, both parents will need a clear explanation of the importance of hand washing and they should be encouraged to be proactive in ensuring that all social visitors wash their hands on entering and leaving the cubicle.

Mary

Gloves are unnecessary except where contact with blood, faeces, vomit or other body fluids is possible.

Tony

As stated earlier, gloves are not necessary at all.

Learning outcome 4:
Show awareness of the materials commonly used in the manufacture of disposable gloves, their relative values and costs

Activity

When next in the clinical area take note of the different types of gloves available to practitioners.

You may discover the following
There are three main types of disposable gloves:

- Latex, which is derived from the sap of the Brazilian rubber tree
- Vinyl – PVC (polyvinylchloride)
- Polythene – plastic (ethylene copolymer).

Research indicates that latex gloves generally offer more protection than vinyl or polythene (Johnson 1997; O'Toole 1997; Ross 1999). However, all gloves may perforate and should therefore be checked for defects. Hands should be hygienically washed before donning gloves and after removing them, finger-nails should be kept short to avoid perforations and gloves should never be reused (Brookes 1994; O'Toole 1997). Disposal of used gloves should be carried out in such a way as to avoid skin contamination and the gloves should be placed in the appropriate bin.

Latex contains a large number of different proteins, some of which can be allergenic. Hypersensitivity is increased due to residual accelerators (chemicals added to latex in order to assist the manufacturing process). The starch powder used in certain gloves can also cause allergens to leak from the rubber and bind to the starch. For these reasons patients, staff and visitors should be educated about the potential problem of allergic reactions and alternative gloves should be made available (Ross 1999).

The cost of gloves varies considerably. In very general terms, non-sterile gloves are half the price of sterile gloves. However, this difference may be increased where sterile gloves are produced to a very high quality using expensive materials. The cost of gloves is an important consideration in an age of spiralling health-care costs.

Learning outcome 5:
Discuss when plastic aprons should be worn, stating the rationale

Activity | Make a list of those occasions when you have seen plastic aprons used by nurses in practice settings.

You might have seen aprons worn:
- When handling body fluids and in other aspects of direct patient/client care, such as bathing, assisting with elimination and bed making.
- When food is being handled and when people are being fed.
- In operating theatres and maternity units.
- When cytotoxic drugs are being prepared and administered.

Plastic aprons provide an impermeable barrier between the nurse's clothes and the patient, and therefore help to protect both parties and reduce cross-infection. Prior to the use of plastic aprons, cotton aprons or gowns were used.

After reviewing the literature, Gould and Chamberlaine (1995) conclude that use of cotton gowns cannot be justified, and that plastic aprons carry fewer bacteria than cotton ones. However, Callaghan (1998), in a study that examined the use of plastic aprons during direct patient contact, found no significant reduction in levels of uniform contamination. There were also serious misunderstandings among nurses concerning the ability of bacteria to cling to plastic aprons. The perception that bacteria do not adhere to plastic is not supported by the data. The study found that nurses rely on plastic aprons to keep their uniforms uncontaminated. Consequently uniforms were worn for more than one day and became heavily contaminated with a variety of bacteria.

In community settings, such as small staffed residences, there is an emphasis on social aspects of care and **normalization** and therefore the use of plastic aprons is likely to be greatly reduced. However, when dealing with body fluids, they are still advisable.

Within hospital settings, Curran (1991) suggests that as plastic aprons are cheap, they should be used as intended by the manufacturers, and disposed of frequently. Callaghan (1998) explains how Curran's guidelines were expanded to form a colour co-ordinated protocol:

Normalization

A concept that has seen much development over the past thirty years. Currently it is viewed as a system that seeks to value positively devalued individuals and groups (*see* Emerson 1992; Swann 1997).

- White plastic aprons for handling body fluids, for toileting, and for direct care. These must be used only for individual patients and then discarded.
- Blue for food related activities. The apron should be discarded following the completion of the food handling.
- Green aprons for the operating theatre and maternity units, as single use items and then discarded.
- Yellow for cytotoxic drug treatment, again for single use and then discarded.

Using such a protocol may help to reduce contamination levels on aprons and the transmission of bacteria between nurses and patients. Some hospitals use different coloured aprons when caring for people who are being source isolated in side rooms, to ensure that the same apron is not worn when caring for other patients. You will need to ensure that you become familiar with any local policies about the wearing of aprons.

Summary
- The appropriate use of gloves and aprons is an important infection control measure. However, they must be removed with care, and disposed of appropriately. Hand washing should always follow.
- Nurses need to understand when to use gloves and aprons and to advise other staff and visitors accordingly.

NON-TOUCH TECHNIQUE

Definition

Non-touch technique involves avoiding direct contact between the skin of one person, normally the hands, and an 'at risk' site in another person. The idea is to avoid contamination through transferring bacteria from the nurse to the patient, or from the patient to the nurse. Non-touch technique acknowledges that even with effective hand washing, hands cannot be sterile. If a non-touch technique is used, then the nurse's hands will not come into contact with the patient or with sterile equipment. Non-touch technique is usually used in procedures that require asepsis, for example, catheterization, venepuncture, tracheal suction and wound care. It is therefore often referred to as 'aseptic technique'.

Learning outcomes

By the end of this section you will be able to:

1. Assess when non-touch technique is required and discuss some key principles.
2. Prepare the patient and the appropriate equipment for this technique, with special reference to wound dressings.
3. Understand the technique and its underpinning rationale, with special reference to wound dressings.

Learning outcome 1:
Assess when non touch technique is required and discuss some key principles.

Activity

Re-read the definition of non-touch technique. In order to maintain asepsis can you identify what might be the single most important action you can perform prior to performing non-touch technique?

Answer:

Hand washing. Take this opportunity to revisit the section concerned with hand washing. Non-touch technique is a prime example of when thorough hand washing is of utmost importance.

Activity

To perform non-touch technique, a nurse can use either gloves or forceps. What do you think might be the advantages and disadvantages of each of these?

You may have thought of the following:
Because hands are not sterile, forceps were traditionally used to perform non-touch technique. However, forceps are awkward to use, and do not prevent the transfer of bacteria from wound to hands (Thomlinson 1987). With a

patient who could move suddenly they might also be dangerous. The relatively new use of disposable gloves has the advantage of greatly aiding dexterity, but can be more costly. Additionally, good gloving technique is required to prevent contamination of gloves. In some situations it may be helpful to use forceps as well e.g. for removing excess moisture from swabs.

Activity

For the following list identify whether it is true or false that a non-touch technique is required:

1. Feeding patients
2. Administering eye drops
3. Taking a patient's temperature
4. Assisting with teeth cleaning
5. Inserting urinary catheters
6. Wound dressings
7. Removal of sutures or clips

You should have identified the following:

2, 5, 6, 7 are true. Note that when instilling eye drops, it is possible to use a non-touch technique without using gloves (*see* Chapter 11 for details about instillation of eye drops). For the three remaining procedures the nurse's hands should be socially clean and non-touch technique is not necessary.

Procedures may vary widely between clinical settings but they should be rational and take account of relevant research. Generally, non-touch technique should be employed following surgery when skin integrity has been interrupted, following trauma to skin tissue, such as experienced by Mrs Wrights, and during invasive procedures such as catheterization. Tiffany would require non-touch technique during any invasive techniques that may be performed as part of her investigations and treatment. **Note**: it has been suggested that a clean, rather than sterile, technique is sufficient in some wound care situations (e.g. chronic wounds) (Hollinworth and Kingston 1998). *See* Chapter 10, Principles of wound care, for a discussion on when to use a clean, rather than a sterile, technique.

Learning outcome 2:
Prepare the patient and the appropriate equipment for this technique, with special reference to wound dressings.

Activity

Discuss with a colleague how you would prepare Mrs Wrights to have her cuts dressed.

Now check your answers:

You would need to explain to Mrs Wrights what you hope to achieve and gain her consent and co-operation. Think about how difficult this might be if the person is anxious or confused. The patient's comfort and privacy should be carefully guarded at all times. It would be important to explain to her that her dressings should be changed as soon as exudate is visible on the surface, as the dressing will no longer act as an impermeable barrier preventing bacteria from the outside reaching the open wound. Note also that if a wound is already infected, then the moist exudate on the surface of the dressing will contaminate any surfaces it comes into contact with.

Activity How might you prepare the environment before embarking upon Mrs Wrights' dressings?

Good lighting, and the comfort and privacy of patients are factors that need to be taken into consideration. Traditionally it has been recommended that cleaning and bed making should cease before wound dressings are carried out, or invasive procedures undertaken. However, according to Ayliffe *et al.* (1999), even when substantial disturbance of bed linen occurs, the increase in airborne counts would be unlikely to greatly increase the risk of infection. Cleaning however, can raise dust, so you should avoid carrying out a wound dressing in the close vicinity of cleaning. Hollinworth and Kingston (1998) report on the successful use of a central treatment suite, with positive pressure controlled air changes, for carrying out wound dressings. This is probably an ideal environment, but many hospitals may not have this facility.

Activity Make a list of the equipment you think you will need to prepare for carrying out Mrs Wrights' dressing.

Compare your list with that in Box 3.2.
The cleaning of the dressing trolley has been a source of debate. Traditionally it was cleaned between patients, with alcohol wipes or spray. There is no evidence that bacteria on the trolley are transferred into the wound or

---

- A dressing trolley or surface that can be used for the equipment.
- A sterile dressing pack.
- If cleansing is assessed as necessary, sterile cleansing solution.
- Additional dressing material. These can be classified as primary contact, low-absorbent or non-absorbing, semi-permeable, alginates, hydrogels and foam dressings (Williams 1998) (*see* Chapter 10, which covers wound care in detail).
- Hypoallergenic tape and clean pair of scissors (if needed for the dressing).
- Clean disposable apron.
- Receptacle for any equipment that will need to be re-sterilized in the Central Sterile Supplies Department (CSSD).
- Alcohol hand rub.

Box 3.2 Equipment for carrying out a wound dressing

vice-versa, and the routine cleaning of trolleys between patients probably serves no useful purpose (Thomson and Bullock 1992). However, the trolley should be free from any visible soiling or dust.

Dressing packs can vary in content with, for example, some containing forceps and some gloves. They usually also contain a gallipot (for solution), gauze swabs, a sterile towel, and a disposal bag. Commercially manufactured packs will often state the content on the wrapper. Whatever the content you should check all packs for integrity. If the pack is damaged, or torn, it should be discarded as the contents can no longer be guaranteed sterile. You should also check that the pack has been sterilized and ensure that the expiry date has not elapsed.

A sterile solution, such as normal saline, can be used to clean/irrigate the wound if indicated. *See* Chapter 10, Principles of wound care, for a discussion on when, and how, wound cleansing should take place. Normal saline is available in sachets, but it is also produced in an aerosol can. Great care must be taken to avoid contamination of the aerosol when used. In many settings it may be advisable for each patient to have his own can, and certainly if the wound is known to be infected or contaminated (Williams 1996). The actual dressing for the wound will depend on many factors, including the condition of the wound. You will need to discuss wound assessment with your assessor/facilitator in practice who will guide you towards the appropriate dressing. Wound assessment and choice of dressings are covered in detail in Chapter 10, Principles of wound care.

If tape is to be used, it should be hypoallergenic tape, in good condition and clean. A clean apron to protect the nurse and the easy availability of a receptacle for used CSSD equipment completes the list.

Learning outcome 3:
Understand the technique and underpinning rationale, with special reference to wound dressings

Before looking at guidelines for non-touch technique for a wound dressing, we will first practise the opening of a dressing-pack, use of forceps, putting on sterile gloves and pouring solution

Activity

If you have access to a skills laboratory and equipment, collect a trolley, alcohol handrub, a dressing pack and a sachet of normal saline, and then wash your hands. Carefully open the dressing pack and slip the inner package onto the surface without contaminating the equipment inside. Now open out the sterile field.

Note: It is important not to touch (and potentially contaminate) the inner surface of the pack (which is your sterile field) other than at the corners, and with fingertips. Most dressing packs will include either forceps or sterile gloves. If forceps are supplied, use a pair to arrange the equipment on your sterile field. If no forceps are supplied, use the sterile disposal bag over your hand to arrange the equipment. The disposal bag is then attached to the trolley. If forceps were used, they can now be discarded. Having done this, you can then practise pouring sterile fluid into a gallipot, but first clean the outside of the sachet with an alcohol swab. Try not to splash the fluid onto your sterile field as this provides a potential focus for bacterial transfer.

Activity

If gloves are not included in the dressing pack, add them now. Wash your hands (or use the alcohol hand rub) and put on the gloves.

Note: You will need to put the gloves on without contaminating the outer surface. Open the pack carefully, handling corners only. Using the inner surface of the folded cuff, push your hand into the glove. If you line up your thumb with the thumb of the glove you will find that the glove goes on more easily. Remember that 'practice makes perfect'. The second glove is easier to put on as you can use your other, gloved, hand to help.

Box 3.3 outlines a set of guidelines you could use to change a wound dressing. These guidelines are intended for use when alone. If you have a second nurse available then this person can, after hand washing, prepare the pack, be available to observe and support the patient throughout the procedure and open additional items onto the sterile field when required. When aseptic procedures are being performed with children, parents can provide support and encouragement.

Hollinworth and Kingston (1998) advise against excessive hand washing during wound dressings, suggesting that the frequency with which hand washing is performed should be based on individual assessment. Note that an alcohol hand rub can be used instead, and if taken to the bedside on the trolley, would mean that you will avoid leaving the patient during the procedure.

The guidelines in Box 3.3 can be adapted as long as the underlying principles are maintained. The important principles of all aseptic/non-touch techniques when applied to wound dressings are that the open wound should not come into contact with any item that is not sterile and that any items that have been in contact with the wound should be discarded safely or decontaminated (Wilson 1995). This same principle applies to any other aseptic procedure. For example, during catheterization (*see* Chapter 6) the sterile catheter, which will be inserted into the sterile bladder, must not be contaminated by anything that is non-sterile. Tony's injection must also be carried out using aseptic technique. The needle will be piercing

1. Explain the procedure and gain consent and co-operation. Throughout observe patient's condition and take into account comfort and privacy.
2. Prepare the environment, including trolley/surface.
3. Collect equipment and place on bottom of trolley.
4. Wash hands and put on apron.
5. Position the patient and adjust clothing to expose required area.
6. Open the outer packaging of the pack and slip the inner package onto the trolley top.
7. Loosen the dressing covering the wound.
8. Wash hands.
9. Open the dressing pack using corners only, and avoiding sterile inner surfaces and content.
10. Open any additional equipment onto the sterile field
11. **Now** if using **forceps**:
    - Use one pair to arrange the equipment on the sterile field.
    - Attach the disposal bag to the trolley.
    - Pour solution, if using, into the gallipot.
    - Then remove the dressing with the forceps and discard them into the bag.
    - Wash hands, and pick up the second pair of forceps.

    Or, if using **gloves**:
    - Use the disposal bag over one hand to arrange the equipment.
    - Then remove the dressing with your hand inside the bag, invert the bag and attach it to the trolley.
    - Pour solution, if using, into the gallipot.
    - Wash hands and then put on sterile gloves.
12. Place sterile towel around wound if required.
13. Carry out wound cleansing/irrigation if indicated.
14. Apply new dressing, or undertake required procedure.
15. Discard gloves or forceps, taking care not to contaminate skin with outer surface of gloves.
16. Secure dressing and make patient comfortable.
17. Dispose of all equipment safely as per waste disposal policy.
18. Remove apron and wash hands.
19. Document the care, reporting any significant findings or effects on the patient.

Box 3.3 Guidelines for using non-touch technique, applied to a wound dressing

the skin (the protective barrier) and entering the sterile muscle. Therefore, the needle, syringe and drug must be sterile and should be prepared and administered using a non-touch technique (*see* Chapter 11: Drug administration).

Summary
■ There are many situations where non-touch technique is necessary in order to prevent cross-infection during invasive procedures.
■ Effective non-touch technique requires good hand washing, sterile equipment and the correct use of gloves or forceps as appropriate.
■ Understanding the underlying principles of non-touch technique enables guidelines to be adapted safely to each individual situation.

SPECIMEN COLLECTION

Laboratory tests can assist with the diagnosis of an infection, and successful laboratory diagnosis depends on effective collection of a specimen. This requires appropriate and timely collection of specimens, the correct technique and equipment, along with rapid and safe transport (Meers *et al.* 1995). The sooner a specimen arrives at a laboratory the greater the chance of organisms surviving and being identified. In general, the greater the quantity of material sent for laboratory examination, the greater the chance of isolating causative organisms. Specimens can be contaminated by poor technique giving rise to confusing or misleading results. Ideally samples should be collected before the beginning of treatments such as antibiotics or antiseptics, or the laboratory should be informed. Both antiseptics and antibiotics will affect the outcome of laboratory results.

Learning outcomes

By the end of this section you will be able to:
1. Identify the general principles relating to the collection of any specimen.
2. Understand the principles of MRSA screening.
3. Be aware of the general principles underpinning the collection of wound swabs and pus.

N.B. The collection of urine and stool specimens is included in Chapter 6, Meeting elimination needs, and collection of sputum specimens is included in Chapter 8, Respiratory assessment and care.

Learning outcome 1:
Identify the general principles relating to the collection of any specimen

General principles of collecting any specimen include:

- Explaining the procedure to the person.
- Maintaining privacy whilst the procedure takes place.
- Ensuring that hands are washed before and after the procedure.
- Wearing non-sterile gloves if handling of body fluids is likely.
- Ensuring that specimens and swabs are placed in the appropriate and correctly labelled container. The microbiology laboratory may be the provider of the correct specimen container. N.B. Do not label the container until after the specimen is collected, to prevent contamination of the label, and mistakes.

If specimens cannot be sent to a laboratory immediately they should be stored in a specimen refrigerator at 4°C. Blood cultures, however, go in an incubator at 37°C.

> **Activity**
>
> Without full information it is impossible to examine a specimen adequately or to report it accurately. Can you make a list of the information that you think it would be essential to document and accompany the specimen?

You may have identified the following:
- Patient's name and location (e.g. address, ward).
- Hospital number and date of birth.
- Consultant's name.
- Date collected.
- Time collected.
- Clinical details of relevance to the specimen e.g. signs of infection.
- Date of onset of the illness.
- Any antibiotic therapy being taken by the patient. Failure to provide this information could lead to a false report (Donovan 1998).
- Type of specimen and site.
- Name and bleep number of the doctor requesting the investigation, as it may be necessary to telephone the result before the report is despatched.

Collection of specimens is potentially hazardous, as staff could be exposed to body fluids of people. Health care workers should make themselves familiar with the health and safety regulations which apply to their individual area of work. Equally, it is the responsibility of managers to provide safe working conditions and ensure that rules are adhered to. All members of staff should be aware of the hazards which they may be exposed to and

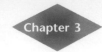

understand the relevance of the measures designed to protect them (Meers *et al.* 1995).

Learning outcome 2:
Understand the principles of MRSA screening

MRSA screening is becoming increasingly prevalent (*see* section on Source isolation, later) and is likely to be performed:

■ Prior to transfer of patients to another hospital.
■ When admitting a patient from another hospital or a nursing home.
■ When other patients in the environment have been found to be infected or colonized with MRSA.

The results will indicate whether or not source isolation is required (see later section).

■ *Activity*	Have you encountered MRSA screening in the practice setting? If so, what sites were swabbed and how was this performed?

After extensively reviewing the literature, the MRSA Working Party Report (1998) advises that choice of screening sites depends on clinical and epidemiological indications. Their recommendation is that initial screening should include the nose, the throat (if a denture wearer), the perineum/groin, skin lesions such as wounds, ulcers, eczema and dermatitis, and invasive sites, e.g. intravenous and stoma sites. Additionally if the patient has an indwelling urinary catheter, a specimen of urine and a urethral swab may be taken, sputum if available, and sometimes the axilla is swabbed too.

You will need to act in accordance with local policy when collecting specimens but the following procedures have been recommended. A transport medium e.g. charcoal, is required. Swabs taken from dryer areas, e.g. the nose and skin, should be moistened first by dipping them into saline.

Nasal swabs

The patient should sit facing a strong light source with her/his head tilted back. The moistened swab is inserted into the nostril and drawn along the floor of the nose with a gentle rotating movement. Care must be taken when inserting the swab, especially in babies.

Throat swabs

A tongue depressor and a good light source are needed. The swab should be quickly but gently rubbed over the pharyngeal wall and/or the tonsillar fossa. This procedure is unpleasant and may cause the patient to gag.

Perineal swabs

This is inconvenient to access for routine screening, but on normal skin, the perineum is the main carriage site. As an alternative, the groin can be swabbed but it may be less sensitive (MRSA Working Party Report 1998).

Learning outcome 3:
Be aware of the general principles underpinning the collection of wound swabs and pus

Collection of a wound swab would be indicated when signs of infection (e.g. purulent discharge, swelling, redness, pain, pyrexia, delayed healing) are present. The swab should be obtained at the beginning of the dressing procedure, after the dressing has been removed and prior to wound dressing. Donovan (1998) reviews the literature on how best to take a wound swab, and her recommendations can be found in Box 3.4. The swab should be taken from the infected site, avoiding surrounding skin and mucous membranes, and then placed in transport medium. If possible, pus should be sent to the laboratory in a universal container, rather than on a swab. Other methods such as filter paper techniques seem not to confer additional advantage (Lawrence and Ameen 1998). The site of the wound must be stated on the request form so that the appropriate culture media can be set up. Different areas of the body have different natural flora, which can be pathogenic elsewhere (Donovan 1998). One swab only should be taken from a wound on any one occasion.

- Irrigate the wound with a gentle stream of normal saline at body temperature (Lawrence 1997), to remove surface contamination.
- Moisten the wound swab with normal saline (Rudensky *et al.* 1992) or transport medium (Wound Care Society 1993).
- Move the swab across the whole wound surface, by using a zigzag movement across the wound while rotating the swab between the fingers (Cooper and Lawrence 1996).
- Sample the whole surface area (Gilchrist 1996) or 1 cm squared if the surface is large (Levine *et al.* 1976).
- Place the swab straight into the transport medium.

Box 3.4 Wound swabbing technique (references cited by Donovan 1998)

Note: Miller (1998) dismisses reliance on wound swabs for diagnosing wound infections, highlighting that many wounds are colonized rather than infected, and that micro-organisms grown from the swab may not in fact be the causation of infection.

Summary

- Collection of specimens can be important diagnostic aids, and should be carried out carefully, as their result will impact on the patient's management.
- Prevention of cross-infection and contamination of the specimen are essential.
- Specimens should be labelled accurately, and full accompanying information is necessary.

SOURCE ISOLATION

Definition

The term source isolation is used to define the steps that are taken to prevent the spread of an infectious agent from an infected or colonized person – the source – to another person. Briefly the precautions used for source isolation include protective barriers such as aprons and gloves, an emphasis on hand washing, and possibly the use of a single room. Strict attention is paid to decontamination of equipment and to the disposal of contaminated linen and waste materials. In some instances, a group of patients with the same infection can be nursed together e.g. in a bay, and this is termed **cohort nursing** (Simpson 1998). This might be used if, for example, there is a group of patients with MRSA, or on the children's ward, a group with RSV. This is appropriate as long as they do not have another transmissible infection, and reinfection is possible (Parker 1999). The MRSA Working Party Report (1998) advises that cohort nursing a group of MRSA patients together in one ward, is preferable to having siderooms occupied by MRSA patients on many different wards.

Learning outcomes

By the end of this section you will be able to:

1. Identify when source isolation is necessary and when universal precautions alone will be sufficient.

2. Discuss the implications of being MRSA positive.
3. Consider the importance of communication and be aware of whom to inform when source isolation is required.
4. Be aware of the preferred requirements and equipment for isolation, and understand the principles underpinning care.
5. Explain the principles underlying the terminal cleaning and disinfection policy of the room.

Learning outcome 1:
Identify when source isolation is necessary, and when universal precautions alone will be sufficient

Activity   Both Mrs Wrights (who is MRSA positive) and Tiffany (who has RSV) require isolation to prevent cross-infection with others. From this, what general principles can you identify about when source isolation is necessary?

These special infection control measures are recommended for patients who are known, or suspected to be, carriers of easily transmitted pathogenic organisms. The precautions used will depend on the type of infection, and care should be based on interpreting the specific route of transmission. Check back to Table 3.1, 'Routes of transmission', if you need to recap on these. It is normally advised that patients with airborne infections, for example, should be nursed in a side room (Simpson 1998; Parker 1999).

In relation to Tiffany and Mrs Wrights:

■   RSV may be transmitted by direct contact with respiratory secretions, or indirect contact with secretions or objects contaminated with the virus (Suviste 1996).
■   The MRSA Working Party Report (1998) states that MRSA infected patients, and where possible carriers, should be isolated in a single room (preferably with an air extraction unit), as airborne particles containing staphylococci are released into the environment.

Patients with blood-borne or enteric infections can be managed in the open ward using protective clothing for handling and disposal of body fluids/blood (Simpson 1998). However, the circumstances of each individual and the environment will need to be taken into account, when deciding whether to isolate in a side room. Parker (1999) suggests that a single room is advisable if:

■   The patient has poor personal hygiene.
■   Is likely to contaminate the ward environment because he has diarrhoea, severe vomiting or bleeding.

However, sometimes the person's clinical condition may prevent isolation or there may not be side rooms available (MacKenzie and Edwards 1997). In most cases, when a single room is necessary, the door should be kept shut, but the infection control team can advise concerning individual cases. For example, with MRSA, the door should be kept closed, unless this is likely to jeopardize patient safety, e.g. with a confused patient (MRSA Working Party Report 1998).

In many situations, adherence to universal infection control measures will be sufficient to prevent transmission, as discussed at the start of this chapter. Many gastrointestinal infections can be managed by using universal precautions (Wilson 1995). For example, in her small staffed residence, Mary would not require isolation, as universal precautions alone should be sufficient to care for her safely.

| **Activity** | To prevent spread of infection to other residents or staff, what precautions should be taken in Mary's residence? |

You might have identified the following:
Points which staff in Mary's unit should consider are:

- Allocate Mary her own toilet if possible.
- Reinforce good personal hygiene, particularly hand washing before eating and after using the toilet.
- Normal crockery and cutlery are usually sufficient. Bacteria are easily removed by washing in hot water and detergent. However, cleaning of crockery and cutlery is best done in a machine at high temperatures; possibly there will be a dishwasher in Mary's residence. If dishes are washed by hand, then clean hot water should be used with detergent. The items should be rinsed and left to drain, rather than being dried with a cloth, as these are easily contaminated (Wilson 1995). Dishcloths should be disposable.
- If there is a suspected outbreak of gastrointestinal illness, defined as when two or more clients or staff are affected by unexplained diarrhoea or vomiting, then further action may be needed, particularly if there are other vulnerable clients sharing Mary's residence. Other residents' GPs, and the infection control team, would need to be informed. Stool specimens should be obtained from those affected even if they no longer have symptoms.

In a small staffed residence, such as Mary's, the above precautions should be enough to prevent cross-infection. However, if gastroenteritis occurs in an institutional setting, such as a hospital, affected patients must be transferred to single rooms where at all possible. Standard isolation procedures should then be put in place and the infection control department informed (Wilson 1995).

Learning outcome 2:
Discuss the implications of being MRSA positive

Mrs Wrights is an example of a patient with MRSA who, as a potential source of infection to other hospital patients and staff, needs to be isolated. Since 1981, a particularly resistant strain of *Staphylococcus aureus* (MRSA) has been causing an increasing number of problems in hospitals throughout the world. *Staphylococcus aureus* is a micro-organism commonly found on normal skin, particularly warmer parts such as the axillae, groins, perineum and nose. This carriage is termed **colonization**, rather than infection; about 80% of people with MRSA are colonized rather than infected with it (Public Health Medicine Environmental Group 1996). The organism referred to by the initials MRSA is a strain of *Staphylococcus aureus*, which has become resistant to the antibiotic methicillin, hence the name methicillin resistant *Staphylococcus aureus*. Strains of MRSA are usually resistant to all penicillins and all cephalosporins. In addition, they may be resistant to other first line antibiotics.

Activity | Why do you think it is important to try to prevent the spread of MRSA?

While as stated above, many people are colonized rather than infected with MRSA, it can result in a range of superficial infections of the skin and can cause hospital acquired wound infections. *Staphylococcus aureus* can also cause more serious infections, such as osteomyelitis, septicaemica, endocarditis and pneumonia (Wilson 1995). The MRSA Working Party Report (1998) presents substantial data to support the clinical importance of MRSA. Unfortunately, the few drugs currently available that have reliable activity against MRSA are very expensive and difficult to administer. They necessitate blood levels being monitored since they are highly toxic.

Staphlococcus aureus and MRSA are usually carried silently. The organism is most likely to be spread on the hands of staff as transient organisms. If staff have certain skin conditions, such as eczema or dermatitis, or have cuts on their skin, then they may harbour the organism and spread it to other staff and patients. The organism can also be carried on skin scales from an infected patient or member of staff and may contaminate uniforms or clothing especially if the clothing is damp. Hand washing, adequate cleaning and patient isolation are considered to be of particular importance in the control of MRSA (MRSA Working Party Report 1998).

Note that patients with MRSA are not considered to be a risk to the community at large, and MRSA is not a contraindication to living at home or being admitted to a home (Public Health Medicine Environmental Group 1996). Indeed, infection control teams may recommend that patients with MRSA, such as Mrs Wrights, are discharged as soon as possible, to minimize risk to other susceptible hospitalized patients (Orchard 1998).

Learning outcome 3:
Consider the importance of communication and be aware of who to inform when source isolation is required

> **Activity** List the key people you may have to communicate with when the decision was made to isolate Mrs Wrights.

You may have identified the following:
Mrs Wrights herself, her relatives and friends, domestic staff, the Infection Control Nurse, or member of the infection control team, and possibly other departments, e.g. X-ray. Further details about these will now be discussed.

Explanations to patients and relatives:

Infections cause emotional as well as physical distress, and care should be taken to explain and reassure patients and their relatives as to the rationale underpinning isolation. Providing information to patients about being isolated has been found to reduce the negative psychological effects (Gammon 1999a). Some clinical areas ask that visitors only enter isolation rooms after permission and instruction from the nurse in charge. While children and susceptible visitors should be discouraged, for most infections the risk to visitors is minimal, as they do not have contact with body fluids (Wilson 1995). If a child is being isolated, visits from family members including young siblings are no problem, but visits from other young children are inadvisable (Simpson 1998). It is common for young babies to be infected with RSV by older school age siblings (Isaacs 1995). Therefore Tiffany's brothers are not at risk from her. As Mrs Wells may also pose an infection risk to others, ward staff may need to sensitively discourage her from close contact with other young children on the ward. Patient information leaflets are available for certain infections, such as MRSA. It is essential that patients understand the rationale behind isolation so that they can fully co-operate with the restrictions.

Explanations to domestic staff

The domestic supervisor should also be informed of any patients who are being isolated. A mop, bucket and disposable cleaning cloths will be provided for the room. The domestic will need to wear apron and gloves when cleaning and these must be discarded into a yellow plastic bag before leaving the room. Most micro-organisms are not able to survive on dry surfaces for long periods of time (Wilson 1998) and therefore the environment need not be a major factor in the transmission of infections. The normal standard of cleaning should be maintained and domestic staff should be reassured that the risks to their own health are minimal if protective clothing is worn and careful hand washing takes place (Wilson 1998).

Infection control team

The clinical area will often have a list of communicable infections which indicates if isolation is necessary and highlights which material from the patient is infectious. If in doubt, the infection control team can offer advice. The infection control team must be contacted if a patient has MRSA, or has been infected, colonized, or transferred from a ward with MRSA cases in the recent past (usually defined as 6 months). Those patients isolated because of other infectious diseases should also be notified to the infection control team. Certain infectious diseases are notifiable to the Medical Officer for Environmental Health. It is the legal responsibility of the doctor, in clinical charge of the patient, to do this (Wilson 1998).

Activity
When next in the practice setting find out who the members of the local infection control team are and where they are located.

The infection control team generally comprises an infection control doctor (ICD) and an infection control nurse (ICN). Their roles include planning, implementing and monitoring the infection prevention and control programme. They are available to offer advice on all matters relating to infection control and the patient. They also provide education to health-care personnel and develop policy. An infection control committee (ICC), from a variety of hospital departments, provides advice and support for the infection control team (ICT). Many community health-care trusts also now employ infection control nurses who work closely with the consultant for Communicable Disease Control. The consultant is responsible for monitoring and controlling the spread of infection in the community (Wilson 1998).

Visits to departments

Departments and staff in areas which the patient may need to visit, need to be informed so that any special arrangements can be made. They may be able to carry out the investigation immediately, to avoid the person waiting in receptions or corridors (Parker 1999), or at the end of the list if appropriate. Porters need not wear protective clothing, but should be advised to wash their hands on completion of the journey (Wilson 1995). As Mrs Wrights has MRSA, any transporting staff with skin abrasions should wear gloves. The trolley or chair should be cleaned with detergent and hot water, or in accordance with local policy, and linen use should comply with local guidelines. Hot water and detergent should be used for hand washing at the conclusion of any contact (MRSA Working Party Report 1998).

Learning outcome 4:
Be aware of the preferred requirements and equipment for isolation, and understand the principles underpinning care

> ■ **Activity**   Construct a list of equipment you think might be required to implement source isolation, and subsequently care for the patient.

Now check your answers:
Items you might have listed include hand soap or antiseptic detergent, non-sterile disposable gloves, paper towels, yellow clinical waste bags, plastic aprons, alcohol hand rub, red water soluble bag and red linen bag, sharps box. Masks are only recommended in situations such as infectious or potentially infectious multi-resistant tuberculosis (Department of Health 1998). The room should also have a good communication system and a television set (MRSA Working Party Report 1998). As a general principle it is sensible to remove excess equipment from the room before the patient is isolated. For children, toys will need to be washable, and kept to a minimum (Simpson 1998). Whilst Tiffany is too young to need many toys, older children may have them. Suviste (1996) investigated the role of communal toys in nosocomial infection on a children's ward. Hard plastic toys were identified as being heavily contaminated with normal bacterial flora. The study did not, however, test for viruses. Aprons and gloves should be worn by all staff handling the patient or in contact with their immediate environment (MRSA Working Party Report 1998). These should be discarded before leaving the room into yellow plastic bags. Of key importance, is the washing of hands before leaving the room. Visitors should also be advised to comply with this request as hands are the most likely route for pathogen transmission (Wilson 1998).

> ■ **Activity**   How do you think that you might deal with the elimination needs of the patient who requires source isolation?

Body fluids and materials, such as faeces, urine and vomit, should be discarded directly into a bedpan washer, macerator or toilet. If the patient with an enteric infection does not have a room with an integral toilet, it may be more practical to allocate a commode to this patient for their sole use. It can then be thoroughly cleaned when no longer required. Generally, any equipment that is solely allocated to an individual patient, should be cleaned and disinfected before removing it from the room. The local disinfection policy will indicate precisely how this may be achieved, or the infection control nurse can advise, but hot water and detergent should be acceptable

(Parker 1999). Any equipment that has not been in contact with infected material does not need special cleaning (Wilson 1998).

Activity

How do you think you might deal with Mrs Wrights used crockery and cutlery, and Tiffany's feeding equipment?

Mrs Wrights crockery and cutlery are equipment that rarely come into contact with infectious material associated with this patient. As such, it is unlikely to become contaminated and can be returned to the kitchen or catering department in the usual way (Wilson 1995).

Equipment for tube feeding Tiffany may be kept in a chemical sterilizing tank in her room, or new, sterile tubes and syringes could be used each time and disposed of in the room after use. Chapter 4 (Bottle-feeding the infant) looks at sterilization of baby feeding equipment in detail.

Activity

If you need to use a hoist or other equipment for Mrs Wrights which infection control factors would you need to take into account?

You will need to wear an apron, and gloves for close contact with Mrs Wrights and for dealing with body fluids. As a general principle it is preferable that equipment is not taken out of the room during the period of isolation. However, if it is not possible to allocate a hoist, for example, solely for Mrs Wrights' use, then the hoist frame should be disinfected before use by another patient. Local policy will dictate precisely what you should use for disinfection, but commonly 70% alcohol wipes, or a 5% solution of hypochlorite detergent powder is used. The hoist, and/or other equipment, must be rinsed and thoroughly dried. Mrs Wrights should have a sling for her sole use.

All instruments or equipment such as writing materials, sphygmomanometers, stethoscopes, and moving and handling aids, should be designated for MRSA patients. If this is not possible, such items should be suitably disinfected before use on other patients (MRSA Working Party Report 1998).

Psychological effects of isolation

Activity

Try to imagine:
• How Mrs Wrights might feel, being isolated in a sideroom.
• How Tiffany's mother might feel being isolated in the cubicle with Tiffany.

Compare your thoughts to the points discussed below.

Gammon (1999a) states that source isolation can be an extremely frightening and anxiety provoking experience for both patients and relatives. He goes on to suggest that the psychological effects of source isolation are not well understood and that more research is needed. He does however describe how patients may feel confined, imprisoned and shut in. Moreover, depression, irregular sleep patterns, and even hallucinations, disorientation and regression are described. A small qualitative study by Oldham (1998) cites patients saying 'There are times when I am completely forgotten'; 'I feel very shut out at the moment'.

The literature concerning paediatric isolation is greater in volume (Gammon 1999b), and indicates that children and their parents suffer high levels of anxiety and depression as a consequence of isolation. Tiffany needs to be isolated to protect others from her respiratory tract infection, and the door to her room should be kept closed. Although Tiffany is too young to be aware of this, she is still affected, e.g. would staff hear her if she was crying? Additionally, being in the cubicle, Mrs Wells could feel isolated, at a time when she is very anxious about her new baby.

Nurses should be sensitive to the psychological implications of being labelled infectious and of being isolated. Patients who are isolated may receive less attention and contact from nurses as they are not in immediate view, and because the nurse must don gloves and apron before entering, quick casual contact will be reduced. It will be important for nurses to try to reduce these patients' isolation and ensure that they approach the person in an understanding manner (*see* Chapter 2, The nurse's approach).

Learning outcome 5:
Explain the principles underlying the terminal cleaning and disinfection policy of the room

Activity	Try to work out from the above discussion the important points to take into consideration when the patient is discharged from the isolation room.

The patient and their relatives will need to be closely informed. The usual procedures for the discharge of a patient should be adhered to. Patients who are known to be infected or colonized with MRSA may be subject to additional guidelines, for example, policy may state that if the patient is to be discharged home, the General Practitioner and the District Nurse must be informed in advance. Similarly, if the patient is discharged to another hospital, or a nursing home, then the medical and nursing staff at the hospital should be informed in advance. Local policy may also dictate that the medical records of patients, known to be infected or colonized with MRSA, should carry a clear mark of identification, or will be electronically tagged on the computer patient activity system.

In terms of cleaning the room, you may have considered the following:
■ **Equipment:** Used, or soiled, disposable equipment will need to be placed into a yellow plastic bag for incineration. It is not usually necessary to discard unused packets of disposable equipment. Non-disposable equipment will need to be cleaned and/or disinfected before being removed from the room. Local disinfection policies will advise on solutions. Blythe

et al. (1998), in a study concerned with MRSA and the environment, highlighted the importance of not overlooking electrical equipment such as call bells and television sets, and pointed out that carpets may become more easily contaminated than hard flooring.

- **Bed linen:** This should be placed in an alginate bag and then into a red nylon outer bag to prevent dissemination of micro-organisms to laundry staff.
- **Furniture:** All furniture and surfaces, including bed frames and mattresses, should be cleaned with hot water and detergent. The study by Blythe *et al.* (1998) indicated that mattresses might be a source of cross-contamination even after terminal cleaning. Mattresses and plastic covered pillows should be checked for permeability and tears. Local policy should be adhered to and may indicate that these items should be condemned if damaged. Curtains may need to be sent for laundering.
- **Room cleaning:** When the equipment has been dealt with, domestic staff, wearing plastic aprons and gloves, should clean the floors and surfaces in the usual way with detergent and hot water. The plastic apron, gloves and any disposable wipes should be discarded into a yellow plastic clinical waste bag and the mop head, if not disposable, placed into a plastic bag for laundering. The mop bucket and handle should be washed and left to dry. Room cleaning must be meticulous and all traces of dust should be removed. Once the room has been thoroughly cleaned, it can be re-used immediately (Wilson 1995), but ensure that all surfaces are dry before re-use. This usually requires a 2-hour time lapse.

Summary

- While universal precautions are sufficient to prevent cross-infection in many circumstances, in some situations additional measures are necessary, in the form of source isolation.
- Source isolation requires correct use of hand washing, gloves, aprons, and waste disposal, and usually a single room for the person who is identified as a source of infection.
- The psychological effects of source isolation, have been documented, and it is important for nurses to be aware of the impact, and provide psychological support.

SHARPS DISPOSAL

Introduction

Safe disposal of sharps, such as needles, blood glucose lancets, intravenous cannula and catheter stylets, is important not only in relation to maintaining a

Learning outcome 3:
Identify local procedures for the disposal of sharps containers

Activity

Locate and read the local hospital Trust policy on the disposal of sharps containers. Note down the main points.

You may have identified the following:

- Sharps containers should not be over-filled. Generally, this means that they should be sealed once they are two thirds full.
- Containers should be sealed according to the manufacturer's instructions. On many containers these may be found on the outside of the box. In addition, Trusts may request extra precautions e.g. sealing over the lid with tape marked 'hazard'.
- Sealed containers should be left at identified collection points in the manner prescribed by the local policy, and labelled with date and source.
- Generally, portering staff remove the boxes and take them to a central point for transport to the incinerator.

Note: policies for community Trusts, residential and nursing homes may vary. You will need to ensure that you are familiar with the relevant policy for the areas that you study in.

Activity

List the people who may be harmed if the local Trust policy on the disposal of sharps containers is not followed correctly.

You may have thought of the following:

- The nursing staff
- The medical staff, and professions allied to medicine
- The portering staff
- Transport drivers
- Staff at the incinerator.

Learning outcome 4:
Identify the actions required following needle stick injury

Activity

With a colleague, discuss what you think should be done following a needle stick injury.

All health-care employers are required to develop mechanisms for dealing with sharps injuries. These mechanisms include identifying the employee's responsibility to report the injury and her subsequent entitlement to be provided with counselling and testing services. However, before this stage is reached, emergency action should be taken. Now check your ideas with Table 3.2.

Table 3.2 Action after a needle stick injury. Note that you should consult and follow your local policy throughout

Emergency action	• Encourage bleeding at the site • Wash wound with fast flowing water, and for splashes to eyes, mouth or into broken skin, rinse thoroughly • Call for assistance • Cover wound with waterproof dressing.
Reporting	• Complete accident/incident form • Inform clinical line manager • Identify patient source, inform manager.
Follow-up	• Make use of counselling if required • Attend for testing if indicated • Follow medical advice.

Note: although the evidence suggests that vigorous washing of the wound is beneficial following a sharps injury (Geberding and Henderson 1992), there is no evidence to indicate that promoting bleeding at the site is effective in 'cleaning' the wound (Fahey *et al*. 1993). Nevertheless, current practice is based upon the apparent logic of this idea.

The policies outlined above are also used if blood or body fluid is splashed into the eyes or mouth, or onto broken skin.

Activity

During your next practice placement, seek out and read the local clinical policy on the action to be taken following a sharps injury.

Summary

■ Sharps pose a potential hazard to nurses, other staff and the public.

■ All nurses must follow Trust or local policy and handle and dispose of sharps safely in order to prevent the risk of needle stick injury to themselves and colleagues.

■ All Trusts have agreed procedures to follow in the event of a needle stick injury and these should be adhered to carefully.

WASTE DISPOSAL

Definition

Definitions of clinical waste vary in different countries, but usually refer to potentially hazardous, toxic or infectious material emanating from patient or animal diagnosis and treatment, or from medical research. This can include dangerous drugs and radioactive substances (Ayliffe *et al.* 1999). Nurses have a responsibility, along with other employees, to dispose of waste safely. The Control of Substances Hazardous to Health (COSHH) regulations, which came into force in 1989, covers all potentially hazardous substances (Dimond 1995), and obviously applies across all health-care settings.

Learning outcomes

By the end of this section you will be able to:

1. Discuss the importance of the correct disposal of clinical waste for the environment and for individuals, including health-care workers.
2. State the colour coding system for waste bags and the recommended process for disposal of the bag.
3. Discuss the storage of clinical waste.

Learning outcome 1:
Discuss the importance of the correct disposal of clinical waste for the environment and for individuals, including health-care workers

Activity

Discuss with a colleague the issues you believe are of greatest importance concerning the safe disposal of clinical waste with respect to both the environment and to individuals within health-care settings.

Issues which you may have considered are:

• Increasing amounts of waste material are being generated globally and the disposal of this is becoming ever more difficult and expensive.
• Landfill sites are less available than formerly, and environmentally safe incinerators are expensive. If not well maintained they can produce toxic emissions.
• Clinical waste is more expensive to dispose of than domestic waste. It is therefore a source of potential unnecessary expenditure for the health-care provider if not correctly labelled and dispatched. The responsibilities of those who produce waste are described in the Environmental Protection Act 1990.
• For individuals within health-care settings there exists the potential to be harmed by exposure to toxic, hazardous or infected material, and the possibility of transmitting infection to other health-care workers or patients.

Activity

Make a list of the materials which might be considered clinical waste in each of the four practice scenarios.

You may have identified the following:

Excretions, secretions, specimens, used wound dressings, sharps, used disposable and reusable medical and nursing equipment and aids to care, such as gloves and aprons.

Learning outcome 2:
State the colour coding system for waste bags and the recommended process for the disposal of the bag

Activity

Write down or discuss with a fellow student:
1. What colour bag should be used for uncontaminated paper and other household waste and what is the recommended process, or method, to dispose of this bag?
2. What colour bag should be used for material contaminated with blood or body fluid, human or animal tissue and what is the recommended process or method to dispose of this bag?
3. What colour should a sharps bin be? What is the recommended process, or method for its disposal?

Now check your answers:

A colour coding system for waste bags has been adopted nationally (Health Services Advisory Committee of the Health and Safety Executive 1992).

Uncontaminated material

Uncontaminated paper and other household waste should be placed in black bags and the recommended process for disposal is landfill.

Contaminated material

Material contaminated with blood or body fluid, human or animal tissue should discarded into yellow bags and treated as if infected. The bags should be separated from other waste. If leakage of body fluids is likely to occur a second bag, or impervious container, should be used to prevent exposure to, and possible contamination of, those who handle waste products. In common with sharps containers, waste bags should be properly sealed when approximately two-thirds full. If over-filled, waste bags tend to break open. They should be labelled with the point of origin, in order to identify the source if problems arise during disposal. Incineration is the process recommended for the disposal of this type of waste. When incinerators are in good working order, this method is suitable for most types of clinical waste, but very wet or dense loads may affect the efficacy of the process. In England and Wales, certain categories of clinical waste such as urine containers, incontinence pads and stoma bags can be landfilled if a site is licensed for this use (Phillips 1999).

Sharps bins

A sharps bin should be yellow and incineration is the recommended method of disposal. Incineration reduces the mass and volume of waste and renders it unrecognizable prior to landfill. New incinerator emission standards came into force in October 1995 (84/360/EEC), and alternative methods now being examined for plants which do not meet the new specifications include: autoclaving, chemical methods, gasification, irradiation, microwaving and disinfection by continuous feed auger. The aim of all methods is to render waste unrecognizable, non-hazardous and acceptable for landfill.

Meers *et al.* (1995) state that much money could be saved if it were possible to separate the 90% of waste that can be disposed of in the same way as domestic waste, from the remaining 10% of clinical waste that requires special provision. In practice, this has been difficult to achieve and it appears that many trusts have taken the safe, though costly and environmentally questionable, decision to treat all their waste as clinical waste (Meers *et al.* 1995).

Learning outcome 3:
Discuss the storage of clinical waste

Activity

Try to find out where clinical waste is stored prior to collection in the hospital and community setting.

Each Trust has its own arrangements, but the following points apply generally everywhere. In the hospital setting, clinical waste is often stored adjacent to the main buildings and for considerable periods of time prior to collection. It is therefore important that the storage area is dry and secure and that different coloured bags are kept separately. To prevent cross-infection, the area should not be accessible to animals, insects or rodents. Children in particular must be denied access. Staff handling the waste should be trained to do so, wear protective clothing, and handle bags by the neck only to avoid the risk of injury from protruding items.

In the community setting, waste produced and handled by the client and family can usually be discarded with normal household waste where the duty of care is exempt. The clinical waste then becomes mixed with large amounts of ordinary waste and is not regarded as a hazard (Wilson 1995). However, the increasing tendency for discharging patients early from hospital settings and ventures such as 'hospital at home' schemes may alter this view. In the community setting sharps generated by those such as insulin-dependent diabetics should be placed in sharps bins and some local authorities arrange for the collection of these from chemists. If sharps bins are not available, then other forms of rigid containers are sometimes used and, or, the needle is blunted with needle clippers.

Local authorities have a legal obligation to provide a collection service for infectious waste if requested, but this often applies only to patients known to be infected with blood-borne viruses, or those undergoing kidney dialysis. Some patients feel that collection infringes on their right to confidentiality and for this reason prefer to transport waste to their local GP or health centre for subsequent disposal.

Summary
- The different categories of waste must be disposed of safely and appropriately to prevent hazards to NHS staff and the public.
- Nurses are highly involved in the generation of clinical waste and must, therefore, show understanding of, and responsibility towards, the correct disposal of clinical waste.

CHAPTER SUMMARY

This chapter commenced by explaining the principles behind the concept of using universal precautions to prevent cross-infection, and the remaining sections have focused on the practical skills involved. Having worked your way through this chapter you should now be aware of the fundamental principles which underpin the prevention of cross-infection. These principles are relevant to all other practical nursing skills, and this chapter will, therefore, be referred to within many other chapters in this book. Adhering to the principles discussed within this chapter will also help to protect the nurse and other health-care staff, from cross-infection, which is essential for the maintenance of a safe working environment. The Code of Professional Conduct (UKCC 1992) demands of nurses that no act or omission on your part, or within your sphere of responsibility, is detrimental to the interests, condition or safety of patients. To adhere to this clause, the prevention of cross-infection is paramount, as hospital acquired infection will invariably have an adverse effect on the individual concerned.

REFERENCES

Ayliffe, G.A.J., Babb, J.R. and Taylor, L.J. 1999. *Hospital-Acquired Infection: Principles and Prevention*, 3rd edn Oxford: Butterworth Heinemann

Blythe, D., Keenlyside, D., Dawson, S.J. and Galloway, A. 1998. Environmental contamination due to methicillin-resistant *Staphylococcus aureus* (MRSA). *Journal of Hospital Infection* **38**, 67-70.

Bowell, B. 1992. Hands up for cleanliness. *Nursing Standard* **6** (15), 24-5.

Brookes, A. 1994. Surgical glove perforation. *Nursing Times* **90** (21), 60, 62.

Callaghan, I. 1998. Bacterial contamination of nurses' uniforms: a study. *Nursing Standard* **13** (1), 37-42.

Carr, J. and Wilson, B. 1987. Self-help skills: washing, dressing and feeding. In: Yule, W. and Carr, J. (eds.) *Behaviour Modification for People with Mental Handicaps*. London: Croom Helm, 143-60.

Curran, E. 1991. Protecting with plastic aprons. *Nursing Times* **87** (38), 64, 66, 68.

Department of Health 1990. *Guidance for clinical health care workers' protection against infection with HIV, HBV and other blood borne pathogens in health care settings. Recommendations of the Expert Advisory Group on AIDS*. London: HMSO.

Department of Health 1998. *The interdepartmental working group on tuberculosis: UK recommendations for the prevention and control of HIV, tuberculosis and drug-resistant tuberculosis*. London: HMSO.

Dimond, B. 1995. *Legal Aspects of Nursing*, 2nd edn. London: Prentice Hall.

Donovan, S. 1998. Wound infection and swabbing. *Professional Nurse* **13**, 757-9.

Emerson, E. 1992. What is Normalisation? In: Brown, H. and Smith, H. (eds.) *Normalisation: A Reader for the Nineties*, London: Routledge, 1-15.

Emmerson, A.M., Enstone, J.E., Griffin, M. *et al*. 1996. The second national prevalence survey of infection in hospitals. *Journal of Hospital Infection* **32** (3) 175-90.

English, J. 1992. Reported hospital needle stick injuries in relation to knowledge/skill, design, and management problems. *Infection Control and Hospital Epidemiology* **13**, 259-64.

Fahey, B.J., Beekmann, S.E., Schmitt, J.M. *et al*. 1993. Managing occupational exposures to HIV-1 in the healthcare workplace. *Infection Control and Hospital Epidemiology* **14**, 405-12.

Fletcher, L. and Buka, P. 1999. *A Legal Framework for Caring: An Introduction to Law and Ethics in Health Care*. London: Macmillan.

Gammon, J. 1999a. Isolated instance. *Nursing Times* **95** (2), 57-60.

Gammon, J. 1999b. The psychological consequences of source isolation: a review of the literature. *Journal of Clinical Nursing* **8**, 13-21.

Gerberding, J.L. and Henderson, D.K. 1992. Management of occupational exposures to bloodborne pathogens: hepatitis B virus, hepatitis C virus, and human immunodeficiency virus. *Clinical Infectious Diseases* **14**, 1179-85.

Gould, D. 1994a. The significance of hand drying in the prevention of infection *Nursing Times* **90** (47), 33-5.

Gould, D. 1994b. Making sense of hand hygiene. *Nursing Times* **90** (30), 63-4.

Gould, D. 1995. Hand decontamination: nurses' opinions and practices. *Nursing Times* **91** (17), 42-5.

Gould, D. 1997. Handwashing *Nursing Times* **93** (37), suppl.

Gould, D. and Chamberlaine, A. 1995. *Staphylococcus aureus*: a review of the literature. *Journal of Clinical Nursing* **4,** 5-12.

Haiduven, D.J., DeMaio, T.M. and Stevens, D.A. 1992. A five-year study of needlestick injuries: significant reduction associated with communication, education, and convenient placement of sharps containers. *Infection Control and Hospital Epidemiology* **13**, 265-71.

Hanrahan, A. and Reutter, L. 1997. A critical review of the literature on sharps injuries: epidemiology, management of exposures and prevention. *Journal of Advanced Nursing* **25**, 144-54.

Health Services Advisory Committee of the Health and Safety Executive 1992. *Safe Disposal of Clinical Waste*. Sheffield: HMSO.

Hollinworth, H. and Kingston, J. 1998. Using a non-sterile technique in wound care. *Professional Nurse* **13**, 226-9.

Howells-Johnson, J. 1997. Universal precautions and infection control in the perioperative setting. *British Journal of Theatre Nursing* **7** (8), 18.

Isaacs, D. 1995. Editorial: Bronchiolitis. *British Medical Journal* **310**, (6971), 4-5.

Johnson, F. 1997. Disposable gloves: research findings on use in practice. *Nursing Standard* **11** (16), 39-40.

Kerr, J. 1998. Handwashing. *Nursing Standard* **12** (51), 35-42.

Kesavan,S., Barodawala, S. and Mulley, G.P. 1998. Now wash your hands? A survey of hospital handwashing facilities. *Journal of Hospital Infection* **40**, 291-93.

Kiernan, M. 1997. Disposing of sharps at home. *Community Nurse* **3** (1), 34.

Lawrence, J.C. and Ameen, H. 1998. Swabs and other sampling techniques. *Journal of Wound Care* **7**, 232-33.

Lowbury, E.J. 1991. Special problems in hospital antisepsis. In: Russell, A.D., Hugo, W.B. and Aycliffe, G.A.J (eds.) *Principles and Practice of Disinfection, Sterilisation and Preservation*. Oxford: Blackwell Science.

Mackenzie, D. and Edwards, A. 1997. MRSA: the psychological effects. *Nursing Standard* **12** (11), 49-51.

McDougall, C. 1999. A clean sheet. *Nursing Times* **95** (28), 54-6.

Meers, P., Sedgwick, J. and Worsley, M. 1995. *The Microbiology and Epidemiology of Infection for Health Science Students*. London: Chapman Hall.

Miller, M. 1998. How do I diagnose and treat wound infection? *British Journal of Nursing* **7**, 335-8.

MRSA Working Party Report 1998. Revised guidelines for the control of methicillin-resistant staphylococcus aureus infection in hospitals. *Journal of Hospital Infection* **39**, 253-90.

O'Toole, S. 1997. Disposable gloves. *Professional Nurse* **13**, 184-87, 189, 190.

Oldham, T. 1998. Isolated cases. *Nursing Times* **94** (11), 67-9.

Orchard, H. 1998. Infection with MRSA: why it is still a growing problem. *Nurse Prescriber/Community Nurse* 4 (9), 46-8.

Parker, L.J. 1999. Current recommendations for isolation practices in nursing. *British Journal of Nursing* **8**, 881-87.

Perry, C. 1998. Three major issues in infection control *British Journal of Nursing* **7** (16), 946-52.

Phillips, G. 1999. Microbiological aspects of clinical waste. *Journal of Hospital Infection* **41**, 1-6.

Price, P.B. 1938. The classification of transient and resident microbes *Journal of Infectious Disease* **63**, 301-8.

Public Health Medicine Environmental Group 1996. *Guidelines on Control of Infection in Residential and Nursing Homes*. London: Department of Health.

Pursell, E. and Gould, D. 1997. A common ailment. *Nursing Times* **93** (3), 53-6.

Ross, S. 1999. Rationalizing the purchase and use of gloves in health care. *British Journal of Nursing* **8** (5), 279, 280, 282, 284, 286, 287.

Royal College of Nursing 1997. *Universal Precautions*. London: RCN.

Russell, P. 1997. Reducing the incidence of needlestick incidents. *Professional Nurse* **12**, 275, 276, 278.

Sedgwick, J. 1984. Handwashing in hospital wards. *Nursing Times* **80** (20), 64-7.

Simpson, C. 1998/9. Infection control. *Paediatric Nursing* **10** (10), 30-3.

Suviste, J. 1996. The toy trap uncovered. *Nursing Times* **92** (10), 56-9.

Swann C. 1997. Development of Services. In: Gates, B. (ed.) *Learning Disabilities*, 3rd edn. London: Churchill Livingstone, 39-54.

Thomlinson, D. 1987. To clean or not to clean. *Nursing Times* **83** (9), 71, 73, 75.

Thomson, G. and Bullock, D. 1992. To clean or not to clean. *Nursing Times* **88** (34), 66, 68.

United Kingdom Central Council for Nursing, Midwifery and Health Visiting. 1992. *Code of Professional Conduct for Nurses, Midwives and Health Visitors*, 3rd edn. London: UKCC.

Weltman, A.C., Short,L.J., Mendelson, M.H. *et al*. 1995. Disposal-related sharps injuries at a new York city teaching hospital. *Infection Control and Hospital Epidemiology* **16**, 268-74.

Williams, C. 1996. Irriclens: a sterile wound cleanser in an aerosol can. *British Journal of Nursing* **5**, 1008-10.

Williams, C. 1998. Guide to dressing for success. *Practice Nurse* **16** (4), 220, 222, 224.

Wilson, J. 1995. *Infection Control in Clinical Practice*. London: Balliere Tindall

Wilson, J. 1998. Providing a safe environment - the management and prevention of infection. In: Hinchliff, S., Norman, S. and Schober, J. (eds.) *Nursing Practice and Health Care: A Foundation Text*. 3rd edn. London: Arnold, 363-95.

4 Assessing and meeting nutritional needs

Kay Child and Sue Higham

Sound nutrition is an essential prerequisite for health and well-being, and hence the old adage 'You are what you eat'. In addition, many clients/patients have an increased need for a nutritious diet because of extra demands for nutrients being placed on the body, e.g. for healing. Therefore nutrition should be of concern to nurses working in any setting, and should be regarded as integral and central to patient/client care: 'The provision of food and fluids is a nursing role' (Florence Nightingale 1859, cited in 1980 edition). However nutrition can unfortunately be seen as basic and taken for granted, and it is sometimes even neglected. Research has indicated that up to 40% of patients in acute hospitals are malnourished at any one time (McWhirter and Pennington 1994).

While everybody needs a nutritious diet to maintain health, there can be many barriers to patients/clients receiving adequate nutrition, including physical, environmental and psychological factors. Thus nurses need to be able to recognize the importance of nutrition in their caring role, and prioritize both assessment and appropriate interventions. This chapter will start with a section which highlights the contribution of nutrition to health and considers what factors may prevent good nutrition being achieved.

Included in this chapter are:
- Recognizing the contribution of nutrition to health
- Assessing clients' nutritional status and developing a plan of action
- Promoting healthy eating
- Preparing and presenting food hygienically
- Assisting the client with oral feeding
- Bottle-feeding the infant
- Supporting the breast-feeding mother.

■ Identifying appropriate nursing strategies to improve clients' nutritional status.

The chapter will end by identifying additional nursing strategies to improve clients' nutritional status

> **Recommended biology reading:**
>
> These questions will help you to focus on the biology underpinning this chapters skills. Use your recommended text book to find out:
>
> • What is a balanced diet?
> • What macronutrients and micronutrients should it contain?
> • Why do we need these nutrients? What are their roles?
> • How are macronutrients digested? Once digested, where do they go?
> • What are the consequences of under-nutrition and over-nutrition?
> • How do requirements for nutrition alter with ageing?
> • What aspects of different age groups (e.g. neonates, infants, children, teenagers, adults and the elderly) may impinge upon nutritional status?
> • How does a 'health need' alter our nutritional demands (or supply)?

PRACTICE SCENARIOS

As already stated, nutrition is relevant for everybody. However, the following practice scenarios highlight some situations where nutritional issues would be particularly important, and they will be referred to throughout this chapter.

■ **Adult**

Mr Miles Jacobs is a 72-year-old man who has been admitted via the Accident and Emergency Department for investigations of dizziness and confusion. He fell over in his home and sustained a fracture to the humerus of his right arm, for which a collar and cuff sling has been applied. On admission he appears to be unkempt with many grazes on his body from the fall. He has poorly fitting dentures, his weight is 64 kilograms, and he is 1.90 metres tall. He says he has no appetite for food or life.

■ **Child**

Alex Billings is 6 months old and is his parents' second child. His mother has been concerned that Alex has not been gaining weight, although he has no other symptoms. Alex appears thin, but is lively and active. There are no concerns about his development.

Cerebral palsy
A motor disorder caused by non-progressive brain defect or lesion, present at birth or shortly after. This may cause a lack of co-ordination in chewing and swallowing, and/or unco-ordinated movements, making it difficult to feed oneself.

Makaton
The Makaton Vocabulary Language Programme is one of the most frquently used methods of communication for people with learning disabilities and comprises signs, symbols and speech (Ferris-Taylor 1997).

■ **Learning disability**

Mandy Weston is 30 years old and has mild **cerebral palsy**. She has been admitted to a small staffed residence for respite care because her mother has been admitted to hospital for an emergency operation. Mandy has no verbal communication, but can make her basic needs known using gestures and some **Makaton** signs. She can walk unaided but is unsteady on her feet. She can feed herself but has difficulty chewing her food. When drinking she needs some assistance to regulate the flow of liquid.

■ **Mental health**

Mrs Beryl Atkins is a 70-year-old woman who has a history of depression and an eating disorder. She has been admitted to the acute ward for the elderly mentally ill with a depressive illness. She lives with her husband, who also has some depressive symptoms, and the community psychiatric nurse visits them regularly. Beryl has been neglecting herself over the past 4 weeks, and has gradually lost interest in food, now only eating a slice of bread and butter with a small cup of tea. As her depression persisted she has lost weight rapidly. She also thinks that her food is being poisoned, so she is reluctant to eat. She prefers to be called Beryl.

RECOGNIZING THE CONTRIBUTION OF NUTRITION TO HEALTH

Health promotion is a statutory requirement of the registered nurse (Statutory Instrument No. 1455 1989), and as we have already established, nutrition plays an essential role in health. It is therefore important to understand the key components of a nutritious diet, and be able to identify the factors which might prevent good nutrition from being achieved.

Learning outcomes

By the end of this section you will be able to:

1. Recognize the major nutrients and their contribution to health.
2. Discuss factors which might influence a healthy individual's nutritional needs.
3. Identify situations in which an individual's nutritional status might be impaired.

Learning outcome 1:
Recognize the major nutrients and their contribution to health

In order to sustain life the body needs a constant supply of certain nutrients from the diet (Edwards 1998). Note that the term diet usually refers to the total food eaten, while nutrients can be defined as 'chemical substances necessary for the correct function of the body' (Piper 1996). The following exercise is designed to help you to check your fundamental knowledge of nutrition. It should be easy if you have worked through the biology questions!

Activity

List the groups of nutrients you can remember. Can you identify what each of these is used for within the body?

Check your answers now, against Table 4.1. Note that most foods contain combinations of different nutrients.

Table 4.1 Nutrients and their role within the body

Nutrient	Function
Proteins	Used for building, growth or recovery of cells and tissues (Pender 1994)
	Major constituent of hormones, enzymes and antibodies (Edwards 1998)
Fats	Source of energy (Pender 1994)
	Component of cell membranes (Edwards 1998)
Carbohydrates	Source of energy and fibre to aid digestion and bowel function (Pender 1994)
Vitamins	Essential in small quantities for the normal growth and functioning of the body (Pender 1994)
Minerals	Important building substances (e.g. calcium in bone) and for the normal functioning of the body (Pender 1994)
Water	Used for building tissues, as a solvent for carrying nutrients and waste, involved in temperature regulation (Pender 1994)
Fibre	Dietary fibre is not, strictly speaking, a nutrient, but its presence in the diet is necessary for the movement of food through the gastrointestinal tract (Hinchliff, 1988)

Activity

Beryl at present only likes to eat bread and butter with a cup of tea. Which of the nutrients listed in Table 4.1 would this diet be including, and which would be particularly missing?

Discussion

Beryl has been eating a very limited diet and is likely to have been having an inadequate intake of energy (calories), protein, vitamins, minerals and fibre. She may have constipation from lack of fibre if she has only been eating white bread. She has lost weight because her energy and protein intake has been insufficient, causing her body to break down fat and muscle to meet its needs. Vitamins and mineral deficiencies may present in various ways. For example, vitamin C normally helps absorption of iron from the diet (Hinchliff 1988); therefore, if it is lacking, iron absorption will be decreased. As Beryl's diet is deficient in both vitamin C and iron, she is at risk of iron deficiency anaemia.

Learning outcome 2:
Discuss factors that might influence a healthy individual's nutritional needs

The amounts of various nutrients required for health vary from individual to individual and throughout life.

> **Activity**   What factors can you think of which might influence a healthy individual's nutritional needs?

You may have identified the following:

Age
Children have higher metabolic rates than adults, and therefore require relatively more energy; they also need to consume sufficient food to support growth (Livingstone 1997). Periods of rapid growth such as infancy and adolescence in particular result in increased energy and nutrient requirements (Piper 1996). In adulthood, as age increases, the energy requirement decreases as older people have a lower metabolic rate than younger adults (Pender 1994).

Sex
Men require more energy because their relatively greater muscle mass results in a higher metabolic rate than in women (Pender 1994)

Height and build
The bigger the body the greater amount of nutrients are required to maintain cells (Piper 1996).

Amount of physical activity
As energy is used as fuel, the greater the physical activity the more energy is used up (Pender 1994).

Pregnancy
During the second and third trimesters of pregnancy, rapid growth of the foetus alters the woman's nutritional needs, although the exact demands made on the mother by the foetus vary from individual to individual. In particular the need for energy, protein, and vitamins A, B, C and D are likely to increase (Wardley et al. 1997). 'Eating for two' is not however necessary. The increased energy required by the foetus is often compensated for in part by decreased maternal activity towards the end of pregnancy, and the average

British diet generally contains sufficient protein to meet the increased demands (Wardley et al. 1997).

Lactation

A breast-feeding woman requires increased energy (as much as 500 calories/day more), increased calcium and increased vitamin A, C and D intake (Wardley et al. 1997).

Being aware of factors affecting nutritional demands in the healthy individual is important, prior to considering factors which can compromise nutritional status.

Learning outcome 3:

Identify situations in which an individual's nutritional status might be impaired

■   *Activity*   What do you think might prevent Alex, Mr Jacobs, Mandy and Mrs Atkins from meeting their nutritional needs?

Some of the points which you might have considered are:

■ **Alex** may be receiving insufficient nutrients from his feeds, either because he is not being fed enough, is being fed the wrong food, or because he is unable to digest and absorb all the nutrients from his diet (malabsorption). Alex has no symptoms such as diarrhoea or vomiting which would suggest that he has malabsorption.

■ **Mr Jacobs** may not be physically able to feed himself, due to his broken arm, which would make it difficult for him to manipulate eating utensils. When he is discharged, handling cooking equipment could be difficult, and if he lives alone, there may be no-one to help him. While his broken arm affects his ability to eat, the healing process will also increase his nutritional demands. His dentures do not fit properly and this will affect his eating. Mr Jacobs is confused, and so he may not recognize the need to provide food for himself. From what he has said, it also appears that he has lost interest in food.

■ **Beryl's** nutritional intake is being affected mainly by psychological factors: her fears of being poisoned making her afraid to eat, and her depression which is causing a lack of appetite. Now that she is in the unit, both the food and the meal times may be unfamiliar, which could make her even more reluctant to eat.

■ **Mandy** has difficulty chewing so she needs food that she can cope with. This food could either be cut up or finely chopped, according to the severity of her chewing difficulties. Whilst her mother is evidently familiar with her needs, the staff in the home will need to ensure the food she is offered is suitable, and that she is given the appropriate assistance with fluids. As

Mandy has been living at home with her mother, she may be very dependent on her to meet her needs. Her appetite may be poor due to the effects of separation anxiety.

These examples illustrate that an individual may be unable to meet his nutritional needs as a result of inadequate intake, inappropriate intake, increased nutritional demands, or any combination of these factors. These factors will now be considered in more detail. Note that if nutritional requirements are unmet for a prolonged period, malnutrition may result. Malnutrition can be defined as a state where there is an imbalance between nutritional intake and nutritional requirements (Harvey 1993, cited by Edwards 1998).

Inadequate intake

There are numerous factors which may lead to an inadequate intake.

Appetite
The psychological stimulus to eat which may be connected with and triggered by emotional stimuli (Pender 1994).

- **Loss of appetite**: Appetite loss may be caused by the pain, stress, reduced physical activity and fatigue which often accompany illness (Pender 1994). Some medications may suppress the appetite. Anxiety can also suppress appetite.
- **Stress**: Some individuals may neglect their diet as a result of busy, stressful lives (Edwards 1998).
- **Lack of knowledge and skills for feeding**: The individual may not understand the importance of eating, and may be unable to buy suitable food and prepare it.
- **Confusion**: People who are confused may not recognize the need, or remember, to eat.
- **Paranoia**: As in Beryl's case, some clients may not eat because of fear of being poisoned.
- **Nausea and vomiting**: Symptoms such as these will prevent individuals from eating even if they feel hungry.
- **Nil by mouth**: Some clients may be unable to eat for prolonged periods as a result of their condition (for example if they are unconscious) or treatment (for example following some types of surgery).
- **Physical factors**: These may interfere with a client's ability to eat and include decayed teeth or ill-fitting dentures causing pain, limited dexterity causing difficulty in manipulating cutlery, or difficulty in swallowing (e.g. some children and adults with cerebral palsy). Difficulty in swallowing is termed **dysphagia**. The physical effort of eating may be too great for some people with chronic diseases such as heart failure or **emphysema** (Edwards 1998), or children with congenital heart disease.

Emphysema
Over-inflation and destructive changes leading to a lack of elasticity in the alveolar walls of the lungs.

- **Dependency**: Individuals who are dependent on others and unable to express their needs are at risk of inadequate intake. Examples would be very young children and people unable to communicate as a result of intellectual or neurological impairment, or dementia.

- **Lack of finance**: Low-income individuals and families often have many demands on limited funds, and nutrition may not be the top priority. There is evidence that parents in these circumstances sacrifice their own nutrition to meet the needs of their children (Graham 1984).

Inappropriate intake

- **Over-eating**: Some people may turn to food as a source of comfort during periods of insecurity, depression or loneliness (Edwards 1998).

- **Incorrectly made up feeds**: Lack of knowledge may result in inappropriate intake; for example errors in making up bottle feeds for infants may result in over-concentrated feeds which may cause harm, or weak feeds, resulting in a failure to gain weight.

- **Restricted diets**: Fad diets and erroneous health beliefs may lead a person to follow a diet that is too restricted to meet their needs. For example, the low-fat, high-fibre diet recommended as healthy eating for adults is inappropriate for very young children who need a diet which is relatively dense in calories because of the smaller volumes consumed (Willis 1997).

Increased demands

In some illness states, the body has an increased requirement for certain nutrients.

Basal metabolic rate
The amount of energy needed by the body for essential processes when at complete rest but awake (Brooker 1998)

The physiological stress of surgery results in increased **basal metabolic rate** and therefore nutritional requirements (Edwards 1998). Nutritional requirements are also increased when undergoing wound or bone healing. Some neurological conditions, such as some types of cerebral palsy, can cause excessive body movements using up energy and thus increasing nutritional demands.

Summary

- An adequate intake of the correct balance of nutrients is essential to maintain health, and prevent malnutrition.
- Many individuals whom nurses encounter have increased nutritional demands but their ability to meet these demands is compromised due to an inadequate, and sometimes inappropriate, dietary intake.

ASSESSING CLIENTS' NUTRITIONAL STATUS AND DEVELOPING A PLAN OF ACTION

Assessment is the collection of information about a patient/client, and would include, for example, gaining a nutritional history and taking physical measurements. Nurses are in a unique position to assess a person's nutritional status, identify clients at risk of malnourishment, and give appropriate advice. As recognized already in this chapter, there are many factors that can interfere with nutritional status. If the nurse does not carry out nutritional screening carefully, then she can put the client at unnecessary risk of suffering from the effects of malnourishment.

Learning outcomes

By the end of this section you will be able to:

1. Identify key nursing skills required for successful assessment.
2. Understand the purpose and use of nutritional assessment tools.
3. Carry out a nutrition screening assessment and recognize if your client is at risk.
4. Discuss a plan of action for your client.

Learning outcome 1:
Identify key nursing skills required for successful assessment

Activity	Assessment comprises measuring, observing and questioning. With reference to the scenarios, how might you assess a client's nutritional status by measuring, observing and questioning?

Measuring

Weighing
All the patients/clients in our scenarios could be weighed, using appropriate weighing scales. This may help, for example, Mr Jacobs or Beryl, to recognize whether he or she has lost or gained any significant weight, assuming that they are aware of their previous weights. The weights can act as a baseline for future weight measurements, as if there is cause for concern, weekly weighing may be indicated. A greater than 10% loss in body weight in the past 3 months signifies that the person is malnourished and should be referred to the dietician.

Body mass index (BMI)
The BMI is determined by considering a person's weight in relation to height, and it indicates healthy ranges for body weight. This calculation is not suitable for use with babies and children.

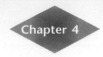

To calculate the BMI, you need to use the formula:

$$\frac{\text{Weight (kg)}}{\text{Height(m}^2)}$$

Thus, Mr Jacobs BMI is:

$$\frac{64}{1.9 \times 1.9} = 17.7$$

McWhirter and Pennington (1994) suggest that a BMI of less than 19 indicates undernourishment, whilst a BMI in the 20–25 range is classed as healthy or normal (*see* Fig. 4.1.). Therefore Mr Jacobs is clearly undernourished.

Growth charts

For children, the most useful guide to nutritional status is the pattern of growth. Eveleth and Tanner (1990, cited by Power 1995) suggest a child's growth rate is the best single index of his health, state of nutrition and sometimes psychological well-being. It is likely, therefore, that Alex's weight, height and head circumference will be plotted on a growth chart. These are widely available for boys and girls of different ages. The chart consists of a graph with age on the horizontal axis, and either height, weight or head circumference on the vertical axis. A series of lines are marked on the graph, representing 'centiles'. These centiles are based on serial measurements taken on 25 000 children between the years 1978 and 1990 (Moules and Ramsay 1998). The value given to a centile represents the percentage of children who are below this height or weight at a given age. This means that 90% of children weigh less than the weight indicated by the 90th centile, whereas 97% of children weigh more than that represented by the 3rd centile. Therefore, a child whose weight falls near, for example, the 90th centile may be considered 'big' for his age, as only 10% of his peers will be heavier than him.

Children are expected to demonstrate steady weight gain, and broadly, to follow the pattern of the centiles marked on the chart. The growth of children whose weight is plotted below the third centile or above the 90th centile is considered outside normal parameters (Moules and Ramsay 1998). It can therefore be seen that weight, height and other measurements must be accurate. **It is common practice for a child's weight to be checked by two nurses**. Professionals trained to perform them accurately (Holden and MacDonald 1997) may also take other anthropometric measurements such as skinfold thickness. Wardley *et al.* (1997) provide a more detailed discussion of the use of growth charts.

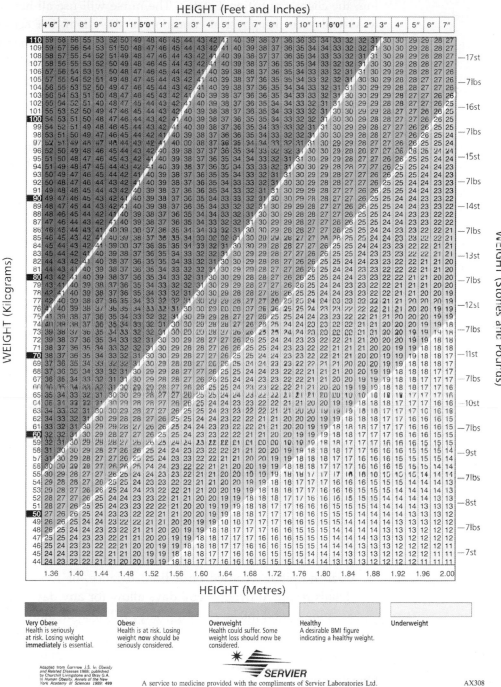

Figure 4.1 The Body Mass Index. © Servier Laboratories Limited 1991

Observing

By using a range of observational skills the nurse will be able to gain insight into the client's nutritional status. The nurse will use all her senses: her eyes to visually see the physical condition of the client, her sense of smell will identify unusual odours, and the nurse can also use her hands to touch the client's skin. You may have identified many of the aspects listed below; most would be useful in assessing the patients/clients in the scenarios.

- Observe if clothing, rings and dentures are fitting comfortably. If not, this could suggest an alteration in weight.
- The skin should be observed for excessive dryness, scaling and temperature.
- The eyes are observed for brightness and to check that they are not sunken into their sockets which could indicate dehydration.
- Note the smell of the breath. Halitosis could indicate poor dental health or dehydration. This could lead you to review the state of the mouth, and aid in determining if there is a problem with the teeth or gums. A sore mouth may be indicative of a poor diet.
- Observe the level of mobility which the client has, for example, whether he can move his arms adequately to feed himself, and can walk or manoeuvre to get access to food.
- Observe for drooling which could be a sign of poor swallowing, as well as poor lip seal.
- Whilst the person is feeding, observe the sequence of breathing and swallowing.
- Observe for non-verbal signals, gestures or signs which the client may use to communicate her wishes, e.g. pushing the dish away.
- In clients' own homes, community nurses can observe what food there is around and whether it is within the sell-by date. Out of date food could indicate that food is being bought but not actually eaten.
- Observe the client's food intake, which will give an indication of the amount of food that is being consumed. For example, a record of Alex's intake over a 24-hour period is a useful indicator of his general feeding pattern. This may be completed by the parents at home as a food diary, or in hospital, recorded on a fluid balance, or food intake, chart. Such details recorded over several days allow for any day to day fluctuations. Keeping a food intake chart for Beryl will also be important in her assessment.

Questioning

The nurse may use a range of questioning techniques to acquire information from the client, including closed, open and probing questions (see Chapter 2).

Closed questions, for example 'are you hungry?' are useful for controlling the interview and for collecting factual information from the client. The closed question is also appropriate to use for a client who has speech or breathing difficulties. However, replies may not always be accurate particularly if the person is confused. The open question, for example 'how are you feeling?' invites the client to give a choosing response, which can provide more detail. Questions like 'What is your favourite food at the moment?' may be useful, if then followed up by asking probing questions, e.g. 'When did you last have this to eat?'

Activity What questions do you think the nurse should ask Alex's parents?

Initially a dietary history should be taken from his parents.
Questions should cover:

- His birth weight and previous pattern of weight gain: this information may be available from Alex's parent held health records.
- His present feeding regime: details of whether Alex is breast or bottle fed, how often and how much and what additional fluid he has.
- Whether weaning has commenced, and if so, what foods are given.
- A description of Alex's feeding behaviour, such as his appetite, and whether he completes his feeds.

Weaning

The term weaning is used to describe the time when semi-solid foods are added to a diet which has previously consisted wholly of breast or formula milk (Gilbert 1998). Alex, at 6 months old, should have begun to eat solid food in addition to his milk feeds. It is important to find out what additional foods he has and how he responds to them. At this age, milk alone – either breast or formula – does not provide sufficient energy, vitamins and minerals to meet the body's needs (Gilbert 1998). Delayed weaning and the introduction of 'doorstep' milk before the age of 12 months can result in iron deficiency anaemia, which may be associated with developmental delay (Daly *et al*. 1998). However, Daly *et al*. (1998) found best practice guidelines were frequently ignored and that weaning practices tended to be passed down from family and friends. This would suggest that culture is a strong factor influencing the choice of weaning foods. The nurse should respect such factors when offering advice, unless weaning practices are deleterious to health. The nurse must also ensure that she is familiar with current guidelines regarding weaning practices before offering advice (e.g. see Department of Health 1994).

Feeding behaviour

Livingstone (1997) suggests that the best single indicator of adequate energy intake is an infant's appetite, and parents who pay attention to their child's cues will avoid under or over-feeding. The emotional atmosphere surrounding feeding and mealtimes, and the response to his own behaviour, will also influence the child's behaviour.

Learning outcome 2:
Understand the purpose and use of nutritional assessment tools

Nutritional screening is the process of identifying clients at risk of malnourishment. It is envisaged that screening is carried out routinely the first time the nurse meets the client, and subsequently at regular intervals in either acute or long care settings, hospital or community areas. A nutritional screening tool is designed to prompt questions to the client or carer about nutrition intake and status. It should be simple and easy to use by the carer and acceptable to the client (McLaren 1998)

Nutritional status is defined using a simple scoring system which, when totalled, identifies risk categories (Bond 1997). Nurses and dieticians have developed a number of screening tools. Although they vary in content, depending on the client group they are intended for, they all have core themes, for example, body mass changes (weight), evidence of dietary consumption, mobility and capability, physical symptoms, and psychological state. The dietician or doctor may use more comprehensive assessment tools to carry out a more detailed nutritional assessment. Klein (1997), cited by McLaren (1998) suggests that the goals of nutritional assessment are:

- To identify clients who are at risk of protein-energy malnutrition, or specific nutrient deficiencies.
- To quantify clients at risk of developing malnutrition-related complications.
- To monitor accuracy of nutritional therapy.

■ *Activity*   Within your own practice area seek out what nutritional screening tools the nurses use to determine nutritional status.

Box 4.1 shows the Adult Nutritional Screening Tool, which was adapted from the Derby Nutritional Score, by the Bucks Nutrition Project. A score of 0–10 = low risk, 10–12 = moderate risk, 12+ = high risk of malnutrition. Compare this with any that you accessed in practice. You should find that the key features are the same. Note that this tool was developed for adults; similar tools for children are not widely available.

Name –	Hosp. No. –
DoB –	Consultant –

✎ Calculate nutritional risk score on admission

✎ Please complete all sections

✎ Please enter a score for each section – even if it is zero

A. Body weight for height (max score 4)		B. Mobility/capability (max score 4)	
Acceptable	0	Fully independent	0
Over-weight	3	Ill-fitting dentures	3
Under-weight and severely under-nourished	4	Needs help with feeding	4
Section score:	☐	Section score:	☐
C. Skin type (max score 5)		**D. Symptoms (max score 6)**	
Healthy	0	Nausea	2
Oedematous and/or discoloured	3	Vomiting	2
Pressure sore/ulceration	5	Constipation and/or diarrhoea	2
		None of the above	0
Section score:	☐	Section score:	☐
E. Appetite and dietary intake (max score 5)		**F. Psychological state (max score 2)**	
Normal	0	Fully orientated	0
NBM (pre-operatively)	0	Mildly confused and/or depressed	2
Reduced (no appetite)	5		
Section score:	☐	Section score:	☐
		Age – If over 65 years score 2	☐
		Total score (maximum total score 28)	

Recent weight loss?   Kg (approx)   Over how long?

Date	Nutritional score							Patient weight	Dietetic referral ✔ or ✗	Nurse signature
	A	B	C	D	E	F	Total			

Box 4.1 The Adult Nutritional Screening Tool (adapted from the Derby Nutritional Score). Reproduced with permission of the Bucks Nutrition Project and the Nutritional Dietetics Department, Derby General Hospital

Learning outcome 3:

Carry out a nutrition screening assessment and recognize if your client is at risk.

Nutritional screening tools have been designed to enable nurses to make an accurate and quick assessment of patients/clients.

Your assessment should have clearly identified Mr Jacobs as being at high risk. Compare your scoring to that below:

- **Bodyweight for height**: On his BMI, Mr Jacobs is under-weight so he scores: 4.
- **Mobility/capability**: He has both ill-fitting dentures, and needs help with feeding so he scores the maximum: 4.
- **Skin type**: As he has abrasions, he scores: 5.
- **Symptoms**: None of these are mentioned, so he scores: 0.
- **Appetite and dietary intake**: This is reduced, so he scores: 5.
- **Psychological state**: Mr Jacobs is confused, so he scores: 2.

As he is over 65 years he scores a further two points, giving him a total score of 22, which is in the high-risk category.

There will be a scoring system incorporated into all nutritional screening tools which will help the nurse to categorize the client's risk status.

You have now practised using the screening tool with several individuals. If you accessed a different screening tool, you might like to try using this too.

When the nurse has determined the category which the client is in, she will be required to act upon the findings. With direction from the qualified nurse a plan of care will be prescribed.

Learning outcome 4:
Discuss a plan of action for your client

Once you have established that a client is at risk, you will need to develop a plan of action. Note that if the client is at high risk, like Mr Jacobs, he will need referral to a dietician for a more in-depth nutritional assessment, and additional nutritional support may be needed. There are a range of ways in which the nurse can help the client to meet nutritional needs. From your individual assessment you will need to identify appropriate helping strategies. Examples of how you can help are:

■ Positioning the client. The client needs to be positioned so that he can eat comfortably. The most appropriate position is the upright position, as this position will lessen the risk of food passing into the respiratory tract, causing choking. Sitting out of bed in a comfortable chair will be preferable to sitting up in bed. There may be circumstances when it is not possible to have the client in the upright position, and then a side lying position may be substituted. It is advisable to use a pillow or similar support, placed behind the back to prevent the accidental rolling into the supine position (Shanley and Starrs 1993).

■ Giving food choices. Tell the client what the choices of food are, and ensure that an appropriate size meal is served. A person with depression could feel overwhelmed if served a large portion.

■ Positioning of food. Ensure that the food is within reach of the client, and actually tell him that the food is in front of him.

■ The clock method. If the client is visually impaired, make her aware of the position of the food on the plate, using the clock method to explain (*see* Fig. 4.2). Ensuring that the plate is of a different colour than the table is also helpful for the visually impaired person, as this helps identification of the plate.

■ Providing the correct equipment e.g. appropriate handled cutlery, lipped plates. You may need to liaise with the occupational therapist here. **Non-slip mats** prevent the plate from moving around, and are useful for people who can only use one hand. **Lipped plates** are high-rimmed plates and bowls that prevent the food from being pushed off or over the side. This allows clients with erratic hand and arm movements to manage with a degree of independence. This might be particularly helpful for Mandy. **Plate guards** work in a similar way.

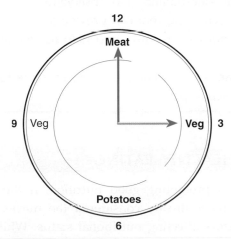

Place the food on the plate roughly at the quarter hours. Explain to the person that the meat is at the 12'o clock position on the plate and the vegetables are at quarter past and quarter to the hour, and the potatoes are at the half past position. Ensure that you keep the foods separate.

Figure 4.2 The clock method. This is a means of helping the visually impaired person to find the food.

■ Eating with clients. This enables the nurse to encourage and prompt the client to eat. For the paranoid client, it may dispel fear of poisoning if the nurse is eating the same meal from the same source.

■ Encourage the client to get her own snacks. In some settings facilities to make snacks, e.g. sandwiches, will be available. For a person with paranoia it may be less frightening to make her own food, from raw materials, than to eat cooked food, which she may be fearful has been poisoned. Alternatively, the client may accept food brought in by her own family.

■ Correct consistency. Food of the correct consistency (e.g. a soft diet) should be provided. Clients with swallowing problems may be recommended thickened fluids by the speech and language therapist which will help to prevent the choking that may occur with liquid.

■ Assisting with feeding the client orally. This might range from cutting up food, and giving verbal encouragement and reinforcement, to total feeding for someone unable to feed himself at all. This will be discussed in detail later in this chapter. Note that Mandy could take up to three times as long to eat because of her cerebral palsy. She would need some assistance to ensure that she can safely regulate the flow of liquid. You should observe for signs of fatigue and offer to help when necessary.

Summary

■ An effective and accurate assessment of nutritional status is essential in order to identify people at risk of nutrition, and their level of risk.

■ To assess systematically and comprehensively requires skills in measurement, questioning, and observation.

■ A nutritional screening tool can provide a more consistent method of assessing nutritional status, and help to identify the at risk individual.

■ Once the assessment is complete, this must be followed up by an appropriate action plan.

PROMOTING HEALTHY EATING

An important part of promoting good nutrition, is the encouragement of healthy eating. We have already considered the nutrients necessary for a healthy diet and factors affecting nutritional status. Whilst, there are many factors which might influence whether a healthy diet can actually be achieved, in a care setting there are particular issues which might make this difficult.

Learning outcomes

By the end of this section you will be able to:

1. Identify the factors which influence the food we eat.
2. Discuss the difficulties in maintaining a healthy diet in a care setting.
3. Select a day's meals appropriate for a client from a menu, in accordance with healthy eating recommendations.

Learning outcome 1:

Identify the factors that influence the food we eat

Activity

Make a list of the food you ate yesterday, and think about what led you to eat what you did.

In thinking about why you ate these particular foods, you might have included:

- Hunger
- You liked the food
- Time of day, e.g. meal times
- Your environment
- Financial situation
- Your emotional state
- How you were feeling physically
- Culture and religion
- Boredom
- Lifestyles.

Note that much of the above are linked to personal choice, but such choices may be restricted within care settings.

Food intake is affected by many factors, which can be divided into categories: physical, psychological and socio-economic. See Table 4.2 for factors that adversely affect healthy eating and therefore nutritional status.

Table 4.2 Factors that adversely affect healthy eating and can affect nutritional status

Physical	*Psychological*	*Socio-economic*
Physical disability/reduced mobility	Confusion	Poverty
Impaired/poor appetite	Depression	Poor cooking skills
Dental problems	Loneliness	Poor eating habits learned in hard times
Poor vision	Institutionalization	
Deafness	Mental frailty	
Sore mouth		
Illness		
Iatrogenic diets		

Learning outcome 2:
Discuss the difficulties in maintaining a healthy diet in a care setting

Activity

With reference to the scenarios, now consider what might cause difficulties for these patients/clients who are now in hospital or residential settings.

Compare your points to those below:

■ In acute settings there are a number of limiting factors. Carers will have limited access to food due to the food hygiene regulations. Cook chill facilities in many areas now mean that meal times are inflexible and therefore the client has to eat at that time or go without. Staffing levels at meal times are often at their lowest because of staff breaks, and there are frequently other activities going on at the same time e.g. medication administration, ward rounds (Kowanko et al. 1999; Edwards 1998). The clients' likes and dislikes, and or cultural and religious diets may be a determining factor in maintaining a healthy diet, but can sometimes be difficult to cater for in the acute setting.

■ All the above issues could affect Mr Jacobs, who, as we have already assessed, is at high risk of under-nutrition. Similar issues could apply if Alex is admitted to the children's ward for investigation, and his mother is breast-feeding. Her nutritional intake must be adequate too but being in an acute setting, this may be hard to achieve if she is staying with Alex in hospital.

■ In the unit where Beryl has been admitted to there may be more flexibility over meal times and food provision, but again, being an institutional setting, this will be limited. Snacks may be available, but there will probably be little flexibility over hot meals. It would be hoped that bread and butter, which is currently all that is acceptable to her, would be readily available. There may well be facilities for families to bring food in, and to heat in a microwave. All food brought in should be labelled and dated. Some mental health units may have canteen facilities, which might provide more choice for clients.

■ As Mandy is in a much smaller unit, there may be greater opportunity to provide meals that she will enjoy. However, it could be difficult for her to communicate her preferences, and as her mother has been admitted to hospital as an emergency, it may be difficult to access information from her.

■ Generally, nurses in many care settings may not have access to sufficient information regarding the client's nutritional preferences and needs, but even if they do, actually catering for them within an institutional setting may be very difficult (Perry 1997). Access to appropriate equipment to help clients with feeding may be limited too.

Learning outcome 3:

Select a day's meals appropriate for a client from a menu, in accordance with healthy eating recommendations

■ **Activity**   With reference to the menu in Box 4.2, think about how you might assist each of the three adults in the scenarios to choose a healthy menu.

Breakfast	Lunch	Supper
Orange juice	Steak and kidney pie	Mushroom soup
	Fish pie	
Cornflakes	Ham salad	White roll
All-Bran	Leeks in cheese sauce	Wholemeal roll
Rice Krispies		
Porridge	Carrots	Egg and cress sandwich
	Green beans	(wholemeal bread)
Scrambled egg		Egg and cress sandwich
on toast	Creamed potatoes	(white bread)
Wholemeal bread	White rice	Ham and tomato
White bread		sandwich
		(wholemeal bread)
	Cheese and biscuits	Ham and tomato
		sandwich
Butter	Apple crumble	(white bread)
Polyunsaturated	with custard	
margarine	Fresh fruit	Tuna fish salad
	Ice cream	
Marmalade		Fresh fruit
Jam		Yoghurt
		Cheese and biscuits

Box 4.2 A daily menu

The first thing you might have considered is the client's choice. It would be good practice for you to spend time with the person discussing likes and dislikes and if the client requires help in filling in the menu, you would be available to assist. If you are with the client, you can direct him/her towards the correct foods to choose, ensuring that there is a balance of the important food groups. For example, Mr Jacobs will require foods that are not only nourishing but also weight-inducing, so you may be encouraging him to eat more carbohydrates and dairy products. With Beryl you will be encouraging her to order a balance of all the groups, not just the breads/carbohydrates. You should consider the client's culture, as some clients' diets may be related to religious beliefs. It is essential in that case that we provide the appropriate foods for the client, e.g. Hallal. Other clients' diets may also be dictated by their beliefs, and a vegetarian or vegan diet may be required.

As well as the client's food intake we need to ensure that sufficient fluid is consumed on a daily basis. Two to three litres of fluid daily is considered adequate for an adult.

There is little on this menu that is suitable for Alex or other young children. Proprietary infant food in jars or packets may be available. Many hospitals have special children's menus, which include traditional favourites such as baked beans, spaghetti, fish fingers and sausages. Whilst these menus do not reflect the best of healthy eating, children who are unwell and in an unfamiliar place may be more willing to eat these, rather than less familiar foods. On most wards, parents can bring in food from home, so long as it is eaten straight away, and any leftovers discarded. Parents may also be willing to supply the child's favourite take-away food!

Summary
- There are a wide range of factors which affect people's food choices.
- When promoting healthy eating, nurses need to try to find out clients' food preferences.
- Within care settings, choice relating to what is eaten and when, can be limited by a number of factors.
- Nurses should be able to guide patients/clients regarding appropriate food choices, with respect for individual preferences, culture, values and beliefs.

PREPARING AND PRESENTING FOOD HYGIENICALLY

Chapter 3 focused on 'Preventing cross-infection', and when involved with food, nurses' adherence to the principles discussed is paramount. This is important with all clients and age groups, but babies, as discussed in this chapter, are particularly vulnerable to cross-infection, as are the immunocompromised and the elderly.

Learning outcomes

By the end of this section you will be able to:

1. **Identify the need for sterilization of infant feeding equipment.**
2. **Clean and sterilize infant feeding equipment using the chemical method.**
3. **Identify good hygiene practice when serving food.**

Learning outcome 1:
Identify the need for sterilization of infant feeding equipment

Activity   Can you think of some reasons why hygiene is particularly important for infant feeding equipment?

You may have been aware of these important points:

- Milk and food residues could provide good growth mediums for bacteria (Dare and O'Donovan 1998).
- A baby is vulnerable to infection, as the immune system is not fully functional at birth. The bottle-fed infant does not receive protection against infection in the form of antibodies in breast milk (Piper 1996). Therefore it is recommended that all infant feeding equipment is sterilized, ideally until the baby is at least 9 months old (Dare and O'Donovan 1998).

How, then, can we ensure that infant feeding equipment is sterile?

Learning outcome 2:
Clean and sterilize infant feeding equipment using the chemical method

Activity   Find out what sterilization methods are available to sterilize infant feeding equipment, in hospital or community.

You may have identified that sterilization tanks containing either a dilute sodium hypochlorite solution or dissolvable tablets are widely used. In the home, however, many families use either the microwave or steam sterilization method. In hospital, single use disposable teats and bottles are often used.

Remember that nothing made of metal should be placed in sterilization tanks, as the chemicals may react with the metal.

Now note the following important points:

- All utensils, including cups, bowls and spoons, must be thoroughly cleansed and rinsed to remove all food and milk residues before submersion.
- Salt is sometimes used as an abrasive to ensure that teats are thoroughly cleansed. If it is, it is essential to ensure all traces of salt are rinsed off, as there is a risk of causing salt poisoning (Moules and Ramsay 1998).
- Utensils must be carefully placed in the tank to ensure that no air bubbles are trapped and everything is totally submerged. This ensures that the entire surface is in contact with the solution. Utensils will be fully sterilized after the time stated by the manufacturer of the sterilizing agent. The tank should be thoroughly washed and the solution renewed daily (Dare and O'Donovan 1998).

Refer to the scenarios and decide what help each client will require. You will identify that all the clients need help but in different ways.

Alex, because of his age, is totally dependent on others to fulfil his nutritional needs and will require either bottle or breastfeeding (*see* section on feeding a baby). However the advice below is relevant for his solid food intake.

Mr Jacobs with his broken right arm may require help with feeding. He is likely to need a non-slip mat for his plate, and cutting up food would be difficult for him. As he has ill-fitting dentures he might need a soft diet as chewing will be a problem.

Mandy has difficulty with chewing so she may need a soft diet that is easily manipulated in the mouth, and she will also require some help with her fluids. Depending on her manual dexterity aids such as a non-slip mat and special utensils might also help her.

Beryl will not require help with feeding but will need supervision and encouragement to ensure that she is eating the food presented to her. This could entail a nurse, who has built up a trusting relationship with her, giving her constant verbal reinforcement, and praising her if she eats. Her husband might be able to visit at meal times to encourage her, and possibly to eat with her. She will need to have her food intake documented on a food chart. Small portions are likely to be more acceptable to her.

When feeding a client the following aspects are essential:

- Preparing the client
- Food presentation
- Feeding the client
- Reporting/evaluating/documenting.

Preparing the client

Ensure that the patient is comfortable before you begin to assist with feeding, for example, that he has been to the toilet, washed his hands, and that his mouth is clean or that the dentures have been washed. Many people will leave dentures in soak over night so prior to feeding breakfast, it would be essential to ensure that they have been cleaned and rinsed, and reinserted. For people with swallowing problems it is essential for the nurse to think about the position of the client in order to prevent aspiration or choking. Correct anatomical alignment will help the passage of food through the pharynx and oesophagus. Clients who can be out of bed should be supported in a chair with their head and trunk flexed slightly forward (Davies 1999). Because eating is a social occasion it will be important that the environment is conducive for eating in. The nurse should remove any unpleasant odours and sights and the table should be cleaned.

Food presentation

To make mealtime a pleasant experience for the person, food presentation will be important. For a person with a poor appetite, particularly if depressed, presentation will influence whether the food will be eaten. The food should be prepared on a tray that is clean with an appropriate drink, a napkin and cutlery. Try to set the meal out so that it tempts the appetite and is enticing to eat. Where food needs to be liquidized, each item should be liquidized separately to preserve distinctive flavours. If appetite is poor, a large meal could be overwhelming, so a small portion is better. Do open cartons, remove lids, and cut up food, because for some clients this is all that is needed to eat independently.

Assisting the client with eating

When an individual is unable to feed himself it becomes the nurse's duty, and privilege, to assist with this essential activity of living. The nurse will need to draw up a chair or stool and sit at eye level with the client, because sitting with the person will convey a relaxed approach.

With the food prepared to the client's likeness the nurse should:

■ Protect the client's clothing with a napkin. Avoid using plastic bibs or paper towels because this will reduce self-esteem and dignity.
■ Ask the client in what order he would like the food. He may communicate this through non-verbal rather than verbal communication, and it is important to observe reactions closely. Food should be cut into bite-sized proportions. If a soft diet is being given, adjust the portion according to the size of the client's mouth.
■ Use normal cutlery/crockery appropriate to the food e.g. a fork for the main course, a spoon for the pudding.
■ Allow time for the person to chew and swallow the food and drink, before offering the next mouthful. **Do not hurry the client**.
■ Talk to the client during the meal, but avoid asking questions.
■ Observe for any signs of choking e.g. coughing, poor colour, and stop feeding if this is suspected. Be especially vigilant if you know that the client has a history of swallowing problems. This may accompany neurological impairment.
■ When the person indicates that he has finished, remove the equipment, and offer the client further drink and the opportunity to clean his mouth and teeth. Particles of food left in the mouth may cause dental decay, or sores can develop around the gums (Nicol *et al.* 1999).

Activity

With a willing colleague feed each other, using a variety of food and drink, e.g. cold, hot, soft, and chewy. When you have experienced being fed, try some of the following positions:

- Sitting in a scrunched up position.
- Sitting on your hands with a blind-fold covering your eyes.
- Lying fairly flat on your side and pretending that you cannot move. **Note**: as discussed above, this is not the recommended position for eating. It should only be used for a person who, for medical reasons, has to lie flat.

Now ask your colleague for feedback about your feeding technique: what did she feel you did well? What does she feel you could do better?

Then reflect on the experience:

- How did it feel to feed/be fed?
- What would have made the experience better?
- What have you learnt from this activity?

Reporting/evaluating/documenting

After assisting a client to eat, you need to complete any relevant documentation e.g. fill in the food chart, and/or fluid balance chart. Remember to report any unusual occurrence to the nurse in charge.

Summary

■ When assisting with feeding, the nurse should prepare the client and the food carefully, and try to promote mealtime as an enjoyable and relaxed event.

■ The nurse's approach to feeding should ensure that the person feels valued and does not feel rushed.

■ Good hygiene should be maintained, including hand washing and oral care for the patient.

■ Monitoring and recording food intake is also important, especially when the client has been assessed as at high risk of malnutrition.

BOTTLE-FEEDING THE INFANT

Parents are encouraged to be active partners in the care of their child in hospital and therefore frequently continue to feed their child as at home. However it is important for the nurse to know how to bottle-feed a baby so that she can step in if parents are unable to, and also, so as to be in a position to offer advice if needed. It may be necessary for a nurse in a mental health setting to supervise a mother caring for her own baby, or to give direct care if the mother is temporarily unable to do so. A learning disabilities nurse may instruct and supervise a client in caring for her own baby. A baby's usual feeding regime should be maintained wherever possible, that is, the same formula, quantity and frequency. The baby may also have preferences as to whether the feed is given tepid, warm or cold, so it is useful to obtain this information from the parent.

Learning outcomes

At the end of this section you will be able to:

1. Make up a formula feed.
2. Feed a baby in a safe manner.

Learning outcome 1:
Make up a formula feed

Activity

> Find out about the variety of infant feeding formulae by either looking in the unit feed kitchen or looking on the shelves of a local supermarket or chemists. Write down the names of the formulae that you find.

There is a wide range of formulae available. Some are suitable for use from birth, while others, called follow-on milks, are designed to meet the different nutritional needs of babies over 6 months. You may also have identified formulae based on soya rather than cow's milk. Ready to use cartons of some milks are available, and all come in tins of powder for reconstitution with water. In hospital, pre-packed individual bottles of many formulae are readily available.

It is important for the nurse to be able to make up a feed, as it may be necessary to instruct a parent. In their study of a deprived inner city area, Daly *et al.* (1998) found frequent errors were: adding powder before liquid; adding an extra scoop to help the baby sleep; warming feeds in a microwave oven.

Feeds may be made up one bottle at a time or sufficient can be made for 24 hours, providing the formula is then cooled immediately and refrigerated until use (Moules and Ramsay 1998). Equipment that is needed for preparing a formula feed can be seen in Table 4.3. Note that some items must be sterile, while others should be clean. Box 4.3 outlines the key points in preparing a formula feed.

Look now at Box 4.3 and note that throughout steps 1–8, touching of the sterilized equipment which will come into contact with the feed should be avoided whenever possible, to reduce the risks of contamination. In hospital, use of a sterile disposable teat, cover and attachment ring units, ensures that the nurse does not need to touch the teat at all, as once the paper seal is removed, the unit can be securely attached to the bottle without removing the cover.

Table 4.3 Equipment required for preparing a formula feed

Clean equipment	Sterilized equipment
Tin of formula	Infant feeding bottle with marked measurements (or measuring jug)
Measuring scoop for that tin of formula	Teat and attachment ring (or attachment ring and disk if feed is to be stored)
Dry knife	Teat cover
Freshly boiled water that has been allowed to cool slightly	Large spoon for mixing if using jug

To make one bottle of formula:
1. Wash hands.
2. Ensure that you have a clean surface to work on, and wear a plastic apron.
3. Collect equipment (*see* Table 4.3).
4. Wash hands again.
5. Measure desired volume of boiled water into bottle or jug. Water is always measured first and the appropriate quantity of milk powder added to this volume.
6. Add correct number of scoops of feed for the volume. Check manufacturer's instructions on tin or packet. The scoops should be level and not packed full. Use the back of the knife to level the powder in the scoop before adding to the liquid. Remember to keep count!
7. If using a jug, stir with the sterile spoon to ensure the powder is fully dissolved. Cover, cool and store.
8. If using a bottle, attach teat or disk to bottle using ring. Ensure the connection is not loose. Cover teat with the teat cover. Shake bottle to ensure powder is fully dissolved.

Box 4.3 Preparing a formula feed: key points

The feed may now be cooled further before feeding to the baby or cooled and completely and refrigerated until required. In hospital, infant feeds should be stored in a refrigerator used solely for infant feeds. When ready to feed the baby, the feed may be re-heated.

Learning outcome 2:
Feed a baby in a safe manner

The baby should be clean and comfortable before commencing the feed. It is common for babies to be fed on demand. This means that the baby is fed when he is hungry and allowed to take as much as he wants. The scenario does not state whether Alex is breast or bottle-fed. As he is failing to gain weight, if he is bottle-fed it will be important to establish how much milk he has each day and whether the formula is made up correctly. It may be necessary to observe Alex's mother making up feeds to ensure that she is following the instructions properly. It is therefore important to know the correct procedure. Note that babies should **never** be left unsupervised with a bottle propped in their mouths, as this represents a choking hazard. It also denies the baby pleasurable intimate physical contact. Box 4.4 outlines the steps in bottle-feeding, and Figure 4.3 shows the position of the teat in the baby's mouth. Any milk remaining when the baby has completed a feed must always be discarded, not saved and reheated later.

The procedure is as follows:
1. The feed should be prepared as in Box 4.3 or a pre-packed bottle used.
2. Wash hands, and wear apron.
3. Collect the correct feed and teat.
4. Warm the feed to the baby's preference, by immersion in a jug of hot water. **Note the need for safety precautions when carrying the jug of hot water**. Baby feeds should never be microwaved, as the heat distribution within the feed is uneven, so the baby is at risk of being severely burnt by the milk (Moules and Ramsay 1998). Check the temperature of the milk. It should feel comfortably warm when sprinkled on the inside of the nurse's wrist.
5. Position the baby comfortably and securely on the nurse's lap, in a semi-upright position.
6. Touch the corner of the baby's mouth with the teat and allow the baby to find the teat and open his mouth
7. Position the teat in the mouth as illustrated in Figure 4.3. Allow the baby to feed until satisfied. The baby may need to be winded periodically by removing teat and either sitting upright or resting baby against nurse's shoulder and gently massaging his back.
8. Ensure that the baby is clean and comfortable on completion of the feed.
9. Record the volume taken and any special comments.
10. Tidy away all equipment.

Box 4.4 Steps in bottle-feeding a baby

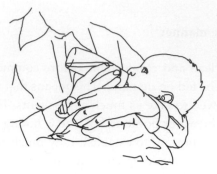

Note the fluid level: The bottle is held so that the teat remains full of milk, to prevent the baby swallowing air.

Figure 4.3 Bottle-feeding the infant

Summary
■ All nurses should be able to prepare a formula feed and bottle-feed a baby.
■ Key principles to adhere to include:
  – scrupulous attention to hygiene
  – following manufacturer's instructions carefully
  – ensuring that the feed is at the correct temperature
  – holding the baby comfortably, and the bottle carefully, to minimize intake of air
  – observing and recording intake.

SUPPORTING THE BREAST-FEEDING MOTHER

It is possible for nurses from all branches to care for either women who are breast-feeding, infants who are breast-fed, or both. A Community Psychiatric Nurse may visit a woman who has post-natal depression. A learning disabilities nurse may visit a family where there is a newborn child with a congenital disability, or may be supporting a mother with learning disabilities learning to care for her child. The adult branch nurse may care for a woman in hospital with an acute condition, who has brought her breast-feeding infant with her.

A world-wide campaign – the Baby Friendly Initiative – has been organized by the World Health Organization and the United Nations Children's Fund to improve hospital practices so that health-care professionals are able to support mothers who choose to breast-feed (Radford 1997). It is therefore important that all nurses are aware of current recommendations with regards to breast-feeding.

In the UK, 63% of women breast-feed their newborn infants, whilst only 26% are still fully breast-feeding at 4 months (Wardley et. al. 1997). It is outside the scope of this book to consider breast-feeding in detail. See further reading for greater discussion of socio-political, cultural and other influences on breast-feeding practice.

Learning outcomes

At the end of this section you will be able to:

1. Identify the health benefits of breast-feeding for babies.
2. Provide an appropriate environment for a breast-feeding woman in a care setting.
3. Access sources of advice for health-care professionals and mothers.

Learning outcome 1:
Identify the health benefits of breast-feeding for babies

Activity

What do you think might be the benefits of breast-feeding to the baby?

The health benefits to both mother and child are widely known (Royal College of Nursing 1998). Infants who are breast-fed are less likely to develop gastrointestinal disorders and allergic reactions; breast milk also contains antibodies to protect against infections and is perfectly balanced to the needs of the infant (Shore 1996). The composition of breast milk changes over time to meet the changing needs of the infant (Wardley *et al.* 1997). If Alex is breast-fed, it will be important to maintain breast-feeding whilst he is in hospital. A period of observation may clarify any problems that might be causing him to fail to gain weight. The frequency and length of breast feeds should be recorded.

Learning outcome 2:
Provide an appropriate environment for a breast-feeding woman in a care setting

Activity

Lactation is the production of milk during breast-feeding (Piper 1996). Find out about the physiology of lactation. Now, from your reading, identify factors that might support breast-feeding in a care setting.

Discussion

You will have found that breast-feeding is a complex process. Earlier in this chapter, the increased nutritional needs of the lactating woman were discussed, and these should be borne in mind. A crucial element in successful breast-feeding is the 'let-down' reflex, resulting from the release of oxytocin from the posterior pituitary gland in response initially to the physical stimulus of the baby's contact with the breast (Henshel and Inch 1996).

Over time this reflex becomes conditioned so that even thinking about her baby can cause a woman's breasts to leak (Henshel and Inch 1996). Once conditioned the reflex can be affected by physical stress (for example caused by painful nipples), emotional stress (e.g. embarrassment), lack of confidence, worry and shock (Henshel and Inch 1996). You can see from the scenario, that many of these factors may potentially influence Alex's mother's milk supply. It is therefore essential that the care environment is supportive to her.

Whilst breast-feeding is evidently natural, it is not entirely instinctive and is at least in part, a skill which has to be learned by both mother and child. A number of factors contribute to successful breast-feeding.

- In order for lactation to become established, the baby must attach properly to the breast. Correct positioning is vital. The mother should be in a comfortable well-supported position and the baby should face the mother's breast (*see* Fig. 4.4).

- It is important to ensure that the baby opens his mouth wide and grasps the whole of the nipple, including the areola, into his mouth. Correct positioning in this way reduces the risk of sore or cracked nipples (Shore 1996).

- The mother should be encouraged to respond to the baby's needs and put him to the breast frequently. Weight gain and a contented baby are dependent upon unrestricted demand feeding (Shore 1997). Therefore mother and child should be kept together at all times.

- A suitably comfortable and private environment should be provided, and respected by all members of the health-care team.

- The breast-feeding woman should have access to a balanced diet and regular fluids.

- If unable to feed the baby for a short time (e.g. because of surgery to mother or child), the mother should be encouraged to express milk, and comfortable, private facilities made available for her to do so. The milk may be stored safely and given to the baby by cup in her absence. In this instance, the nurse should seek advice about the correct procedure for the storage of human milk. If the baby is unable to breast-feed for any reason,

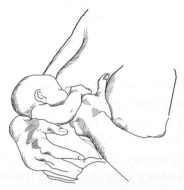

Figure 4.4 Correct position for breast-feeding

encouraging the mother to express milk will help maintain milk production until the baby is able to feed again. It is now recommended that a breast-feeding baby should not be given a bottle-feed or dummy, as sucking on a teat requires the baby to use a different technique from feeding at the breast (Radford 1997).

Note that if a mother is on some medications, these may either interfere with breast-feeding or contraindicate breast-feeding. The British National Formulary carries details of these drugs in an appendix.

Activity

Find out what provision is made where you work for breast-feeding women. Consider the wider environment, such as Outpatients Departments, reception areas or Accident and Emergency Departments. How might the recommendations outlined above be achieved in these areas?

If you are working on a paediatric unit, you might like to carry out the audit suggested in the Royal College of Nursing's *Guidance for Good Practice* (1998).

Learning outcome 3:
Access sources of advice for health care professionals and mothers

If difficulties with breast-feeding arise, staff should know to whom to refer. A hospital may have a designated person to provide support and advice across departments to breast-feeding women. In the community, midwives and health visitors may be available for advice. There are also a number of support groups whose volunteers may be available (see Box 4.5).

National Childbirth Trust Breast-feeding Promotion Group, Alexandra House, Oldham Terrace, Acton, London W3 6NH. Tel: 020 8992 8637.

La Leche League, Breast-feeding help and information. BM3424, London WC1 6XX. Tel: 020 7242 1278.

Association of Breast-feeding Mothers, ABM, PO Box 207, Bridgwater TA6 7YT. email: ABM@clara.net

Box 4.5 Breast-feeding support groups

Summary
- Breast-feeding has clear health benefits for babies, and thus all health-care professionals should understand how they can support the breast-feeding mother, and know where to access advice.
- All care settings should provide facilities for the breast-feeding mother, including a conducive environment and access to food and drink.

IDENTIFYING ADDITIONAL NURSING STRATEGIES TO IMPROVE CLIENTS' NUTRITIONAL STATUS

Nurses have a responsibility to assess systematically their clients' nutritional status and needs, and to assist and support their clients in meeting those nutritional needs.

This section will consider the nurse's role when a client is unable to meet her nutritional needs fully from a normal dietary intake.

Learning outcomes

At the end of this section you will be able to:

1. Identify other health-care professionals who may be involved in the nutritional care of clients.
2. Discuss strategies to enhance the nutritional value of a client's oral intake.
3. Be aware of appropriate interventions if a client is unable to meet their nutritional needs orally.

Learning outcome 1:
Identify other health-care professionals who may be involved in the nutritional care of clients

Activity

Think back to the patients/clients in our scenarios, and list other health-care professionals who you think might be able to help them in meeting their nutritional needs.

Your list may include the following:

- **Physicians**: clients may have an underlying medical problem, which needs to be treated. Some dietary supplements may need to be prescribed by a doctor. Alex may need some investigations to find out if there is a physical cause for his lack of weight gain.
- **Pharmacists**: may have a role in advising physicians; they may also be involved in aspects of enteral and parenteral nutrition (*see* Learning outcome 3).
- **Dentists**: may assist clients with dental or denture problems. If Mr Jacob's dentures fitted properly, this could help considerably with his eating.
- **Health visitors**: are able to offer general advice on healthy eating, particularly for the under fives. The health visitor will be an important source of support for Alex's mother, and will help with monitoring his growth and weight gain. Some health centres have health advisors for the elderly.
- **Psychologists**: a referral would be appropriate if the person has an eating disorder, for example.

■ **Dieticians**: are experts in nutrition, able to perform comprehensive assessments of a client's nutritional status and needs. They are able to offer general healthy eating advice, guidance for the use of dietary supplements and specific advice for the dietary management in relation to medical disorders e.g. diabetes mellitus. As Mr Jacobs has been assessed as at high risk of malnutrition he must be referred to the dietician. Depending on Beryl's nutritional score, she will probably need to be referred to the dietician too.

■ **Speech and language therapists**: are able to assist clients of all ages and abilities with chewing and swallowing problems (for example, an infant with a **cleft palate**, or an elderly person with dysphagia following a cerebrovascular accident). The speech and language therapist may be able to help with Mandy's swallowing problems. It would be particularly important to refer Mandy if she was experiencing frequent coughing and/or chest infections, which might indicate that food was being aspirated.

■ **Physiotherapists**: may also be able to assist clients with motor problems, such as cerebral palsy, and help with positioning. This is likely to be helpful for Mr Jacobs and Mandy.

■ **Occupational therapists**: may be able to help by identifying suitable feeding or positioning aids to promote independence. Mandy and Mr Jacobs would be likely to benefit from this help.

■ **Social worker**: would be involved in arranging home care packages, including home-carers to serve meals and shop, and meals on wheels. This may well be essential to enable Mr Jacob's nutrition to be maintained after discharge.

Cleft palate

A congenital defect characterized by a fissure on the midline of the palate. This may cause difficulty in sucking, as there may be a connection between the nasal passages and the mouth.

Learning outcome 2:
Discuss strategies to enhance the nutritional value of a client's oral intake

Sometimes if appetite is poor or the person is very unwell, food intake may be insufficient to meet nutritional needs. Other individuals might have increased nutritional needs as a result of a higher metabolic rate as a consequence of chronic illness (Moules and Ramsay 1998). A wide range of supplements is available, some of which are designed to be added to the person's normal diet (e.g. powdered glucose polymers such as Maxijul and Polycal), or to be taken as a drink between normal meals (e.g. Fresubin, Fortisip and Enlive) (Holden and MacDonald 1997). The purpose of these is to increase the nutritional value of oral intake; some provide just calories whilst others provide proteins, vitamins and minerals in addition to calories. A dietician can advise which is most appropriate for an individual client following a comprehensive nutritional assessment. There are a wide variety of flavours available, and for a client such as Beryl, it may be possible to find some acceptable to her.

Even with the use of supplements, it may not be possible for some clients to fully meet their nutritional needs with oral intake. This may be for a temporary period (for example if the person is unconscious) or for a much longer time, even permanently.

Learning outcome 3:
Be aware of appropriate interventions if a client is unable to meet their nutritional needs orally

Activity   If you were unable to eat, how might you be helped to meet your nutritional needs? Have you seen any methods used in practice, to provide nutrition for people unable to eat and drink?

You might have seen enteral or parenteral feeding used for the person who is unable to meet his nutritional needs orally.

Enteral feeding

This may be used to supplement or completely replace oral intake. Enteral feeding may be achieved via a nasogastric tube (a tube passed via the nose down the oesophagus and into the stomach) or via gastrostomy (an opening in the abdominal wall, through which a tube is passed to allow feeds to enter the stomach directly). Nasogastric tubes may be used for short-term problems, e.g. a baby with a respiratory infection who is too breathless to feed normally. Gastrostomy tubes are used when the problem is longer term or permanent (Arrowsmith 1996), for example to maintain adequate nutrition for a client with severe neurological impairment, for whom swallowing is extremely difficult or hazardous.

Parenteral feeding

Parenteral feeding may be used when the client is unable to use the gastrointestinal tract for nutrition, either temporarily or long-term. An example would be a client who had major surgery to the gastrointestinal tract. Parenteral nutrition involves the administration of all the substances needed to meet nutritional needs directly into the circulation via a device in the client's vein (Moules and Ramsay 1998).

Summary
- A multidisciplinary approach to promoting nutrition will optimize specialist skills and knowledge, giving patients and clients the best chance of having their individual nutritional needs met in full.

■ If nutritional needs cannot be met through the client's usual oral diet, other alternatives must be found. These could be oral supplements, enteral feeding or parenteral feeding. The dietician's input and advice will be essential in these situations.

CHAPTER SUMMARY

This chapter has highlighted throughout the importance of nutrition for the maintenance of health. As has been suggested nurses are in an excellent position to screen clients for nutritional risk as part of their assessment, and should work collaboratively with other health-care professionals to identify and implement strategies to meet the differing nutritional needs of individuals. This chapter has included general principles which apply across a range of ages and settings. Nutrition is, however, a vast subject, and readers are encouraged to access further reading if wishing to enquire into specialist areas in more depth. To conclude, all nurses should recognize the importance of nutrition, and be able to promote nutrition in their everyday practice.

REFERENCES

Arrowsmith, H. 1996. Nursing management of a patient receiving gastrostomy feeding. *British Journal of Nursing*, **5**, 268–73.

Bond, S. 1997. *Eating Matters*. Newcastle: Centre for Health Services Research University of Newcastle upon Tyne.

Brooker, C. 1998. *Human Structure and Function*, 2nd edn. London: Mosby.

Daly, A., MacDonald, A. and Booth, I.W. 1998. Diet and disadvantage: observations on infant feeding from an inner-city *Journal of Human Nutrition and Dietetics* **11**, 381–89.

Department of Health 1992. *The Nutrition of Elderly People. Report 43 on Health and Social Subjects.* London: HMSO

Department of Health 1994. *Weaning and the Weaning Diet Report on Health and Social Subjects no.45* London: HMSO.

Dare, A. and O'Donovan, M. 1998. *A Practical Guide to Working with Babies*, 2nd edn. Cheltenham: Stanley Thornes.

Davies, S. 1999. Dysphagia in acute strokes. *Nursing Standard* **13**(30), 49–55.

Edwards, S. 1998. Malnutrition in hospital patients: where does it come from? *British Journal of Nursing* **7**, 954, 956–58, 971–74.

Ferris-Taylor, R. 1997. Communication. In: Gates, B. (ed.) *Learning Disabilities*, 3rd edn. London: Churchill Livingstone, 195–224.

Gilbert, P. 1998. Common feeding problems in babies and children: 2 *Professional Care of the Mother and Child* **8** (3), 63–6.

Graham, H. 1984. *Women, Health and the Family*. London: Harvester Wheatsheaf.

Henshel, D. and Inch, S. 1996. *Breastfeeding: A Guide for Midwives* Cheshire: Books for Midwives Press.

Hinchliff, S.M 1988. The acquisition of nutrients. In: Hinchliff, S.M. and Montague, S.E. (eds.) *Physiology for Nursing Practice*. London: Balliere Tindall, 395–440.

Holden, C. and MacDonald, A. 1997. Nutritional care: the nurse's role. *Paediatric Nursing* **9 (4)**, 29–34.

Kowanko, I., Simon, S. and Wood J. 1999. Nutritional care of the patient: nurses' knowledge and attitude in the acute care setting. *Journal of Clinical Nursing* **8**, 217–24.

Livingstone, B. 1997. Healthy eating in infancy *Professional Care of the Mother and Child* **7** (1), 9–11.

McLaren, S. 1998. Nutritional assessment and screening. *Professional Nursing Studies Supplement* **13** (6), S9–S15.

McWhirter, J.P. and Pennington, C.R. 1994. Incidence and recognition of malnutrition in hospital. *British Medical Journal* **308**, 495–98.

Moules, T. and Ramsay, J. 1998. *The Textbook of Children's Nursing*. Cheltenham: Stanley Thornes.

Nicol, M., Bavin, C., Bedford-Taylor, S. *et al*. 1999. *Essential Nursing Skills*. London: Mosby.

Nightingale, F. 1980. *Notes on Nursing: What It Is and What It Is Not*. Edinburgh: Churchill Livingstone.

Pender, F. 1994. *Nutrition and Dietetics*. Edinburgh: Campion Press.

Perry, L. 1997. Nutrition: a hard nut to crack. An exploration of knowledge, attitudes and activities of qualified nurses in relation to nutritional nursing care. *Journal of Clinical Nursing* **6**, 315–24.

Perry, A. and Potter, P. 1994. *Clinical Nursing Skills and Techniques*. Missouri: Mosby.

Piper, B. 1996. *Diet and Nutrition: A Guide for Students and Practitioners*. London: Chapman and Hall.

Power, C. 1995. Children's physical development. In: Botting, B. (ed.) *The Health of Our Children: Decennial Supplement*. London: OPCS, 28–41.

Radford, A. 1997. The baby friendly initiative – supporting a mother's choice. *Paediatric Nursing* **9** (2), 9–10.

Royal College of Nursing. 1998. *Breastfeeding in Paediatric Units: Guidance for Good Practice*. London: Royal College of Nursing.

Shanley, E. and Starrs, T. 1993. *Learning Disabilities: A Handbook of Care*, 2nd edn. Edinburgh: Churchill Livingstone.

Shore, C. 1996. Successful breastfeeding. *Paediatric Nursing* **8** (9), 32–5.

Statutory Instrument No 1455. 1989. Competencies for pre-registration nursing programmes. Approved Amendment no. 9, 18A. Nurses', Midwives' and Health Visitors' Rules.

Wardley, B., Puntis, J. and Taitz, S. 1997. *Handbook of Child Nutrition*. Oxford: Oxford University Press.

Willis, J. 1997. Food fads and scares: the nutritional health of the nation's children. *Health Visitor* **70** (9), 354–55.

FURTHER READING

Bond, S. 1998. Eating matters-improving dietary care in hospitals. *Nursing Standard* **12** (17), 41–2.

Palmer, G. 1993. *The Politics of Breastfeeding*, 2nd edn. London: Pandora Press.

Royal College of Midwives 1999. *Successful Breastfeeding*, 3rd edn. Edinburgh: Churchill Livingstone.

Meeting hygiene needs

5

Chrissie Major

Assisting patients/clients to meet their hygiene needs is a fundamental and vital part of nursing care. It contributes greatly to comfort, gives an opportunity for observing physical and psychological needs, and provides a chance to build a trusting relationship, which is at the heart of good nursing. Henderson's definition of nursing emphasized this point, stating that 'the unique function of the nurse is to assist the individual . . . in the performance of those activities contributing to health . . . that he would perform unaided if he had the necessary strength, will or knowledge' (Henderson, 1960). Hygiene is one of those activities which most people learn to perform for themselves. However disability, and physical and mental health problems, may lead to the necessity for assistance, on either a temporary or permanent basis. For babies and small children, parents will usually be resident and will attend to their child's hygiene. However, if parents are unable to be present, the nurse would need to meet the child's hygiene needs. As with any procedure, hygiene care must be discussed with the person beforehand, and consent obtained.

Included in this chapter are:
- Rationale for meeting hygiene needs and potential hazards
- Bathing a person in bed
- Washing a person's hair in bed
- Bathing and showering in the bathroom
- Facial shaving
- Oral hygiene

The principles of care (e.g. observation, comfort, communication, safety and prevention of cross infection) which are discussed in this chapter are generally relevant to anyone of any age. How they are carried out for each individual will, however vary, and will of course, for a child, take developmental stage into account. Note that young babies' immune systems are not yet fully developed, and therefore prevention of cross-infection (see Chapter 3) is of particular importance (Simpson 1998). Specific care relating to the hygiene needs of babies, e.g. baby bathing, top and tailing, are not discussed in this chapter, but are covered in some detail by Kay (2000).

Recommended biology reading

You are advised to revise the layers of the skin. In addition, these questions will also help you to focus on the biology underpinning this chapter's skills. Use your recommended textbook to find out:

- The skin and oral cavity plays host to a range of micro-organisms. Which of these are potentially pathogenic?
- What is saliva composed of, how is it produced, and what is its role in maintaining a healthy mouth?
- What protective mechanisms do eyes have which help to prevent them from becoming infected?
- Distinguish between transient and resident bacteria found on the skin. Which of these cannot be removed with hand washing? (Chapter 3, Hand washing, will help you).
- Why does the skin on the palm side of the hands and sole side of the feet wrinkle when soaked in water?
- Why do we sweat and what does sweat contain?
- What is the 'acid mantle' and how can it be destroyed?

PRACTICE SCENARIOS

The following practice scenarios will be referred to throughout this chapter, in relation to meeting hygiene needs.

Body Mass Index
Is explained in Chapter 4 in the section 'Assessing clients' nutritional status and developing a plan of action'. A BMI of 16 indicates a person is underweight.

■ **Adult**

Miss Gladys Bradshaw, a retired schoolteacher aged 73 years, has been admitted for investigation of weight loss. She is weak and her general condition is poor. She has a **body mass index (BMI)** of 16, and complains that her dentures are ill-fitting, so that she is unable to eat properly. Her tongue appears coated and her mouth is dry. Investigations confirm that she has an inoperable carcinoma of the colon.

■ **Child**

Kevin O'Riordan, aged 14 years, has undergone an emergency appendicetomy for a perforated appendix, leading to **peritonitis**. He has an abdominal wound, is receiving intravenous fluids, and is nil by mouth. He seems quiet and uncommunicative. Kevin has two younger sisters. His parents spend part of each day at the hospital with him.

■ **Learning disability**

Robert Brown is a 30-year-old man with a learning disability who lives in a small staffed unit. Due to accompanying physical disabilities he uses a wheelchair for mobilizing. Joint deformities make it difficult to position him comfortably in the wheelchair. He is underweight and incontinent of urine and faeces; his skin tends to be dry. He has a poor appetite and is unable to feed himself or manage his own hygiene needs. He likes to be called Bob. Note: in Chapter 9, we will consider Bob's needs in relation to his mobility.

■ **Mental health**

Mrs Dora Mills is a 67-year-old woman with a long history of schizophrenic type illness. Her psychotic episodes are delusional in nature, and she is paranoid towards other people, believing that they want to poison her, the air and the water supplies. Her hygiene is very poor. She does enjoy having a bath, but when psychotic, becomes verbally and physically abusive when it is suggested. She has no teeth or dentures in her mouth and does not own a toothbrush.

Peritonitis
Inflammation of the peritoneum, the membrane lining the abdominal cavity. Results in pain, tenderness and fever.

RATIONALE FOR MEETING HYGIENE NEEDS AND POTENTIAL HAZARDS

Learning outcomes

By the end of this section you will be able to:

1. Identify why facilitating patients/clients to meet their hygiene needs is a beneficial nursing action.
2. Discuss possible hazards associated with meeting hygiene needs.

Learning outcome 1:
Identify why facilitating patients/clients to meet their hygiene needs is a beneficial nursing action

Activity

Many benefits have been associated with bathing patients (Whiting 1999). Why might it be important for nurses to assist with hygiene needs? Consider how you might feel if you were incapacitated, and unable to attend to your hygiene.

Points which you may have included are:

- Feeling clean and comfortable is an important social need for most people; to feel well groomed and not offensive to others can help to maintain self-esteem (Rader 1994).

- The act of assisting a client with personal hygiene needs allows the nurse to build up a trusting relationship (Tracey 1992), and to make a number of valuable observations, e.g. the condition of the skin.

- Cleansing the skin removes potentially harmful micro-organisms and also sweat, dead skin cells and the bacteria which produce body odour.

- Washing stimulates the circulation; the movement associated with this and the effect of warm water on the skin is beneficial, both physiologically and psychologically (Sloane *et al.* 1995).

- It is a private time where communication may be facilitated.

As identified above, whilst assisting with hygiene needs, an observant nurse can learn a great deal about the person.

■ *Activity*	Make a list of the things you can observe while assisting a person with hygiene. Looking at the scenarios might give you some clues.

You may have thought about the following:

- Condition of the skin: e.g. redness, any breaks in the skin, skin infections or bruising. This will be important for Miss Bradshaw because of advancing disease, and for Bob whose mobility is much restricted. *See* Chapter 9: Pressure sore risk assessment, for how pressure sore risk can be identified.

- Hydration and nutrition: does the skin feel dry and loose, or oedematous? You might identify that any of the patients/clients in this chapter's scenarios could potentially become dehydrated due to poor fluid intake, and their skin could become dry. Chapter 4: Assessment of nutritional status, emphasizes that visually observing skin is important in assessment.

- The person's mental state: is the person anxious, calm, depressed, demotivated, cheerful, or confused? This would be an important observation with all the people in this chapter's scenarios.

- Physical ability: to what extent can the person do things for him/herself? Does activity cause breathlessness or fatigue? Is there any apparent limb weakness or difficulty/discomfort on movement?

- Condition of any wound, drain or IV sites: this could apply to Miss Bradshaw, and to Kevin in particular. You could note oozing, or inflammation of surrounding skin, for example.

Learning outcome 2:
Discuss possible hazards associated with meeting hygiene needs

As discussed above, meeting hygiene needs should be a therapeutic activity, and yet there are a number of potential problems.

■ *Activity*	What could be possible hazards associated with hygiene care?

You might have identified the following:

- Bathing may cause disturbance to a very ill patient (such as Miss Bradshaw) who has limited reserves of energy. Kevin may still be sleepy post-anaesthetic, and be feeling uncomfortable, and therefore not want to have a wash. As stated in the scenario, depending on Mrs Mills' mental state, she may fear bathing, and be angry if it is suggested.
- The person may become chilled if large areas of the body are exposed. Both Bob and Miss Bradshaw are underweight, and thus are even more likely to become cold if care is not taken. Small babies are also susceptible to the cold (Kay 2000).
- Rather than removing harmful micro-organisms, the procedure may actively contaminate the skin by redistributing micro-organisms from heavily colonized areas such as the perineum, to other areas (Gould 1994). Cross-infection from other patients may be facilitated if the nurse is careless about infection control procedures, such as hand washing between patients.
- Excessive washing and the use of harsh soaps, may remove essential oils and the protective natural flora of the skin (Thaipisuttikul 1998; Skewes 1997).
- Having to allow other people, strangers, to perform intimate personal tasks can be a source of shame or embarrassment. There may be cultural differences in the gender and relationships of who is permitted to perform these procedures, so you will need to be aware of this and be sensitive to each individual. You should also take into account age; a teenager, such as Kevin, may be very uncomfortable about having personal care performed by a nurse or a parent. Consider how each of the patients/clients described in the scenarios may feel under these circumstances. How would you feel?

Many of the above hazards can be minimized by careful assessment of the individual.

BATHING A PERSON IN BED

Bathing a person in bed may be the preferred option to meet hygiene needs when the person is unable to get out of bed for medical reasons (e.g. after certain surgery or injuries), or when the person is too unwell or weak to be able to get out of bed. Miss Bradshaw and Kevin may need this option at present. Note that whilst this section focuses on bathing in bed, some patients, who are unable to wash in the bathroom, may be able to sit out in a chair to wash, using a bowl. The nurse may need to give assistance according to individual needs, and the principles discussed in this section can be adapted in this situation.

Learning outcomes

1. Discuss ways of maintaining patients' dignity and enhancing comfort.
2. Describe the procedure for this activity.

Learning outcome 1:
Discuss ways of maintaining patient's dignity and enhancing comfort

Activity	How might you maintain dignity and comfort for people while bathing in bed?

Points which you might have identified include:
-   Ensuring privacy by drawing cubicle curtains.
-   Encouraging people to do as much as possible for themselves and allowing sufficient time to do so.
-   Not exposing any more of the patient's body than is necessary for the task being carried out.
-   Remember, also, that your communication and approach to the individual will do much to promote dignity (*see* Chapter 2: The nurse's approach).

Learning outcome 2:
Describe the procedure for this activity

Before commencing the bathing of a person in bed, you will need to make an assessment of the individual.

Activity	What items should you include in your assessment? Consider Kevin and Miss Bradshaw, for example.

You may have thought of the following:
-   The person's usual hygiene routine – some people bath in the morning, others in the evening. Not everyone baths every day. If possible, try to maintain the person's usual routine. For a child in hospital, this will provide comfort and reassurance (Kay 2000). Consider: can you fit the routine to the patient, rather than the patient to the routine?

■ How does the person feel today? For example, is Miss Bradshaw anxious to be clean and groomed, or feeling so ill and fragile that the bare minimum will suffice until she feels more comfortable? Is Kevin too tired or uncomfortable to be bothered with a wash at present? A sick child is better left undisturbed unless there is a good indication otherwise (Kay 2000). Particularly when the person is unwell or fatigued, try to combine other care with hygiene needs, so that the person can then be left to rest, e.g. if the person needs turning for pressure relief, bathing can be timed to coincide with turning. Ensure that pain is controlled as bathing inevitably involves movement, which would cause further pain.

■ How much assistance is needed? Can you promote independence in any way, or is some time and care needed to re-establish self esteem?

■ Does the person want the nurse to help, or is there a relative coming in who she would like to help her? Kevin's family visit for part of each day. Would Kevin rather they helped him to wash? With children, it is important to negotiate with parents to what extent they would like involvement in their child's care (Kawik 1996; Coyne 1995a). A small study conducted by Coyne (1995b) suggested that parents all expected to carry out everyday care such as bathing. However, they may need assistance or guidance, particular when their child has dressings in place, and movement is impaired. Note that Kevin, as a teenager, may or may not want his parents to help him. For some parents of chronically sick children, it may be a relief for the nurse to carry out their child's hygiene care (Kay 2000). This may also be the case with informal carers of adults.

■ Does the person need to empty his bladder or bowels before commencing the bath? Offer this facility. Chapter 6 discusses assisting with elimination in detail.

■ What toiletries does she usually use? It might be interesting to make a list of your own requirements, and compare it to a friend's.

■ What time is available – do you have the time now, or will you have more later? Will you need another nurse to help you? Other health-care professionals, e.g. physiotherapists, dieticians, etc. may need access to the patient too.

Equipment

Having made this assessment, you will be ready to gather the equipment needed. Always try to think ahead and collect all that you will need at the start, thus avoiding having to leave the person during the procedure. Box 5.1 lists equipment which you will need.

- Patient's own washing bowl
- Soap or liquid skin cleanser
- Disposable flannels
- Towels
- Comb and/or brush
- Toiletries as required
- Clean bed linen and nightclothes
- Linen skip
- Plastic apron and disposable gloves.

Box 5.1 Preparing to bath a patient in bed: equipment required

Procedure

Below, is a suggested procedure for bathing a person in bed, which is likely to maintain comfort and prevent the person from becoming cold. Remember that a sensitive and empathetic approach should be maintained throughout. Ensure that you have introduced yourself to the patient, and that you use the bedbath as an opportunity to build further rapport. The patient may be pleased to engage in conversation. However, she may feel too weak and wish for a minimum of interaction, so be sensitive to non-verbal cues. For a child use play, and try to make this a fun activity (Kay 2000).

- Wash your hands and put on the plastic apron (and gloves if needed – *see* Chapter 3, Use of gloves and aprons).
- Fill the bowl with comfortably warm water.
- Remove the top bedclothes, leaving the patient covered by a blanket, sheet or towel.
- Remove the pyjama jacket or nightdress. If the patient has a weak arm or is attached to an intravenous infusion (IVI) like Kevin, remove this arm from the clothing last.

Activity

Practise with a friend or colleague, removing a pyjama jacket from each other, while pretending that one arm's mobility is impaired. Now try replacing it, inserting the affected arm first.

- Can the patient wash her own face? Even quite an unwell person may like to do this for herself. Otherwise, wash the patient's face, using soap if the patient uses this. Never poke inside ears. Take care to wash from the inner to outer corner of the eye (thus reducing risk of contamination). Rinse off soap, if used, and dry carefully.

Activity

With a friend or colleague, practise washing and drying each other's face. How did it feel?

■ Note that people who are unconscious or semiconscious are at risk of corneal damage and eye infections, as the normal protective mechanisms of the eyes (e.g. corneal reflexes) are impaired. Such people therefore require eye care in order to maintain healthy eyes and prevent future problems. A flow chart to assess the type and frequency of eye care required by unconscious or semi-conscious patients, can be found in Laight (1995). Laight (1996) identifies, however, that there has been little research to provide an evidence-based approach to eye care. Key points relating to eye care can be found in Box 5.2.

- Assessment should include checking whether the eyelids are clean, whether the corneas are dry (i.e. dull, no sparkle from reflected light), whether there is any sign of infection (e.g. redness, discharge), and whether the eyes are closed.
- If eyelids are unclean, wash your hands, and cleanse the eyelids with gauze, moistened with sterile water.
- Instillation of hypromellose eyedrops will prevent the corneas drying out. Lucrilube can be prescribed for persistently dry corneas and for open eyes.
- Assessment of eyes and instillation of hypromellose eyedrops should occur at least every 6 hours, but more frequently if corneas are dry.

Box 5.2 Eye care for unconscious or semi-conscious patients, key points (based on Laight 1995; 1996, and further personal communication)

■ Place a towel under the arm furthest away from you, and wash from the hand to the axilla. Rinse off the soap and dry thoroughly, taking care not to dislodge any cannulae or dressings. Repeat with the other arm.

■ Uncover the chest and abdomen and wash and dry this area in the same way, again taking care not to dislodge dressings or attachments. Work gently but quickly to prevent the patient from becoming chilled. Pay special attention to skin folds and under the breasts, as these areas may be moist through sweat and therefore heavily colonized with micro-organisms. A little talcum powder may be applied if liked; shake it into your hand rather than directly onto the patient, as the fine powder can be irritating if inhaled. Cover the chest and abdomen once this is completed. Other toiletries such as antiperspirant or body spray, can be applied as wished by the patient.

■ Change the water at this point, or at any time if it feels cool or becomes excessively soiled.

■ Now remove any lower body clothing, including thrombo-embolic deterrent stockings, cover the leg nearest you, and place the towel under the opposite leg. Wash the leg from toes to groin, rinse and dry. Apply moisturising lotion if the skin appears dry over the shins or feet. Repeat with the other leg.

up the soiled bottom sheet lengthways, close to the patient. Place a towel along the patient's back, wash, rinse and dry as before, noting any skin problems as previously outlined.

■ **Activity**   Which skin areas do you think you should pay most attention to?

Comment: The areas most at risk from pressure damage. These are the sacrum, trochanters, elbow and shoulder tips, base of the skull and heels. (*see* Chapter 9, Pressure sore risk assessment, for more details).

■ For the patient able to sit up, the buttocks can be washed in a similar fashion. Assist the patient to put on clean nightwear. Replace the thrombo-embolic deterrent stockings if worn and change the bottom sheet. To do this, roll or concertina fold a clean sheet close to the patient, without contaminating the clean sheet with the soiled one. Assist the patient to roll back towards you, and support him while your assistant removes the soiled sheet, pulls though the clean one and secures it.

■ **Activity**   Consider what might be the infection control issues in disposing of the soiled sheet.

Look back to the principles outlined in Chapter 3, Preventing cross-infection. Note that Health Service Guidelines have established a national colour coding standard for disposal of linen (NHS Management Executive 1995). Used linen (soiled and foul) should be disposed of in white or off-white bags. Infected linen should be placed into a water soluble bag and then into a red bag.

■ **Activity**   You will need two friends/colleagues for this exercise, and access to a bed in the skills laboratory. Practise changing the bottom sheet, taking it in turns to be the 'patient'.

Consider: did you feel vulnerable during this? What reassured you?

Finally:

■ Assist the patient into an appropriate and comfortable position, as determined by his/her condition and care plan. Recall safe moving and handling methods for this.

■ Brush or comb the patient's hair into their preferred style.

■ Assist with make-up if required by patient, and with oral hygiene (*see* later section).

■ Place the locker and call bell within reach.

■ Wash and dry the bowl, and dispose of soiled equipment appropriately (*see* Chapter 3, Waste disposal). Note that wash bowls should be stored upside down to reduce colonization by micro-organisms, which prefer horizontal surfaces.

■ Document any observations made, and the care given, in the care plan or nursing notes.

Summary

- It is important to assess the suitability of a bed bath for the individual patient, and negotiate involvement by the patient and family, as desired.
- Respect for the individual's privacy and dignity, and maintenance of comfort, should be promoted.
- Adhering to infection control procedures is paramount.

WASHING A PERSON'S HAIR IN BED

Learning outcomes

By the end of this section you will be able to:

1. State the circumstances under which this activity may be carried out.
2. Describe the procedure, considering infection control, and patient comfort and safety needs.

Learning outcome 1:
State the circumstances under which this activity may be carried out

Many people will not be confined to bed for long enough for hair washing to become a problem, and will be able to visit the bathroom where hair washing may be more easily accomplished. In the short term, a dry shampoo may be brushed through the hair, to absorb grease, sebum and remove dead skin cells. However, if a patient is to remain in bed for long periods of time, his/her hair will become in need of washing.

Activity	Recalling the scenarios, which of the patients is this most likely to apply to?

Comment: Miss Bradshaw, as her disease becomes more advanced, might need to have her hair washed in bed.

Some hospitals may actually have a hairdresser who will visit the ward and wash the patient's hair in bed. Find out if this facility is available in your area.

Activity	You may have been introduced to Roper *et al.* (1996) model of nursing. Which activity of living might hair washing be associated with?

Comment: 'Personal cleansing and dressing', and also 'Expressing sexuality'; in many cultures, hair and hairstyles play a large part in defining and advertising sexual identity. Hair can be an important part of a person's body image, and its condition may improve or lower self-esteem. You will note that these issues are considered in Chapter 2.

Learning outcome 2:
Describe the procedure, considering infection control, and patient comfort and safety needs

As with bathing in bed, try to think ahead about what you will need. Suggested equipment is in Box 5.4

> - Plastic bowl, shampoo guard
> - Plastic sheeting
> - Large jug or bowl of hand hot water
> - Empty bowl
> - Small jug
> - Shampoo and conditioner, as requested by the patient
> - Towels
> - Flannel
> - Brush/comb and hairdryer
> - Plastic apron.

Box 5.4 Preparing to wash hair in bed: equipment required

Positioning

First remove the head of the bed, and assist the patient to lie flat.

Activity

Consider patient safety and comfort – what patients might not be able to lie in this way?

You might have considered:
Patients who are very breathless, those with arthritis of the neck, or patients on skull traction, among others. It is therefore very important before commencing hair washing to assess the individual. If the patient cannot lie down, hair can be washed over a bowl on a bed table.

Procedure

- Place the empty bowl on a chair or bed table at the head of the bed, at a lower level. Consider your own comfort at this point; is the bed at a comfortable height for you to work without stooping?
- Arrange the plastic sheet to protect the mattress, and a towel to protect the patient's shoulders.
- Move the patient, using a glide sheet, so that her head is over the bowl. An assistant may be required to support the patient's head.
- Having checked the temperature of the water, wet the hair using the small jug. The patient may like to protect her eyes with a flannel.

■ Apply shampoo, massage gently into the scalp, and rinse off. Repeat this if desired. Apply conditioner, if used, comb through, leave for a minute or two, and rinse off until the hair feels clean. You may have to empty the bowl at intervals, before it gets too full.

■ Be aware of health and safety issues – mop up any spills immediately.

■ Wrap the patient's hair in a clean towel and empty the bowl.

■ Slide the patient back onto the bed, and remove the plastic sheet. Make sure the bottom sheet is not damp; replace if necessary.

■ Replace the head of the bed, and assist the patient to sit up if able, using a safe moving and handling technique.

■ Towel the hair dry, and style the hair as desired, using a hair dryer if necessary.

■ Activity

What health and safety issues should be considered when using hairdryers?

You may have identified:

- Hair dryer not too hot
- Trailing flexes
- Equipment checked regularly by electricians
- Electrical equipment and water don't mix.

Therefore, do take care to avoid these hazards.

Finally, wash and dry bowls and jug, and dispose of all equipment, in accordance with hospital policy. Leave the patient comfortable, with bed table, locker and call bell within reach. Document the care given in the care plan or nursing notes.

Summary

■ If hair washing in bed is required, carefully assess the patient's suitability first.

■ Be aware of individual preferences in hair care.

■ Maintain health and safety for both yourself and the patient.

BATHING OR SHOWERING IN THE BATHROOM

If a patient is able to visit the bathroom for personal hygiene needs, this is usually preferable for a number of reasons, which will be discussed in this section.

Learning outcomes

On completion of this section you will be able to:

1. State the advantages/disadvantages for bathing in the bathroom.
2. Describe the procedure, discussing health and safety issues.

Learning outcome 1:
State the advantages/disadvantages of bathing in the bathroom

Activity   Which of the people in this chapter's scenarios may be able to visit the bathroom?

Comment: All should be able to at some stage, but as previously mentioned, Miss Bradshaw and Kevin may at some point be too weak, tired or in pain to do so. The presence of a wound is not a contraindication to a shower or bath, as long as the skin edges of the wound are sealed (Briggs 1997), so Kevin, once over the initial acute post-operative phase, will be able to bath or shower. It has been suggested that a shower is preferable to a bath for a person with a wound as there is less risk of cross-infection from a previous user (Gilchrist 1990). Children may prefer to slowly and gently soak off dressings in warm water in the bath or shower, which may be less distressing and cause less damage to the epithelium (Bale 1996). Mrs Mills, depending on her mental state, may need a lot of verbal encouragement in order to go to the bathroom. Nurses will need to build up a trusting relationship with her, so that they can suggest bathing without upsetting her or causing offence. It would be important for all staff to understand Mrs Mills' fears and concerns, and approach her in a consistent fashion. However, if Mrs Mills refuses to go to the bathroom, her wishes must be respected.

Activity   Why might it be preferable for hygiene needs to be met in the bathroom, rather than at the bedside?

You might have considered these points:
The bathroom is a more familiar environment in which to attend to hygiene, which would be important for someone who is confused, or who is preparing for discharge home. Privacy may be more easily maintained, and there is a continuous supply of water, for instance. There may be cultural reasons why bathing in the bathroom may be highly desirable. Muslims, Hindus and Sikhs may prefer to cleanse themselves under running water, as in a shower, or by pouring water from a jug (Henley 1982; Henley 1983a; Henley 1983b). This is easier to achieve in the bathroom. For older people, going into a bath is a familiar activity, and some people, e.g. with muscle spasm, find a bath relaxing and therapeutic, particularly when used with bath water additives (Tarling 1997). For small children, bathtime is usually enjoyable and fun. For some people, actually going in the bath or shower may not be possible or desirable, but they may be able to at least sit and wash at the sink, which is usually preferable to washing in, or by, the bed.

   As discussed above, there are good reasons why a person may be better able to meet his/her hygiene needs in the bathroom. However, you may be able to think of some possible problems.

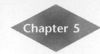
List possible problems with bathing in the bathroom.

Comment: Patients may become chilled if a suitable temperature cannot be maintained. It can also be exhausting for people with few reserves of strength, like Miss Bradshaw. People with special moving and handling needs, like Bob, need suitable equipment to enable them to access baths or showers. These are discussed in detail by Tarling (1997), and occupational therapists can advise. There are shower trolleys available, which can be useful for some individuals, e.g. those with spinal injuries, and other neurological conditions such as cerebral palsy. It is important that sound moving and handling practices are maintained by nurses within the bathroom to prevent injury to the client or nurse.

Learning outcome 2:
Describe the procedure, discussing health and safety issues

As with washing a client in bed, it is important to introduce yourself, and build a rapport prior to assisting with personal care. Assisting with hygiene in the bathroom provides a good opportunity to further the nurse-client relationship, as it involves one-to-one interaction in a private environment. As discussed previously, parents will usually wish to carry on with bathing of their child but may need assistance and support if the child has a physical impairment. The carers of some adults may also wish to continue to be involved in bathing. A person with dementia, for example, may be more comfortable if their usual carer assists. This involvement in care should be negotiated by the nurse and not taken for granted, as some informal carers may be exhausted and, as noted previously, may need a break. Involving relatives in bathing may sometimes be important in preparation for discharge, particularly where a person has become newly disabled. The nurse can take the opportunity to teach relatives about use of equipment and skin care for example.

Equipment

As always, it is important to plan ahead, and gather all equipment likely to be needed. Having to leave the bathroom to fetch items, when the person is undressed, could lead to chilling and exposure. As with bathing a person in bed, the toiletries required will vary between individuals, so always ask about preferences. With some individuals this may be indicated through non-verbal rather than verbal communication. You are likely to need towels, soap/shower gel or other cleansing agent, shampoo/conditioner (if hair washing is to be carried out), clean clothing (of the client's choice), brush/comb, toothbrush and toothpaste, and flannel/disposable washcloths.

Some people may be prescribed specific skincare agents for use in the bath or afterwards. For children, a selection of bath toys should be available, and for babies, a baby bath will be used.

Preparing the bathroom

After assembling the equipment, check that the bathroom is free, and has been cleaned after any previous user.

Activity   Why is it necessary to check the bathroom prior to taking your client there?

Comment: apart from any physical soiling, you need to consider potential risk of cross-infection. Always adhere to the relevant infection control policy for your practice setting, regarding cleaning of baths/showers between clients. You should also check that the floor is not wet or slippery, and that any extra equipment, such as a hoist or shower stool, is in place and in safe working order. Also check the temperature of the bathroom, as some clients, particularly if underweight like Bob, might be susceptible to the cold, as will the very young and the old. Warm the bathroom first if necessary.

Bathing or showering procedure

The following steps are a suggested procedure, which will maintain comfort and safety. As when bedbathing a client, assisting with hygiene in the bathroom requires the nurse to be sensitive and respectful.

- If bathing, fill the bath with warm water, using your elbow or a bath thermometer to check the temperature.
- Assist the person to the bathroom, offering them the opportunity to use the toilet if necessary.
- Assist with undressing, maintaining dignity and comfort, avoiding unnecessary exposure, by the use of towels.
- If the person has a urinary catheter *in situ*, a shower is preferable. However, if a bath is used, then the catheter should be clamped if the catheter has to be lifted above bladder level (e.g. when assisting the person in and out of the bath), to prevent reflux of urine back into the bladder (Getliffe 1997).
- If bathing, check the bath water temperature again, and allow the person to check for him/herself if able.
- Using suitable equipment, if necessary, help the person into the bath, or onto the shower chair. If the shower is being used, check the temperature before use.

■ You should consider enabling the person to maintain independence at this point, by encouraging/enabling him to wash himself as far as possible. Bob may be physically unable to assist, but can be encouraged to co-operate, and his carers will need to be sensitive to his feelings and preferences. He should not be rushed and adequate time should be allowed to enable him to participate to some degree in this activity if he wishes. Mrs Mills will need gentle prompting without being patronizing. Consideration should be given to the client with sensory impairment, e.g. visually impaired. Always take time to orientate the client to the environment, such as where the soap is.

■ As with bathing in bed, particular attention should be given to skin creases, and areas susceptible to becoming sore e.g. under breasts, palms of hands which are fixed in tonic flexion. Note also, as in the earlier section 'Bathing in bed', the importance of foot care for some people, in particular diabetics. Check Box 5.3, to remind yourself of the essential observations and care.

■ You should only leave a person alone in the bath or shower, if safety has been assessed, e.g. a person with epilepsy should not be left alone; neither should a child, or a person who is confused. You would need to carefully assess whether Mrs Mills could safely be left. Always check with the registered nurse, if unsure. If it has been assessed as safe to leave the person, ensure that the call bell is within reach, and working, before leaving.

■ Remember, as discussed earlier, the condition of the skin can be specifically observed, as well as psychological and physical condition e.g. any pain or breathlessness on movement, level of motivation to assist.

■ If hair washing is required, use clean water in a washbasin or bowl, and a jug, or shower attachment. Wet the hair, allowing the patient to protect his/her eyes with a flannel. Apply shampoo, and massage gently into the scalp. Rinse and repeat, if necessary, and apply conditioner, as needed. Rinse again, and dry with a clean towel.

■ Before assisting the person out of the bath, it may be easier to let the water out, and dry the upper body. This minimizes the time for the person to become chilled. Assist the person out of the bath or shower, using equipment as necessary, and give what assistance is needed to dry, again thinking about maintaining comfort and dignity by avoiding unnecessary exposure. Talcum powder and other toiletries may be applied if liked at this point. Can you recall the safety points about applying talcum powder which were discussed in the section on bathing in bed?

■ Assist the person to dress in clean clothes, to clean teeth (*see* oral hygiene section), and to brush/style hair as desired. Once again, assess the person's ability to participate in dressing. Mrs Mills may need verbal encouragement and reinforcement. Bob may be able to indicate clothing preferences, and cooperate in dressing. His incontinence should be managed as per his individual programme plan, which may mean applying a pad and pants during dressing. *See* Chapter 6, Promoting continence and managing incontinence, for detailed discussion on these issues.

■ Dispose of used equipment in accordance with waste disposal policy, and leave the bathroom ready for the next user.

■ Document the care given in the care plan or nursing notes.

Summary

- ■ Meeting hygiene needs in the bathroom is preferable for many reasons, e.g. privacy, availability of running water.
- ■ When assisting with hygiene in the bathroom, always assemble all equipment beforehand, to avoid leaving the individual alone.
- ■ The bathroom is potentially hazardous; it is important to take active steps to avoid accidents, such as falls or scalding, and only leave clients alone, if you have assessed that it is safe.
- ■ Maintain privacy and dignity throughout, and promote independence.

FACIAL SHAVING

Learning outcomes

On completion of this section you will be able to:

1. Discuss the rationale for shaving male patients/clients.
2. List the equipment needed and describe the procedure.

Learning outcome 1:
Discuss the rationale for shaving male patients/clients

Removal of facial hair has important social and cultural meanings. In some cultures, for example Sikhs, neither facial nor hair on the head may be cut. In others, for example, Western European, a wide variety of facial hair is socially acceptable, and plays a part in maintaining self-esteem. For many men, therefore, being clean shaven will be important, and being unable to self-care in this way, distressing.

■ **Activity** Talk to a male relative or friend who is usually clean shaven. Ask him how he would feel if unable to shave himself.

However, there may be some individuals for whom shaving may be hazardous. For example, individuals receiving anti-coagulant medication may be at risk of bleeding from minor cuts which could occur.

Comment: using an electric razor rather than a wet shave will be safer.

Learning outcome 2:
List the equipment needed and describe the procedure

Equipment

You will need:

- Either a razor, with shaving soap/foam and shaving brush, or the person's own electric razor (communal razors pose a high risk of cross-infection).
- Towel and flannel/ disposable washcloth.
- Bowl of hand hot water.
- Aftershave as desired by the client.

The procedure

Assemble the equipment, and assist the person to sit up if possible. Protect the person's chest with the towel. Assess to what extent the person can assist. With some men, careful positioning, provision of a shaving mirror, and having all equipment to hand, may enable independence with shaving. Note that shaving does require very fine motor control and therefore it is unlikely that Bob would be able to safely participate. It is important to always assess the client's capability; consulting the individual programme plan should clarify this, and any particular precautions that need to be taken.

Wet shaving

- Wet the brush and apply the soap to the face, or use the foam, working up a good lather.
- Work in the direction of the hair growth, starting with the cheeks, and moving on to the neck and around the mouth.
- Hold the skin taut and avoid any sores or moles. The client may be able to help by tightening his facial muscles. However this would not be possible for all men, e.g. if facial weakness is present.
- For some clients, e.g. Bob, the facial skin may be hypersensitive, and therefore great care should be taken.
- Rinse the razor after each stroke.
- When you have finished, rinse the face with clean water and dry, apply aftershave if used. Dispose of used equipment safely.

Dry shaving
- The skin should be clean and dry – a little talcum powder may help. Work with circular strokes, keeping the skin taut as for wet shaving.
- Assist the person to rinse his face when finished, apply aftershave if desired, and clean the razor ready for the next occasion.

Document your care in the care plan or nursing notes.

Activity

For this you will need a willing male friend, relative or colleague. Practise this activity – even if you shave yourself, you may find this more difficult than you expect. Ask your 'patient' to comment on your technique.

Summary
- Facial shaving is important to many male clients. The nurse should assist if the person is unable to self-care, thus maintaining self-esteem.
- A gentle and careful technique should be used, using the person's preferred equipment.

ORAL HYGIENE

Maintaining oral hygiene is an important aspect of nursing care, as it can do much to enhance quality of life. Jones (1998) advocates that nurses should include mouth-care as part of daily hygiene for the debilitated, but should also be promoting effective oral hygiene in people who are capable of self-care.

Learning outcomes

By the end of this section you will be able to:

1. Discuss the rationale for the maintenance of good oral hygiene.
2. Identify factors which increase vulnerability to poor oral hygiene, and consider how those at risk can be identified.
3. Understand how oral hygiene can be carried out safely, and based on best evidence.

Learning outcome 1:
Discuss the rationale for the maintenance of good oral hygiene

Oral hygiene aims to maintain a healthy oral mucosa, teeth, gums and lips, by the use of toothpaste, brush or other cleansing agents. Good oral hygiene is an important part of personal hygiene care (Somerville 1999), and a dry mouth has been identified as a symptom causing people considerable distress (Kaye 1992).

What problems may arise if oral hygiene is poor?

You may have considered:
- Mouth and gum infections such as candidiasis (thrush), which is a fungal infection (Torrance 1990).
- Poor appetite and therefore malnutrition (Peate 1993).
- Halitosis leading to social withdrawal.
- Systemic spread of infection in immunocompromised patients (Corbett 1997).
- Loss of self-esteem and poor body image (Somerville 1999).

Learning outcome 2:
Identify factors which increase vulnerability to poor oral hygiene, and consider how those at risk can be identified

■ **Activity**   Consider the people in this chapter's scenarios – do you think any of them are at risk of poor oral hygiene?

Comment: You should have identified that they are all at risk because:
- Miss Bradshaw has ill-fitting dentures, and she is generally debilitated.
- Kevin is nil by mouth.
- Mrs Mills has poor self-caring skills.
- Bob has physical difficulties, and a poor appetite.

There are many factors that can lead to poor oral hygiene (*see* Table 5.1). Looking at this table might indicate further possible risk factors than you had previously identified. For example, Mrs Mills may well be being prescribed a tranquillizer, which would increase her risk as it reduces salivary production. Kevin could be receiving morphine to control his pain which will increase his mouth dryness. Thurgood (1994) notes that most seriously ill people will have mouth problems, which will cause further discomfort and distress.

In order to assess the need for and frequency of mouth-care, an assessment tool can be helpful. One which was developed by Regnard and Fitton (1989) for use in an intensive care unit, could be used in other settings (*see* Box 5.3). This flow chart helps to indicate oral care which might be appropriate in different situations. Note that Bowsher *et al.*'s (1999) systematic review suggests that as yet, there is insufficient evidence to support oral assessment procedures, or how frequently mouth care should be carried out.

Learning outcome 3:
Understand how oral hygiene can be carried out safely, and based on best evidence

Bowsher *et al.*'s (1999) systematic review indicates that evidence-based oral care is not always apparent. For example, there is clear evidence against the

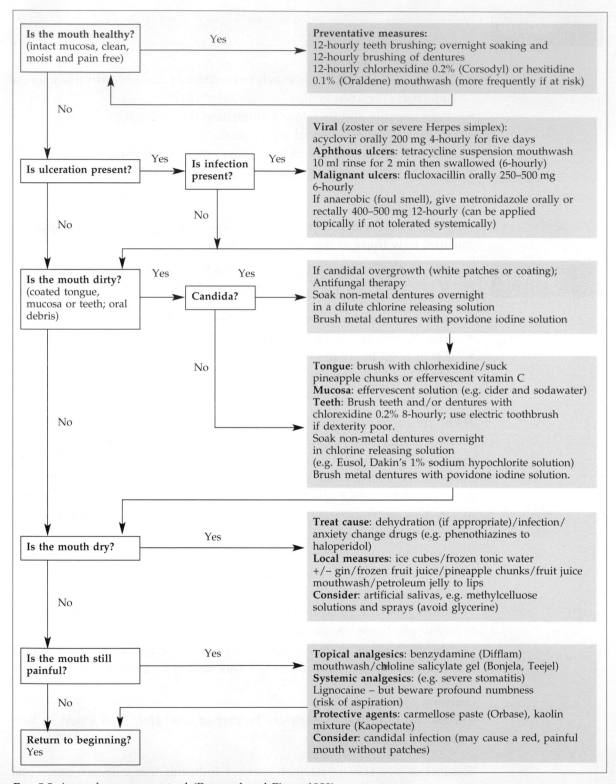

Is the mouth healthy?
(intact mucosa, clean, moist and pain free) — Yes →

Preventative measures:
12-hourly teeth brushing; overnight soaking and 12-hourly brushing of dentures
12-hourly chlorhexidine 0.2% (Corsodyl) or hexitidine 0.1% (Oraldene) mouthwash (more frequently if at risk)

No ↓

Is ulceration present? — Yes → **Is infection present?** — Yes →

Viral (zoster or severe Herpes simplex): acyclovir orally 200 mg 4-hourly for five days
Aphthous ulcers: tetracycline suspension mouthwash 10 ml rinse for 2 min then swallowed (6-hourly)
Malignant ulcers: flucloxacillin orally 250–500 mg 6-hourly
If anaerobic (foul smell), give metronidazole orally or rectally 400–500 mg 12-hourly (can be applied topically if not tolerated systemically)

No ↓   No ↓

Is the mouth dirty?
(coated tongue, mucosa or teeth; oral debris) — Yes → **Candida?** — Yes →

If candidal overgrowth (white patches or coating); Antifungal therapy
Soak non-metal dentures overnight in a dilute chlorine releasing solution
Brush metal dentures with povidone iodine solution

No ↓

Tongue: brush with chlorhexidine/suck pineapple chunks or effervescent vitamin C
Mucosa: effervescent solution (e.g. cider and sodawater)
Teeth: Brush teeth and/or dentures with chlorexidine 0.2% 8-hourly; use electric toothbrush if dexterity poor.
Soak non-metal dentures overnight in chlorine releasing solution (e.g. Eusol, Dakin's 1% sodium hypochlorite solution)
Brush metal dentures with povidone iodine solution.

No ↓

Is the mouth dry? — Yes →

Treat cause: dehydration (if appropriate)/infection/anxiety change drugs (e.g. phenothiazines to haloperidol)
Local measures: ice cubes/frozen tonic water +/– gin/frozen fruit juice/pineapple chunks/fruit juice mouthwash/petroleum jelly to lips
Consider: artificial salivas, e.g. methylcelluose solutions and sprays (avoid glycerine)

No ↓

Is the mouth still painful? — Yes →

Topical analgesics: benzydamine (Difflam) mouthwash/choline salicylate gel (Bonjela, Teejel)
Systemic analgesics: (e.g. severe stomatitis) Lignocaine – but beware profound numbness (risk of aspiration)
Protective agents: carmellose paste (Orbase), kaolin mixture (Kaopectate)
Consider: candidal infection (may cause a red, painful mouth without patches)

No ↓

Return to beginning?
Yes

Box 5.5 An oral assessment tool (Regnard and Fitton 1989)

Table 5.1 Factors predisposing to mouth problems (adapted from Thurgood 1994)

Drugs	Cytotoxic drugs (reduce autoimmune response)
	Corticosteroids (affect tissue healing)
	Antibiotics (alters oral bacterial balance, allowing infection by *Candida albicans*)
	Antihistamines, antispasmodics, anticholinergics, psychotropics, antidepressants, and tranquillizers (reduce salivary production)
	Diuretics (increase fluid loss)
	Morphine (causes mouth dryness)
Treatments	Radiotherapy of head/neck (causes localized inflammation, affects ability to eat/drink normally)
	Oxygen therapy, particularly if given unhumidified at high flow rates (dries oral mucosa)
	Suction (can damage oral mucosa)
	Restricted oral intake e.g. nil by mouth pre or post-operatively (potential for dehydration and dry mouth)
Mental or physical health problems or disability	Diseases: diabetes, thyroid dysfunction, oral disease/trauma, cerebrovascular disease
	Mental health problems: confusion, depression
	Terminal illness
	Acute/chronic breathing problems
	Unconsciousness
	Lack of manual dexterity

use of hydrogen peroxide mouthwashes, lemon and glycerin swabs, and using foam swabs for teeth cleaning, yet they can still be found used in practice. As with any other nursing practice, best available evidence should be used for oral hygiene. A variety of equipment may be needed, depending on the care identified as appropriate for the individual. Box 5.6 lists possible items.

- Spatula and pen torch (to inspect the oral cavity)
- Small soft bristled toothbrush (for teeth cleaning)
- Foam sticks (for moistening oral mucosa)
- Mouthwash, e.g. chlorhexidine (to prevent dental plaque) or water (for teeth cleaning)
- Toothpaste
- Container for dentures, if needed
- Lip lubricant e.g. soft paraffin, to prevent dry lips (Bowsher *et al.* 1999)
- Beaker and receiver (for mouth rinsing)
- Disposable gloves and plastic apron
- Towel, tissues, waterproof sheet.

Box 5.6 Equipment for oral care

Rationale for choice of equipment

A small, soft-bristled toothbrush has been identified as the most effective agent for removing plaque and debris from the mouth, teeth and tongue (Thurgood 1994). Toothpaste is the most pleasant cleaning agent (Roth and Creason 1986). It should always be fluoridated, a low fluoride formulation being used for children (Jones 1998). Jones (1998) advises that toothpaste has a generally drying effect so it should be used sparingly. Sodium bicarbonate 1% is often advocated if the mouth is filled with thick, sticky mucus, as it can break down mucin, but there remains insufficient evidence to support its use (Bowsher *et al.* 1999), and Jones (1998) warns that in a critically ill person, its application could affect electrolyte balance. Most antiseptic mouthwashes have a very transient effect so they are of limited value (Jones 1998). However, those containing chlorhexidine gluconate e.g. Corsodyl, if used for one minute, can reduce bacterial counts by up to 80% (Schiott et al. 1970, cited by Jones 1998). This is therefore worthwhile in the very vulnerable person e.g. immunocompromised, very sick or frail elderly people. Jones (1998) advises that for cleansing and moistening oral mucosa, pH-balanced swabsticks are preferable, but if foam swab sticks are used, they are best when coated with Corsodyl gel, as that is gentler to the delicate oral mucosa. Note that there are saliva substitutes available for people with dry mouths, e.g. luborant (Jones 1998).

> **Activity** ■   How might oral hygiene be achieved for each of the people in this chapter's scenarios? Looking back at the tool in Box 5.5 might be helpful.

Some suggestions:
- For Miss Bradshaw and Kevin, placing equipment within reach and assisting as necessary, may be all that is required. Whilst Kevin is nil by mouth and in bed, mouthwashes should be offered regularly, as well as teeth cleaning facilities twice daily, or more frequently if requested. After vomiting, for example, mouthwashes/teeth cleaning facilities should be offered. Note that young children under 7 years would need their teeth to be cleaned by an adult (Kay 2000) to ensure that plaque is removed effectively. Thus, if parents are unable to be present the nurse should help the young child with teeth cleaning.
- For Bob, teeth cleaning can be carried out at the sink in the bathroom. A soft toothbrush should be used and great care taken with the nurse paying attention to any indications of discomfort. Bob can be encouraged to participate to the best of his ability. However, to carry out effective teeth cleaning requires good physical dexterity, and the nurse should be aware of the need to maintain sound oral hygiene, therefore reducing the risk of tooth decay, which would adversely affect his quality of life. You would

need to consult his individual programme plan, to ascertain his level of participation in his oral hygiene.

■ Mrs Mills is physically able but may need gentle but persistent verbal encouragement and reinforcement to perform this task. As discussed earlier, it will be important for the nurse to have built up a trusting relationship prior to suggesting the need for oral hygiene.

Some people, who are more dependent and debilitated, would require the nurse to carry out oral hygiene on a regular basis by the bedside. When Miss Bradshaw's condition worsens, she would be likely to need this care, which is described below.

Oral hygiene procedure: key points

■ Position: After explaining the procedure and gaining consent, the person should be assisted into a sitting position, or, if unconscious, on his/her side to prevent inhalation of solutions or secretions.

■ Protect the person's chest with a towel, or the bed with the waterproof sheet.

■ Assemble the equipment – any mouthwash solution should be freshly prepared, and renewed after 24 hours. If water is used for immunocompromised patients, it should be sterile.

■ Wash hands, and put on gloves and apron, if required.

■ Lip crusting can be removed by gently sponging with warm water (Jones 1998). Observe for any breaks in the skin or signs of herpes simplex (cold sore), which would require treatment by acyclovir cream.

■ Remove the person's dentures, if worn. They should be brushed well to remove debris, using denture paste – ordinary toothpaste is too abrasive – and rinsed well. Box 5.7 lists key points for effective denture care.

■ If the person has her own teeth, they should be brushed using the toothbrush and paste. Box 5.8 explains how teeth cleaning should be carried out. If the person is able to perform this for herself, it is much better to facilitate this.

■ Gentle swabbing of the mucous membrane with foam sticks moistened with warm water or chlorhexidine mouthwash, will remove debris, and moisten the oral mucous membrane helping to keep it intact (Jones 1998).

■ Observe the condition of the mouth and particularly the tongue. If the tongue is coated, swab gently as above. A whitened appearance indicates a candidal infection (thrush), and this should be reported so that an antifungal infection agent can be prescribed.

■ Assist the person to rinse the mouth thoroughly with the chosen mouthwash solution, or use a rinsed toothbrush to do this if she is unable. Suction can be used to remove excess fluid from the mouth if the patient is unconscious, or has dysphagia (swallowing difficulty), as it is essential to prevent choking or aspiration of fluid (Jones 1998). A conscious person who is nursed flat e.g. after a spinal injury, can use a straw to suck fluid into the mouth to rinse and to spit through afterwards.

- Note that although foam sticks can be used to clean the oral mucosa, they are not so effective at removing debris and plaque from the teeth (Bowsher et al. 1999).
- Replace any dentures, top set first.
- Apply lip lubricant, if lips are dry. Use tissues to blot any excess water or lubricant.
- Leave the person comfortable, and dispose of equipment according to waste disposal policy.
- Document care given in the care plan or nursing notes.

- Wash hands and wear gloves.
- Remove dentures into a container and rinse to remove loose debris.
- Use the person's special denture brush, scrub all surfaces, using denture paste or a little soap, to remove all debris, over a bowl of tepid water.
- Rinse thoroughly.
- When dentures are unworn, store in a marked container filled with clean water.
- Soaking plastic dentures 2–3 times per week in dilute hypochlorite will help to prevent oral candidiasis. Again, always rinse thoroughly before replacing in the mouth.
- Dentures with a metal portion should only be soaked in dilute hypochlorite for about 20 minutes, because of danger of corrosion.

Box 5.7 Denture care (adapted from Jones 1998)

Activity

With a friend or colleague, take turns to clean each other's teeth, using your own toothbrush, and the instructions in Box 5.8. Also, try moistening each other's mouth using foam sticks, dipped in water or mouthwash solution. How did it feel?

Summary
- Effective oral care makes an important contribution to an individual's physical, psychological and social well-being.
- Available research should be utilized by nurses when assessing and implementing oral care.

- Explain procedure and gain consent.
- Wash hands, wear gloves and maintain privacy.
- It may be best to work at the side of the person, cradling the head.
- Remove any partial dentures into a bowl.
- Start at the front of the mouth in the upper jaw.
- Use a soft brush with a small amount of toothpaste pressed into the surface (to avoid it dislodging into the mouth and possible aspiration).
- Place the brush sideways against the teeth (*see* diagram below) overlaying the gum edges with bristles pointing towards the teeth roots.
- Use a side-to-side motion, moving the brush head just a fraction of an inch at a time, using light pressure to squeeze the gum tissue against the teeth.
- Move around the upper teeth, replacing the brush section by section against the teeth.
- Try to use the same action inside the upper jaw.
- Repeat for the outer and inner surfaces of the lower jaw.
- Finally, scrub the chewing surfaces of the upper and lower teeth with a forward and backward motion.
- Ask the person to rinse the mouth with warm water to remove debris, paste etc., or use foam sticks moistened with water to gently sweep away the debris and toothpaste.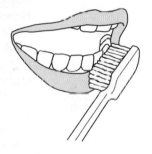
- Wash toothbrush well and leave it to dry in the air. Do not store in a sponge bag or container. Toothbrushes should be replaced every 6–12 weeks.

Box 5.8 Teeth cleaning (adapted from Jones 1998)

CHAPTER SUMMARY

Giving personal care, with attention to the individual's dignity, privacy and personal needs, is a fundamental and essential skill for nurses. Further key principles include cultural sensitivity and prevention of cross-infection. It is important to carefully assess how hygiene needs can be met for each individual, maintaining and promoting independence where possible. People with physical and mental health problems may be able to regain self-care skills with appropriate aids, encouragement and support. Teaching the person to manage personal hygiene and dressing can be an important part of rehabilitation, and should involve the multidisciplinary team, and an individualized approach.

REFERENCES

Adcock, L. 1998. Educating diabetics. *Journal of Community Nursing* **12** (5), 4, 6, 8.

Bale, S. 1996. Caring for children with wounds. *Journal of Wound Care* **5** (4), 177–80.

Bowsher, J., Boyle, S. and Griffiths, J. 1999. Oral care. *Nursing Standard* **13** (37), 31.

Briggs, M. 1997. Principles of closed wound care. *Journal of Wound Care* **6** (6), 288–92.

Clapham, L. 1997. Preventing foot problems in patients with diabetes. *Professional Nurse* **12**, 851–3.

Corbett, C.O. 1997. Mouth care and chemotherapy. *Paediatric Nursing* **9** (3), 19–21.

Coyne, I.T. 1995a. Parental participation in care: a critical review of the literature. *Journal of Advanced Nursing* **21**, 716–22.

Coyne, I.T. 1995b. Partnership in care: parents' views of participation in their hospitalized child's care. *Journal of Clinical Nursing* **4**, 71–9.

Edwards, V. 1998. A multidisciplinary approach to foot care in diabetes. *Nurse Prescriber/Community Nurse* **4** (2), 53–5.

Foster, A. 1999. Diabetes care: getting your patients on a sure footing. *Nursing Times* **95** (37), 51–2.

Getliffe, K. 1997. Catheters and catheterization. In: Getliffe, K. and Dolman, M. (eds.) *Promoting Continence: A Clinical and Research Resource.* London: Ballière Tindall, 281–341.

Gilchrist, B. 1990. Washing and dressing after surgery. *Nursing Times* **86** (50) Supplement, 71.

Gould, D. 1994. Helping the patient with personal hygiene *Nursing Standard* **8** (34), 30–2.

Henderson, V. 1960. *Basic Principles of Nursing Care*: Basel: S. Karger, for International Council of Nurses.

Henley, A. 1982. *Asians in Britain: Caring for Muslims and their Families: Religious Aspects of Care.* London: National Extension College.

Henley, A. 1983a: *Asians in Britain: Caring for Hindus and their Families: Religious Aspects of Care.* London: National Extension College.

Henley, A. 1983b: *Asians in Britain: Caring for Sikhs and their Families: Religious Aspects of Care.* London: National Extension College.

Jones, C.V. 1998. The importance of oral hygiene in nutritional support. *British Journal of Nursing* 74, 76–8, 80–3.

Kawik, L. 1996. Nurses' and parents' perceptions of participation and partnership in caring for a hospitalized child. *British Journal of Nursing* **5** (7), 430–4.

Kay, J. 2000. Hygiene. In: Huband, S. and Trigg, E. (eds.) *Practices in Children's Nursing: Guidelines for Hospital and Community.* Edinburgh: Churchill Livingstone, 131–7.

Kaye, P. 1992. *A–Z of Hospice and Palliative Medicine.* Northampton: EPL Publications.

Laight, S.E. 1995. A vision for eye care: a brief study of the change process. *Intensive and Critical Care Nursing* **11**, 217–22.

Laight, S.E. 1996. The efficacy of eye care for ventilated patients: outline of an experimental comparative research pilot study.*Intensive and Critical Care Nursing* **12**, 16–26.

Litchfield, B. and Ramkissoon, S. 1996. Foot-care education in patients with diabetes. *Professional Nurse* **11**, 510–12.

McConnell, E.A. 1998. Teaching a patient with diabetes how to protect her feet. *Nursing (Horsham)* **28** (12), 32.

NHS Management Executive. 1995. Hospital laundry arrangements for used and infected linen. HSG(95)18. London: HMSO.

Peate, I. 1993. Nurse-administered oral hygiene in the hospitalised patient. *British Journal of Nursing* **2**, 459–62.

Rader, J. 1994. To bathe or not to bathe: that is the question. *Journal of Gerontological Nursing* **20** (9), 53–4.

Regnard, C and Fitton, S. 1989. Mouth care: a flow diagram. In: Doyle, D., Hanks, G. and MacDonald, N. (eds.) *Oxford Textbook of Palliative Medicine.* Oxford: Oxford University Press.

Renwick, P., Vowden, K., Wilkinson, D. and Vowden, P. 1998. The pathophysiology and treatment of diabetic foot disease. *Journal of Wound Care* **7**, 107–10.

Roper, N., Logan, W. and Tierney, A. 1996. *The Elements of Nursing*, 4th edn. Edinburgh: Churchill Livingstone.

Roth, P.T. and Creason, N.S. 1986. Nurse administered oral hygiene: is there a scientific basis? *Journal of Advanced Nursing* **8,** 33–34.

Simpson, C. 1998/9. Infection control. *Paediatric Nursing* **10** (10), 30–33.

Skewes, S.M. 1997. Bathing: it's a tough job! *Journal of Gerontological Nursing* **230** (5), 53–9.

Sloane, P., Rader, J., Barrick, A. *et al.* 1995. Bathing persons with dementia. *The Gerontologist* **35** (5), 672–8.

Somerville, R. 1999. Oral care in the intensive care setting: a case study. *Nursing in Critical Care* **4** (1), 7–13.

Tarling, C. 1997. Washing and bathing. In: *The Guide to Handling of Patients: Introducing a Safer Handling Policy*, 4th edn. London. National Back Pain Association, 172–180.

Thaipisuttikul, Y. 1998. Pruritic skin diseases in the elderly. *The Journal of Dermatology* **25**, 153–7.

Thompson, J. 1999. Foot problems and care of feet: part two – common disorders. *Community Practitioner* **72**, 178–9.

Thurgood, G. 1994. Nurse maintenance of oral hygiene *British Journal of Nursing* **3** (7), 332–53.

Torrance, C. 1990. Oral hygiene. *Surgical Nursing* **13** (4), 16–20.

Tracey, C.A. 1992. Hygiene assistance. In: Bulecheck, G.M. and McCloskey, J.C. (eds.) *Nursing Interventions: Essential Nursing Treatments*, 2nd edn. Philadelphia, PA: W.B. Saunders.

Whiting, L.S. 1999. Maintaining patients' personal hygiene. *Nursing Practice* **14** (5), 338–40.

Young, T. 1997. Diabetic foot ulceration. *Practice Nursing* **8** (9), 24–5, 27.

Chapter 6

Meeting elimination needs

Lesley Baillie and Vickie Arrowsmith

Elimination of urine and faeces is an essential bodily function which we usually become independent in within the first few years of life. Elimination is then usually a private function, but when disability, or physical or mental health problems are present, independence in elimination is often affected. Assistance by nurses may then be needed so that potential problems can be avoided and actual problems can be managed.

Included in this chapter are:
- Assisting with elimination: helping people to use the toilet, bedpans, urinals and commodes
- Urinalysis
- Collecting urine and stool specimens
- Caring for the person with a urinary catheter
- Use of enemas and suppositories
- Promotion of continence and management of incontinence.

Recommended biology reading:
These questions will help you to focus on the biology underpinning this chapter's skills. Use your recommended text book to consider the following:

- What are the stuctures involved in the urinary system?
- Within the kidney, blood is filtered. What forces are involved in filtration? Where does filtration occur? Which substances are not filtered out and why?

- What is the role of the juxtaglomerular apparatus?
- What happens to the glomerular filtrate as it passes along the nephron?
- How and why does the concentration of urine vary?
- Urine is stored in the bladder. How does the bladder expand as it fills up?
- What is micturition and how does it occur?
- What is cystitis? Why is it generally more common in females than in males?
- What factors can increase the risk of urinary tract infection?
- What are the different regions of the digestive tract and their functions?
- How does food move through the digestive tract?
- What is the gastrocolic reflex?
- What do stools/faeces consist of?
- How do we defaecate?
- What is constipation?
- What factors increase the risk of constipation?

PRACTICE SCENARIOS

The following scenarios illustrate situations where assistance with elimination will be needed, and will be referred to throughout this chapter.

■ **Adult**

Mrs Sarah Newton is a 36-year-old former school teacher, who lives with her husband and school age children, and was diagnosed 3 years ago as having **multiple sclerosis**. Her vision has now become affected, she is confined to a wheelchair, and she has a long-term urinary catheter *in situ*. The district nurse visits weekly to assess the situation and attend to the catheter. Unfortunately a urinary tract infection has occurred on several occasions. Mrs Newton has asked staff to address her as Sarah.

Multiple sclerosis
Progressive destruction of myelin sheaths of neurones in the central nervous system. Can cause loss of movement and sensation, and affect elimination.

■ **Child**

Toby Williams, aged 18 months, has arrived in Accident and Emergency, with his concerned parents, with a 24-hour history of diarrhoea and vomiting. After initial nursing assessment and review by the paediatrician, it is decided that Toby needs admission for rehydration and observation. The collection of urine and stool specimens has been requested.

■ **Learning disability**

John Smythe is a 28-year-old client with a severe learning disability. He lives in a staffed group home where he is generally continent, but he is known to be incontinent in unfamiliar environments. He will be going into hospital soon to have a small operation which will require him being an in-patient for about 3 days. Staff are concerned that management of his continence may be an issue.

■ **Mental health**

Mrs Vera Wilson, aged 80 years, has been readmitted to the ward for the elderly mentally ill after a marked deterioration in her mental state. Her mood is low and she appears confused, disorientated, agitated and restless. She also seems frightened, and has a distended abdomen that appears to be causing her much discomfort. Due to her agitated and confused state she is unable to state clearly how she is feeling, but her husband reveals to the staff that Vera has been unable to pass urine over the last day, and that she appears to be in retention. He also says that Vera's appetite is very poor, and that she is prone to constipation.

ASSISTING WITH ELIMINATION: HELPING PEOPLE TO USE THE TOILET, BEDPANS, URINALS, AND COMMODES

Learning outcomes

By the end of this section you will be able to:

1. Identify why a person might need help with elimination, and what equipment you could use to give assistance.
2. Discuss the important principles, which you would need to consider when assisting with elimination.

Learning outcome 1:
Identify why a person might need help with elimination, and what equipment you could use to give assistance

■ **Activity**

Reflect back on your placement experiences and write down all the reasons why a person might need help with elimination.

Discussion points

There are many situations where a person might need help. Part of the assessment of any newly admitted or referred person will be to identify any problems with elimination, and whether assistance is required. An example of when help would be needed is when a person has impaired mobility. This might be someone who is temporarily confined to bed following orthopaedic surgery, someone who has a neurological disorder, or someone who is highly breathless. People who are very weak or unwell e.g. bleeding severely, or confused (like Mrs Wilson), will also need help with elimination.

> **■ Activity**
>
> What equipment is available to assist with elimination? There may be examples of equipment in the skills laboratory or within your practice placement.

Discussion points

The toilet

Whenever possible a person can be helped to reach the toilet. This is a more familiar environment in which to eliminate (particularly helpful if the person is confused and/or disorientated), and it is more private. To eliminate in a ward, behind closed curtains, may not feel very private at all. Noise and smell may be obvious, and this potential embarrassment could lead the person to ignore the need to defaecate, which can lead to constipation (Edwards 1997). You might need to walk with the person, who may need to use sticks, a frame or crutches (*see* Chapter 9, Assisting with mobility), and this could be part of this persons programme of mobilization. For a person unable to walk, you would use the wheelchair to take him to the toilet.

The commode

If the person is very ill or weak it may be unwise for him to leave the bedside. When making decisions about this it is important to check the care plan, and seek advice if you are unsure.

If the person is able to get out of bed, a commode will be preferable to using a bedpan, as it promotes a more conducive position for elimination and will usually feel more comfortable. A commode has a pan underneath, which can be removed after use, and either macerated (if disposable) or put into the washer-disinfector if reusable. There are many types of commode available but those which are a good size, easy to manoeuvre, and have arms which are easy to remove are preferable (Ballinger *et al*. 1996). Tarling (1997) discusses types of commodes and their advantages and disadvantages, with particular reference to moving and handling issues.

Bedpans/urinals/potties

Some people may have to stay in bed for medical reasons, for example, after certain surgery. If a bedpan must be used, you will need to choose between a standard bedpan which the patient will need to sit up on, and a flat 'slipper' pan, which a patient can roll on to – essential when someone is unable to sit up. To pass urine there are both male and female urinals available. Female urinals are particularly useful for women who have to lie flat (for example following back surgery). For a young child, a potty will be used. If the child will be in hospital for long, the family may wish to bring the child's own potty in as this can decrease anxiety.

Reusable equipment

Equipment can be reusable, in which case it may be made from stainless steel or plastic. After use it will need to be put in the washer-disinfector. This first cold rinses, then hot rinses, then disinfects, which includes heating to 80°C for one minute, before being cooled. Disadvantages of this system are that it is not always effective (up to 22% of bedpans need to be reprocessed) and the cycle is slow (Johnson 1989).

Disposable equipment

Disposable equipment is made from paper pulp and so the bedpans and potties need to be placed onto a plastic support. After use, the disposable equipment is put into the macerator which processes them quickly. The plastic supports should be washed with hot water and detergent. Johnson (1989) found that nurses preferred the disposable system, which was also assessed as being cheaper once capital costs were considered.

Learning outcome 2:
Discuss the important principles, which you would need to consider when assisting with elimination

Activity

If you are assisting someone with elimination, what do you think would be important principles of care?

Box 6.1 lists important principles which you could have identified. Adhering to these can enable this practical skill to be a therapeutic action by the nurse (*see* Chapter 1). These principles will now be discussed.

- Approachability and communication
- Privacy and dignity
- Promptness
- Prevention of cross-infection
- Observation
- Prevention of accidents
- Promotion of independence and patient/parent participation
- Promotion of hygiene and comfort.

Box 6.1 Principles to follow when assisting with elimination

Approachability and communication

People who have needed help with their elimination invariably describe it as embarrassing and even distressing. The authors have known patients admit to reducing their fluid intake (thus increasing their risk of complications such as a urinary tract infection), so that they need not call for a bedpan or commode so often. In Koch and Kelly's (1999) study women with multiple sclerosis talked of feelings of 'humiliation' at having to ask for help with elimination. If a nurse does not appear approachable, then people may not feel that they can ask for help. This could lead to discomfort (emotionally and physically), or even to incontinence, retention of urine or constipation. Chapter 2 discusses in detail the nurse's approach to the client. You will need to be aware of non-verbal communication such as proximity to the person, body language, and facial expression/eye contact.

If the person has communication difficulties, the nurse will need to observe for non-verbal cues (such as restlessness), and sometimes a picture board (which could include a picture of a toilet) can be used for the person to indicate his need to eliminate. When John is admitted to hospital for his operation, the staff from his home need to ensure that nurses in the admitting ward know how John will communicate his need to go to the toilet, which may be through signing or symbols. The nurses will also need to understand that if they ask John if he needs to go to the toilet, they will need to give him enough time to answer, as processing information may take much longer for the client with learning disabilities, possibly up to 3 minutes. Verbal communication when assisting with elimination should include clear and appropriate use of language, taking developmental stage into account. Children will often have particular terms, which they may use in relation to elimination, and the nurse will need to know these if parents will not be readily available.

Privacy and dignity

If these important principles are not maintained, the person may feel embarrassed and degraded, and self-esteem may be affected. Remember also that these principles are identified in the Code for Professional Conduct (UKCC 1992). To maintain privacy and dignity always ensure that bedside curtains are pulled shut properly, or the toilet door closed, and that patients are covered up whilst on the bedpan or commode. Note that some people may only want a nurse of the same sex to help them. It is important to approach each person as an individual being sensitive to non-verbal cues and being aware of possible cultural issues, whilst not making assumptions. Within some religions, e.g. Muslims (Henley 1982), Hindus (Henley 1983a) and Sikhs (Henley 1983b), modesty about the body is a requirement, and the exposure of a woman to a man, and physical contact between a woman and a man who is not her husband, are forbidden. The nurse should also speak privately and quietly when assisting with elimination.

Promptness

This is an important principle as people suffering from certain types of incontinence (urge incontinence) will not be able to wait (*see* section on Managing incontinence later in this chapter). Also if patients are not able to attempt to open their bowels when they feel the need, faeces are pushed back into the sigmoid colon or remain in the rectum, where water continues to be reabsorbed. This leads to faeces becoming harder and more painful and difficult to pass, which may lead to constipation (Edwards 1997). The nurse should try to give priority to meeting elimination needs, remembering that the patient is in a powerless position, dependent on the nurse for help with this basic need. When the patient has finished eliminating, again the nurse should respond promptly, to avoid discomfort and maintain safety. Patients should be provided with a call bell with an explanation for use.

Prevention of cross-infection

When helping a person with elimination, cross-infection is a high risk. Patients in an in-patient setting may be particularly vulnerable to infection due to their medical conditions, and some micro-organisms are resistant in nature (*see* Chapter 3). It has been found that a third of reusable bedpans may be contaminated with (mainly Gram-negative) bacteria after having been through a cleaning cycle (Block *et al.* 1990), which could lead to cross-infection between patients. Ayliffe *et al.* (1999) recommend disinfection of non-disposable urinals and bedpans by heat. Careful hand washing is the most important measure when assisting with elimination, as spread is principally via the hands of staff (Gould and Chamberlain 1994). Urine is normally sterile, but will often be contaminated while voiding by bacteria present around the urethral opening (Gould 1994). Urine provides an excellent medium for bacterial growth, especially Gram-negative bacteria (*Pseudomonas, Klebsiella, Escherichia coli (E. coli), Proteus*) which can survive only when water and inorganic ions are present (Gould 1994). Urine passed into a bedpan or urinal should therefore be disposed of quickly, as standing at room temperature will allow any bacteria present to divide approximately once every 30 minutes (Gould 1994) thus becoming a reservoir of infection. When a patient (for example Toby) has diarrhoea which could be infected, prevention of cross-infection is essential. As well as prompt disposal of the diarrhoea and hand washing, it is likely that nurses would employ source isolation techniques, including nursing Toby in a single room and use of gloves and aprons (*see* Chapter 3).

Observation

When assisting with elimination there will be many useful observations which you can make, and these are listed with explanations in Table 6.1.

Table 6.1 Observations to make when assisting with elimination

Observation	Explanation
Ability to move	To lift onto a bedpan, transfer to a commode or toilet, or stand to use a urinal. Whether any apparent discomfort/pain, breathlessness or weakness when moving.
Skin condition	Redness or broken areas on sacrum or buttocks. Soreness of groin, perineum, penis or vulva.
Self-care ability	Physical/mental ability to remove or adapt clothing, before and after elimination, and to carry out hygiene afterwards.
Amount and frequency of urine output	A fluid input/output chart may be maintained if there are concerns about fluid balance. Urine will be measured in a jug and recorded in millilitres. Nappies can be weighed: 1 g = 1 ml. Poor overall urine output could occur in dehydration or shock. No urinary output could mean retention of urine. Frequent small amounts of urine might indicate a urinary tract infection (UTI). Monitoring of frequency and amount may be part of a bladder re-education programme.
Appearance of urine	*See* Urinalysis, next section. Very dark, concentrated urine might indicate dehydration, and smoky offensive urine might indicate UTI. Presence of blood may be due to kidney trauma or disease.
Appearance of stools	Consistency and frequency of stools – hard and infrequent which could indicate constipation, or frequent and loose, termed diarrhoea, which could be infected. A stool chart to record frequency, appearance and consistency might be maintained. If infection is suspected, a stool specimen will be collected and sent (*see* later section).

Prevention of accidents

To prevent damage to either yourself, colleagues or the patient, you will need to do a moving and handling risk assessment, and this should be documented. Questions to consider might be:

- Can the patient move himself onto the bedpan?
- Can the patient weight bear and transfer onto a commode unaided, or with one nurse or two nurses, or is a hoist necessary?

Tarling (1997) advises that if two nurses are needed to support a standing patient, a third will be needed to adjust clothing and clean him. Moving and handling in relation to toileting, is covered in detail by Tarling (1997). If the patient is using the bedpan in bed you will need to assess how you will ensure that she does not topple over. Certainly on a narrow trolley, sides must be put up, and these may be appropriate for some patients who are in bed. Balancing on a bedpan can be difficult, and it may be safer for sides to be up which can be held onto for support. Using the commode by the bedside is potentially hazardous. You will need to ensure that brakes are on securely, and that there are no fluids on the floor or other slippery substances. Is the person safe to leave? Is he confused and likely to try to stand up alone leading to a fall? You may find that there is specific documentation for moving and handling risk assessment, and a fall risk assessment scale can help to identify a person who is at risk of falls. Find out if such risk assessment tools are used in your current or next practice placement.

Promotion of independence and patient/parental participation

You will need to assess the person's abilities, and promote independence whilst also maintaining hygiene and safety. Learning how to use the toilet unaided, after a **cerebrovascular accident** (CVA) for example, may take some time, and both short and long term goals may be necessary. Teaching the person how to manage transfers safely (for example from chair to commode), and how to remove clothing, are situations where education may be needed. For people with learning disabilities, independence will be promoted if they are well orientated to their environment and where the toilet is and are taken to the same toilet by the same route each time. If the nurses on John's admitting ward can take these steps, John may be able to find his own way to the toilet independently. These steps may also be helpful for the person with dementia.

With a child, when the family is present, it should be assessed as to what involvement they want in the care. Are parents comfortable and confident to assist, and to what extent? The nurse will need to ensure that parents know where equipment is kept, and that they are aware of any special requirements, such as the need to measure and record urine output. Kawik (1996) found that there is an assumption that parents will be involved in care, but the extent and scope of involvement is often not negotiated. A review by Coyne (1995a) indicated that there is a wide variation in the level of care which parents are willing to undertake, and that nurses should work in partnership with parents. A subsequent small study conducted by Coyne (1995b) suggested that parents all expected to carry out everyday care such as bathing and toileting, but more technical skills (which included measuring urine) were considered to be the nurse's job.

Promotion of hygiene and comfort

You will need to consider how hygiene can be promoted for the bedside patient when meeting elimination needs, ensuring that you enable the person to wash hands, and the perineal and genital area where necessary. Unfortunately Pritchard and Hathaway (1988) found that offering hand washing facilities to

Cerebrovascular accident

Cerebral damage caused either by decreased blood flow or haemorrhage. Effects vary but often causes paralysis down one side of the body (hemiplegia), speech and swallowing difficulty, and elimination difficulties. Commonly termed a 'stroke'.

bedfast patients after the use of bedpan or urinal was often overlooked. When taking someone to the toilet ensure that he is able to wash his hands at the sink afterwards. Always leave access to toilet tissue, and if the person is unable to wipe himself, then you will need to either do this for him, or give assistance to the person, who may be learning or relearning this skill. With a female patient always wipe the vulval area from top to bottom to prevent transmission of bowel bacterial flora (such as *E. coli*) from the anal area to the urethra (Nazarko 1995). Females have a short urethra (4 cm), which can easily lead to contamination by such bacteria if care is not taken. Note that within Asia, the use of the left hand is reserved for washing underneath after using the toilet, the right hand being used for eating and other activities (Henley 1982; Henley 1983a; Henley 1983b). These rules may also be important to some Asians living in Britain. At all times prevent the person from becoming cold, covering legs with a blanket for example, and ensure that a patient using the bedpan is comfortably supported with pillows. Remember that psychological comfort will be promoted by your attitude and approach (*see* Chapter 2).

Summary

- Many health problems will lead to a person needing help with elimination.
- There is various equipment available to assist the person who is unable to go to the toilet. The nurse will need to assess which is appropriate for each individual.
- There are a number of important principles which need to be followed when helping a person with elimination to ensure that care is therapeutic, effective and safe.

URINALYSIS

Urinalysis is the testing of urine for a variety of substances, which will give valuable and immediate information about an individual's kidneys, urinary tract and liver, and will often influence the patient's subsequent management (Rowell 1998).

Learning outcomes

By the end of this section you will be able to:

1. Understand the process of urinalysis.
2. Show insight into the meaning of the results of a urinalysis, and what action to take if abnormal results are obtained.
3. Identify when urinalysis should be performed.

Table 6.2 Clinical significance of test results (adapted from Bayer, 1998 and Bayer, 1997b with kind permission)

Significance of positive results	*Commonest causes of abnormalities, and possible action to take*
Glucose Not normally detectable in urine. Found when its concentration exceeds the renal threshold.	**In people with raised blood glucose concentration**: diabetes mellitus or glucose infusion. **In people without raised blood glucose concentration**: pregnancy or renal glycosuria. **Action**: If positive, a blood glucose measurement should be performed, and further action may follow.
Bilirubin Presence in urine indicates an excess of conjugated bilirubin in plasma. Note that stale urine may give a false-negative result.	**Liver cell injury**: e.g. viral or drug induced hepatitis, paracetamol overdose, late stage cirrhosis. **Biliary tract obstruction**: e.g. by gall stones, carcinoma of the head of pancreas, biliary atresia in infants. **Action**: Should always be reported as further investigations will be needed.
Ketones Indicates accumulation of acetoacetate secondary to excessive breakdown of body fat. Some drugs e.g. L-dopa, may give a false-positive result.	Fasting, particularly with fever and/or vomiting. Most often seen in children. Diabetic ketoacidosis. Ketotic hypoglycaemia in young children. **Action**: Urgent action is needed if the person is a known or suspected diabetic.
Specific gravity A measure of total solute concentration in urine. In health varies widely according to the need to excrete water and solutes.	**High values** are found in dehydration, or in impaired kidney function e.g. chronic renal failure. **Low values** are found in people with intact renal function and high fluid intake, diabetes insipidus, chronic renal failure, hypercalcaemia, hypokalaemia.
Blood May be haematuria (intact blood cells) or haemoglobinuria (free haemoglobin – excreted from plasma or liberated from red cells in the urine).	**Haematuria**: Due to kidney disorders e.g. glomerulonephritis, polycystic kidneys, tumours. Due to urinary tract disorders e.g. stones, tumours, infection, benign prostatic enlargement. **Haemoglobinuria**: Severe haemolysis e.g. sickle cell disease crisis. Breakdown of red cells in urine (especially when urine is dilute and testing is delayed). **Action**: Should be reported. Follow-up will depend on other tests and clinical picture.

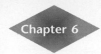

Table 6.2 (Continued)

Significance of positive results	Commonest causes of abnormalities, and possible action to take
pH In health, the pH of uncontaminated urine ranges from 4.5–8.0. **Note:** a high pH will be found if testing stale urine, therefore such specimens should not be used.	**Low values** Found in acidaemia as in diabetic ketoacidosis. Also starvation or potassium depletion. **High values** Found in stale urine, alkalaemia (except when due to potassium depletion) e.g. due to vomiting and consumption of large amounts of antacids, renal tubular acidosis, urinary tract infection with ammonia forming organisms. **Action:** Depends on other test results.
Protein A range of proteins can be detected but the reagent is most sensitive to albumin, so a negative result does not rule out presence of other proteins.	Albuminuria may be found in acute and chronic glomerulonephritis, urinary tract infection, glomerular involvement in systemic lupus erythematosus, nephrotic syndrome, pre-eclampsia, fever, heart failure and postural (orthostatic) proteinuria. **Action:** Transient results are seldom important but persistent positive results will need investigating for underlying cause. Other test results and clinical picture should be considered.
Urobilinogen Urinary excretion of urobilinogen reflects the combined effects of production of bilirubin, conversion of bilirubin to urobilinogen in the gut, and reabsorption into the bloodstream. Note that false-negatives are found in stale urine.	**Increased secretion** May be due to increased production e.g. in red blood cell disorders such as sickle cell disease, or due to decreased uptake by the liver e.g. in viral hepatitis and cirrhosis. **Decreased secretion** May be due to biliary tract obstruction e.g. gallstones, carcinoma of pancreas, or due to sterilization of the colon by unabsorbable antibiotics, e.g. neomycin, which prevents bacterial conversion of bilirubin to urobilinogen. **Action:** Urgent investigation is needed.
Nitrite Most organisms which infect the urinary tract contain an enzyme system which catalyses the conversion of dietary nitrate which is normally present in urine, to nitrite which is not found in urine unless there is a urinary tract infection.	Presence indicates urinary tract infection due to nitrite producing organisms. However absence does not exclude infection, as some organisms are unable to convert dietary nitrate to nitrite. False-negatives are also found if there is insufficient dietary nitrate, or urine has not been in the bladder long enough (4 hours is ideal) for the conversion to take place. **Action:** Specimen should be sent for microscopy and culture.
Leucocytes Will be present when some of the leucocytes which have entered inflamed tissue from the blood, are shed in the urine.	Indicates a urinary tract infection, especially when it is accompanied by acute inflammation of the urinary tract. **Action:** Specimen should be sent for microscopy and culture.

microscopy, culture and sensitivity (MC & S). This laboratory test examines the urine under the microscope, cultures the urine to see whether bacteria grow, and then checks what antibiotics the bacteria are sensitive to. The prevalence of UTI increases with ageing but typical symptoms (such as pain, **frequency** and pyrexia) may not be present in older people (O'Meara 1999). Urine should first be assessed visually and if obviously infected (cloudy and offensive) or blood-stained, then it should be sent for MC & S. If however the urine is clear, a urinalysis will show whether there are leucocytes, nitrites, protein or blood present. A positive nitrite test indicates infection but a few cases may be missed. Positive tests for leucocytes, blood or protein may also suggest UTI. If all four tests (for nitrites, leucocytes, blood and protein) are negative it is highly likely that there is no infection, and therefore sending urine for MC & S is not indicated (Bayer 1997a). This systematic assessment of urine helps to avoid the unnecessary sending of urine specimens (McNaughton and Cavanagh 1998) (*see* flow chart from Bayer 1997a, Fig. 6.2).

Frequency
Passing urine more frequently than about seven times in 24 hours.

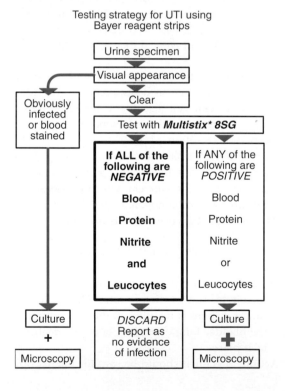

Figure 6.2 Flow chart from Bayer (1997a) showing when to send urine for microscopy and culture (reproduced with kind permission)

Learning outcome 3:
Identify when urinalysis should be performed

For each of the scenarios at the start of the chapter, identify why you would want to do a urinalysis, and how the urine could be collected.

Discussion points

A urinalysis is a simple and non-invasive procedure which gives many clues as to the health and well-being of a person, thus a nursing assessment of a newly referred or admitted patient/client should always include a urinalysis. Urinalysis will also be performed for other people who may be at risk of developing health problems, which can be indicated through a urinalysis. Examples of this can include: during pregnancy (when presence of protein or glucose may be particularly significant), or after an abdominal injury (to screen for blood which might indicate kidney damage).

Both Mrs Wilson and Toby have been newly admitted, and a urinalysis will give insight into their physical well-being. Urinalysis might indicate a UTI (which can lead to confusion, which Mrs Wilson has). Note that as Mrs Wilson appears to be in retention, it will not be possible to test her urine until this is resolved. A short-term measure might be to pass a catheter, to relieve the retention. This would enable a specimen of urine to be obtained (see section on specimen collection) so a urinalysis can be performed and a specimen sent for MC & S if appropriate. Toby would need to have an adhesive bag applied to collect urine in, or his parents can be asked to try to catch some urine into a receptacle when he begins to urinate (*see* next section, Box 6.5, for details about collecting a urine specimen from a child). When John is admitted for his operation, nurses will need to test his urine. If John was unable to respond to the request for a sample, the nurse could take him to the toilet in which a receptacle has been placed. Sarah's urine is also likely to be tested if the district nurse observes signs of a UTI, and then a catheter specimen of urine (*see* Box 6.3) would be collected and tested.

Summary
- Urinalysis is a non-invasive and frequently performed practical skill which can provide very useful information about a person's health status.
- To obtain an accurate result, the steps in a urinalysis must be carried out carefully with an appropriately collected specimen.
- It is important to understand the significance of abnormal results and subsequent action to take.

COLLECTING URINE AND STOOL SPECIMENS

In this section different types of urine specimen and the collection of a stool (faeces) specimen will be discussed. Obtaining such specimens from patients/clients is often necessary as they can provide important diagnostic information, which will impact on management and care. General principles relating to specimen collection were considered in Chapter 3 (Preventing cross-infection), and it is recommended that you relook at this, but key points can be found in Box 6.2.

- Use of universal precautions to prevent cross-infection
- Clear explanations
- Maintenance of patient/client privacy, dignity and comfort
- Avoid contamination of the specimen
- Prompt transportation to the laboratory, or refrigerate for up to 24 hours
- Clear labelling
- Correct and comprehensive accompanying information
- Documentation in patient/client notes of the date and time of the specimen collection.

Box 6.2 Collection of specimens: key points

Learning outcomes

By the end of this section you will be able to discuss:

1. The collection of a catheter specimen of urine.
2. The collection of a midstream specimen of urine, and how this can be adapted with different age groups and different situations.
3. The collection of a 24-hour specimen of urine.
4. The collection of a stool specimen.

Learning outcome 1:
Discuss the collection of a catheter specimen of urine

A catheter specimen of urine is taken for bacteriological examination to ascertain if treatment is required, when symptoms of a UTI are present in the person. As discussed earlier in the chapter, the district nurse may need to collect a catheter specimen of urine (CSU) from Sarah if a UTI is suspected, and if Mrs Wilson has a catheter passed to relieve her retention, a specimen may well be taken. CSUs are nearly always infected after 5 days (Mead 1998a). However the nurse must use aseptic technique and sterile equipment to reduce the risk of contaminating the specimen. This is particularly important since the medical management of the patient is based on the results of the bacteriological examination of the urine. Urine should be obtained from the special sampling port on the drainage system and never taken from the bag, as a fresh specimen is needed. Box 6.3 outlines the key principles to follow.

Equipment

Alcohol swab, receiver, syringe (20 ml) and needle (21 g bore), specimen pot and request form. A gate clamp may be required.

Key points

- Adhere to general points outlined in **Box 6.2**.
- Locate the sample port on the catheter bag tubing. Some drainage bags have a latex port which requires an needle and syringe to aspirate the urine. Others have a needleless port and a syringe can be attached directly to this to withdraw the urine.
- If there is no urine present in the catheter tubing, clamp the tubing below the sample port until sufficient urine collects. Never clamp the actual catheter, as this could damage it.
- Swab the sample port with alcohol swab and allow the port to dry. Insert the needle into the port at an angle of 45 degrees to prevent going straight through the tubing.
- For needleless sampling ports follow the same procedure, but attach the syringe directly to the sampling port.
- Withdraw the required amount of urine, remove the top from the specimen pot and fill the pot with urine. Dispose of the needle and syringe into a sharps box immediately. Replace the cap on the pot.

Box 6.3 Collection of a catheter specimen of urine: equipment and key points

Learning outcome 2:
Discuss the collection of a midstream specimen of urine, and how this can be adapted with different age groups and different situations

The midstream specimen of urine (MSU) is obtained using a clean procedure. If a UTI is suspected, in a non-catheterized patient, an MSU is ideal and will lead to a more accurate result. It is a useful aid in diagnosis and the aim is to collect the midstream which is not contaminated by micro-organisms outside the urinary tract. How the specimen should be collected has been the subject of much research which, according to Brown *et al.*'s (1991) meta-analysis, has still not provided a clear evidence base for practice. Generally, it appears best that the specimen should be collected as soon as possible after waking, when urine is normally available and in concentrated form. Patients have often been asked to undertake perineal cleansing with sterile swabs and saline prior to giving the specimen, to prevent contamination. However, there has been some doubt as to the effectiveness of this (Brown *et al.* 1991). It can be theorized that the first part of the stream should flush away micro-organisms from the first part of the urethra, and that the urine should not flow over the perineum, as long as there is sufficient urine in the bladder to produce a good stream. If there is insufficient urine in the bladder, the specimen should be collected later. The equipment needed and key points of the procedure can be found in Box 6.4.

Equipment

A toilet or commode as appropriate.

A specimen pot and laboratory request form.

Disposable gloves

Procedure

- Adhere to key points in **Box 6.2**.
- Explain to the person to start passing urine as usual, then catch some urine (about 20 ml: – 2.5 cm or 1 inch up the pot) in the specimen pot, and then finish voiding into the toilet or commode. Wear gloves and assist the person if necessary.

Box 6.4 Midstream specimens of urine: equipment and procedure

Note that if a urine specimen is being collected because of suspected tuberculosis (TB) or cancer of the urinary tract, then an early morning specimen, being more concentrated, is most likely to contain the tubercle bacillus or malignant cells (Beynon 1997). Usually, three consecutive early morning specimens will be required.

■ Activity   Read through Box 6.4. As you can see, co-operation and understanding by the person would be needed. Look at the practice scenarios and consider to what extent you might achieve understanding and consent from Mrs Wilson, Toby, and John.

You may have identified that difficulties would exist with obtaining an MSU from all these individuals. It would be very difficult to obtain an MSU from Mrs Wilson as she is confused and disorientated, and at present she is in retention. John may have difficulty understanding and co-ordinating what is expected of him. The nurse could either take him to the toilet, about 30 minutes after a drink, and try to collect the specimen in a clean receptacle in the toilet, or, if possible, catch the mid stream in a pot for him, whilst wearing gloves. This approach could also be used for the person who is confused.

Toby would not be able to produce an MSU as he is too young. An older toilet trained child may be able to produce an MSU however (de Sousa 1996). Disposable nappies are no longer suitable for urine collection since manufacturers have adopted gel-based absorption (Vernon *et al.* 1994).

Alternative methods of collecting specimens from younger children are collecting a non-midstream specimen into a potty, the clean catch method, and a urine bag. See Box 6.5 for details about these methods. Supra-pubic aspiration is an alternative method to obtain urine from an infant (de Sousa 1996). This procedure involves aspiration of bladder contents through a needle and is performed by a doctor.

General principles
- Appropriate explanation to child and family.
- Parents may be able to collect the specimen, or help.
- Use the child's familiar terminology for passing urine (Campbell and Glasper 1995).
- Normal social hygiene e.g. washing genitalia with soap and water and drying carefully is considered sufficient prior to specimen collection (MacQueen 2000).

Clean potty specimen
- Can be used for the potty trained toddler.
- Wash the potty in washing up liquid and hot water.
- Give the child a drink, and offer the potty about 30 minutes later.

A clean catch specimen
- Used for a toddler who is not toilet trained or a baby.
- For a toddler, remove the nappy and then try to catch the urine in a sterile gallipot inside a potty (Vernon 1995).
- Alternatively, for a baby, remove the nappy and ask the parent to try to catch a specimen in a container, perhaps with the baby lying in the cot or up playing.

Adhesive bag
- Used for an infant or toddler who is not toilet trained.
- Uses a single use, sterile adhesive urine bag.
- Remove the nappy, and apply the bag firmly.
- With females, stretch the perineum taut during application to ensure a leak proof fit.
- With males, place the penis and the scrotum inside the bag.
- Check the bag regularly so that it can be removed as soon as a specimen is produced.
- Note that there can be difficulties with fixation and preventing leakage, and 10% of specimens may be contaminated with faeces (de Sousa 1996).

Box 6.5 Collecting a urine sample from a child

Learning outcome 3:
Discuss the collection of a 24-hour specimen of urine

Sometimes it is necessary to collect the total volume of urine passed within a 24-hour period, which is then analyzed within the laboratory. This is so that the 24-hour excretion of a variety of key metabolites (e.g. protein, creatinine) can be assessed (Laker 1994). Box 6.6 outlines the equipment needed and the procedure. Campbell and Glasper (1995) note that a 24-hour urine collection in infants and children is somewhat challenging. For infants and small children, collection bags are required which can include collection tubes so that the bag will not need frequent removal thus causing irritation. Older children will need a clear explanation.

Equipment

A toilet, commode, urinal, bedpan, potty or collection bags (as appropriate for the individual)

A jug, a 24-hour urine collection container, gloves.

Procedure

- Assess the person's ability to participate in the collection. When the person next passes urine, it is discarded. This marks the beginning of the 24-hour period for collection.
- Label the container with the person's details (name, ward and hospital number), and the time and date the collection started.
- Put a sign on the bed or door of the room belonging to the person indicating that a 24-hour urine collection is in place, the date and time it started and when it will finish.
- Every time the person passes urine it is collected and poured into the container, which is stored in the sluice. The person may be able to do this independently or may need assistance. Check compliance and understanding throughout.
- Ask the person to empty the bladder just before the end of the 24-hour collection period, and advise him that this ends the collection period.
- Remove the sign from the door or bed.
- Clean or discard the jug used.
- Record the completion time and ensure that the urine collection and laboratory request forms are dispatched correctly as soon as possible.

Note: if one sample of urine becomes contaminated or is accidently discarded, the test must be discontinued and restarted.

Box 6.6 24-hour urine collection: equipment and key points

Learning outcome 4:
Discuss the collection of a stool specimen

When do you think it might be necessary to collect a stool specimen?

You may have identified that a stool specimen will be needed if a person has complained of abnormal stools, or you have observed (as when assisting the person using the commode) that the person has an abnormality such as diarrhoea. There are many causes of diarrhoea, but these include gastrointestinal infection. Infection is particularly likely if the stool is offensive, and has an abnormal colour such as green. In these instances the stool will be sent for MC & S, to detect the causative micro-organism, and identify any antibiotics which it is sensitive to. Stool specimens are also sent for examination for occult (hidden) blood, if rectal bleeding is suspected but not obvious. Sometimes stool specimens are sent for examination for parasites. The key points in the collection of a stool specimen are outlined in Box 6.7. There are stool specimen collectors available which have a spoon attached to the lid. Although these are easy to use when collecting the specimen, they can be difficult for laboratory staff to handle without getting contaminated.

Equipment

A bedpan, gloves, apron, a sterile stool specimen pot or a sterile specimen pot and a spatula, a specimen bag and the laboratory request form.

Procedure

- Adhere to general points in **Box 6.2**. Note that infection control procedures are essential throughout.
- Ask the person to use a bedpan or commode to catch the specimen. If possible the patient should be helped to a toilet rather than use a commode (Gill 1999). A disposable bedpan can be placed under the toilet lid.
- When the stool is available, take the bedpan to the sluice, open the sterile container and using a spatula, fill the container about a third full with faeces, and then secure the lid.
- Refrigerate the specimen if it cannot go to the laboratory immediately.
- In infections such as amoebiasis, the stool must be be fresh and warm (Mead 1998b), thus special arrangements for collection must be made with the laboratory.
- Remember to complete the stool chart if a record being kept.

Box 6.7 Collection of a stool specimen: equipment and key points

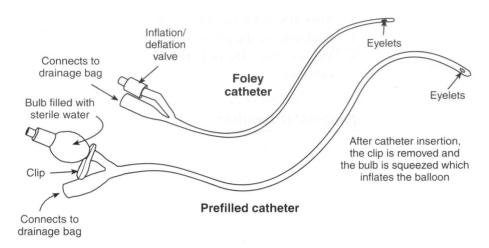

Figure 6.3 Examples of urinary catheters. (Photograph of Biocath™ Foley catheters kindly provided by Bard Limited.) ™Trademark of C.R. Bard, Inc., or an affiliate.

Now read through the following points and relate them to your observations:

Packaging

Catheters are packaged to enable ease of insertion into the bladder, and with only the exception of self-catheterization, strict aseptic technique is employed. The way in which the catheter is packaged, including double wrapping, assists in the maintenance of sterility. It has been estimated that one person in eight has an in-dwelling catheter in hospital and 4% in the community, and problems with infection affect about 50% of patients (Laurent 1998). Note also that there is a batch number and expiry date on the packaging. These are important and will need to be entered into patients' documentation.

Catheter size

You will have noted the size of the catheter. The size is measured in relation to its external diameter, and is measured in Charriere (Ch) or French gauge units (Fg). One Ch unit equals 0.3 mm, and the catheters range in size from 6–8 (for paediatric use) to 30 Ch. A size 12 Ch catheter is 4.0 mm in diameter. The size most commonly used for women is 12–14 Ch and for men, 12–16 Ch (Macauley 1997). As a general rule the smallest size catheter should be used, as large catheters are associated with complications including urethral irritation, urethral trauma, bladder spasm, urinary bypassing, pressure necrosis and increased risk of infection (Getliffe 1996; Laurent 1998).

Catheter length

Catheters are manufactured in two lengths: 30–40 cm to accommodate the male urethra and 23–26 cm for female use. However the longer catheter is often used for women, particularly the obese, because it allows easier access to the junction of the catheter and the drainage bag. (Macauley 1997).

Balloon

The foley catheter is the design most frequently used for in-dwelling urethral catheterization (Getliffe 1996). It has a rounded tip with two drainage eyes and the balloon is an integral part of this type of catheter which, when inflated, holds the catheter *in situ*. There are two channels, one for drainage and the other for inflating the balloon. The balloon sits at the sensitive base of the bladder and can potentially cause irritation, spasm and mechanical damage to the bladder. Retention balloons come in three sizes: 3–5 ml for children, 10 ml for standard adults, and 30 ml for after some urological procedures (Macauley 1997). Catheters for intermittent use are usually a simple tube design and do not have an inflatable balloon as there is no requirement for them to be retained in the bladder. Some suprapubic catheters do not have a balloon, but are secured by a flange and held in place by skin sutures.

Material

The material the catheter is made of is often dependent upon the length of time it is envisaged the catheter will remain *in situ*. For short-term use, plastic, latex (up to 7–10 days) and teflon coated latex (up to 28 days) are commonly used, and these materials are considerably cheaper than long-term catheter materials. Some patients may be allergic to latex, and screening is advisable if latex is to be used (Woodward 1997). Plastic catheters have been found to exert low toxicity because of the inert nature of plastic. Also, the rate that this material absorbs water is low, and so the catheter retains the widest internal diameter, making these catheters a common material of choice for drainage of post-operative blood clots and debris. However, plastic catheters can remain rigid at body temperature and have been associated with bladder spasm, pain and leakage of urine (Blannin and Hobden 1980, cited by Macauley 1997). For long-term use silicone, silicone elastamer-coated latex, and hydrogel coated catheters are all suitable (Laurent 1998). The cost of the catheter should not be the primary factor in the selection process. However, the nurse should be aware of the different costs when selecting.

Did you know?

Prior to the use of closed drainage systems almost 100% of patients developed urinary tract infections within 96 hours (Kass 1957, cited by Macauley 1997). As closed drainage systems have been shown to reduce this rate of infection, they are now accepted as good practice (Macauley 1997). However, urinary tract infections still account for 23% of infection acquired in hospital (Emmerson *et al.* 1996), and the major predisposing factor is the presence of an in-dwelling catheter (Wilson 1995). Therefore the care of the catheterized patient is aimed at preventing infection, as well as promoting comfort, acceptance and understanding, and catheterization is best avoided if at all possible (Ayliffe *et al.*, 1999; Macauley 1997).

Activity

Figure 6.7 shows a diagram of a closed urinary drainage system. Where do you think bacteria could enter into the system?

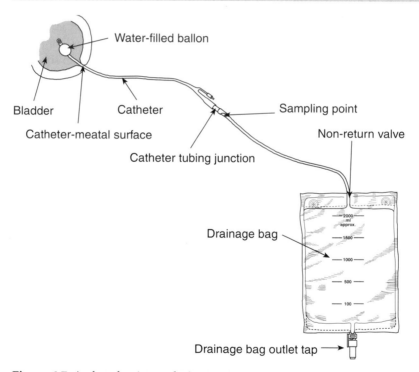

Figure 6.7 A closed urinary drainage system

Compare your answers with the list below.

Potential ports of entry include:

- The urethral meatus around the catheter.
- The junction between the catheter and the tubing to the catheter bag.
- The specimen sampling port.
- The drainage outlet.

Bacteria are also believed to enter the bladder at the time of catheterization via the peri-urethral space.

Learning outcome 3:
State the main complications associated with urinary catheterization

Infection, encrustation and eventual blockage are problems associated with urinary catheterization (Laurent 1998; Burr and Nuseibeh 1997; Wilson 1995). Other complications include urethral strictures, pressure necrosis, spasm, discomfort and pain (Winn 1996).

With a catheter *in situ* the bladder's normal closing mechanism is obstructed and the natural flushing mechanism of micturition is lost. Additionally the close proximity of the catheter to the bowel means that there exists a risk of infection, because bacteria can be mechanically transferred across skin surfaces (Meers *et al.* 1995). Bacteria having entered the urinary system may cling to the surface of the catheter. This creates a living biofilm that is almost impossible to remove. The bacteria can cause the urine to become more alkaline than usual and encrustation on the catheter surface then occurs, which can lead to blockage. This in turn may lead to retention of urine or to leaking, and pain. These outcomes are distressing for patients, and can result in loss of comfort and dignity (Laurent 1998).

Bacteria may colonize the urinary tract without invading the tissues. This is referred to as bacteruria. When tissue is invaded by bacteria, problems include local infection, which may result in foul smelling urine, or systemic infection which can result in pyrexia. If the catheter or drainage tubing is kinked, the build up of urine in the bladder may result in the infected urine entering the ureters or kidneys and causing pyelonephritis (Getliffe 1997; Wilson 1995).

Pyelonephritis
Inflammation of the kidney, usually due to bacteria which have ascended from the bladder, having entered through the urethra.

■ *Activity* To what extent might Sarah and Mrs Wilson be at risk of urinary tract infection, and why?

You may have identified that Sarah is at risk as a result of long-term catheterization, probably due to cross-infection (Ayliffe *et al.* 1999). Urinary retention (as experienced by Mrs Wilson) can be dealt with by using intermittent catheterization (Winn and Thompson 1998), but depending upon circumstances, an in-dwelling catheter may be a necessity whilst the cause of her retention is investigated. Coagulase-negative staphylococci or micrococci may normally be found in the anterior urethra, and these are a common cause of infection immediately following catheterization which could affect Mrs Wilson. Therefore early infections are often endogenous, but cross-infection (exogenous infection) occurs later in patients with in-dwelling catheters (Ayliffe *et al.* 1999).

Learning outcome 4:
Understand the principles underpinning urethral catheterization

■ **Activity**

Before reading the following section refer to Chapter 3 for an explanation and discussion of non-touch technique. It is important that you understand these principles as they underpin the procedure of urinary catheterization.

In addition to the guidelines expressed in Chapter 3, there are a number of other factors to take into account when catheterizing a patient. Note that in many NHS trusts additional training needs to be undertaken by the trained nurse to perform male urethral catheterization. However, many of the principles are synonymous with female urethral catheterization. Suprapubic catheterization is usually a medical procedure, and is not considered here. It is important to note that catheterization is an invasive procedure and the effects on the patient may be many, both psychologically and socially.

Appropriate and effective communication and sensitivity are essential when catheterization takes place (*see* Chapter 2). Care should be taken to explain where the catheter is inserted, and why the procedure is necessary, ensuring that verbal consent is gained. With a confused person such as Mrs Wilson, this will be difficult but as she is in retention, the catheter is necessary to relieve her discomfort. Her husband's support in explaining may help. For a child, the parent can support and comfort the child during the procedure; sedation may be necessary (Mohammed 2000).

Once the catheter has been inserted, dietary advice, including fluid intake and avoidance of constipation, can be an important part of patient education (Getliffe 1996). Further education will be needed if the person will be in the community with a urinary catheter and the district nurse (as in Sarah's case) will be involved. Box 6.8 outlines the equipment needed, and key points, when undertaking female urethral catheterization.

Learning outcome 5:
Discuss the care required for the person with an in-dwelling urinary catheter

■ **Activity**

For Sarah and Mrs Wilson, think about what specific care might be needed in relation to catheter care.

You may have thought of the following:
- Hygiene
- Emptying of the catheter bag
- Appropriate positioning of the bag
- Adequate fluid intake.

These issues will now be discussed.

Equipment

A catheterization pack if available, or a dressing pack and sterile receiver, sterile gloves, an appropriate catheter, sterile soduim chloride, catheter bag and stand or holder, lubricant/anaesthetic gel, syringe and sterile water of appropriate size and amount to inflate the balloon, disposable waterproof absorbent pad, specimen pot (if required), a good light source.

Note a second nurse may be needed to help position the patient who needs to be preferably flat with her legs apart to allow good access and visibility.

Procedure

1. Non-touch technique should be strictly adhered to throughout (*see* Chapter 3: hand washing, use of gloves and aprons and non-touch technique).
2. Place the disposable pad under the patient's buttocks.
3. Open the catheter bag and arrange at the side of the bed, ensuring the attachment tip remains sterile.
4. Open the catheterization or dressing pack, and open the catheter on to the sterile field but do not remove it from its internal wrapping.
5. Draw up the sterile water to inflate the balloon (unless catheter is pre-filled).
6. Pour sodium chloride into the gallipot.
7. Open sterile gloves, wash hands, and apply gloves.
8. Place sterile towels over patient's thighs and between legs.
9. Cleanse the perineal area with the sodium chloride, and then using non-dominant hand, separate labia minora and cleanse the meatus.
10. Carefully locate the urethra, insert anaesthetic gel, and wait for the time recommended by the manufacturer, usually 5 minutes. Anaesthetic gel not only prevents pain, but also opens up and lubricates the length of the urethra, helping to prevent trauma. Manufacturers claim that merely to lubricate the tip of the catheter is ineffective as the lubricant is quickly wiped away on insertion.
11. Place a receiver with the catheter on the sterile towel between the patient's legs. Expose the tip of the catheter by pulling off the top of the wrapper at the serrations.
12. Hold the catheter so that the distal end remains in the receiver and gradually advance it out of its wrapper in an upward and backward direction along the line of the urethra.
13. Advance the catheter 5–7 cm or until urine flows out of the catheter.
14. Advance the catheter a further 5 cm. Never force the catheter. If resistance is encountered stop and seek medical advice.
15. Inflate the balloon with the correct amount of water. Incorrectly filled balloons can inflate irregularly and irritate the bladder mucosa (Wilson 1997).
16. Attach the urinary drainage bag, and make the patient comfortable.
17. Finally, send a urine specimen if indicated, measure and record the urine collected, and document the catheterization in the patient's notes.

Box 6.8 Female urethral catheterization: equipment and procedure

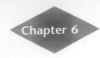

Hygiene

The main aim of cleansing is to remove secretions and encrustation and prevent infection. Where possible patients should be encouraged to attend to their own meatal and perineal hygiene needs, thus reducing the risk of cross-infection whilst promoting self-care and dignity. However, for the person unable to maintain their hygiene, the nurse should carry this out, wearing gloves, and in a gentle and sensitive manner. Regular cleansing with soap and water and clean wash cloths is sufficient (Wilson 1997), and powders and lotions should not be used as they may trap organisms in the area (Nicol *et al*. 1999). In both male and female patients the cleansing of the area surrounding the catheter–meatal junction is particularly necessary after faecal incontinence (Wilson 1997). For female patients, it is important to clean from front to back, thus preventing possible movement of bacteria from the anal area and perineum to the catheter meatal junction. The catheter should be gently wiped in one direction, away from the vulva. In male patients the foreskin should be retracted before cleansing and the same principles of cleaning the catheter away from the catheter–meatal junction should be adhered to. The foreskin must be replaced afterwards. With a suprapubic catheter, once the wound has healed around the catheter, simple cleansing with soap and water is usually sufficient to maintain hygiene.

Emptying the catheter bag

Activity

> You may recall that micro-organisms can be introduced into the drainage system at the junction between the catheter and bag or via the drainage tap. Bearing this in mind try to work out the equipment you would need, and how you would use it, to safely empty a catheter bag.

Compare your answer with Box 6.9.

Unless hands are thoroughly washed between patients and a clean container used, micro-organisms are readily transferred to the next patient. Aycliffe *et al*. (1999) suggest that disinfection of hands with 70% alcohol is rapid and effective. Note that there is no evidence that bags need to be changed at specific intervals, but should be changed when damaged or blocked with deposits. Disconnection of the catheter from the drainage bag significantly increases the risk of introducing bacteria into the system and should therefore be avoided if possible (Wilson 1997).

Appropriate positioning of the catheter bag

Catheter bags should be positioned to avoid reflux and facilitate the use of gravity, and positioned clear of floors or other sources of contamination (McLaren 1997). Drainage bags should always be positioned below the level

---

Equipment

Non-sterile gloves and apron, a heat disinfected or disposable container e.g. a urinal or jug, paper towel to cover, alcohol swab.

Key points

- Explain the procedure to the patient. Some patients may prefer to be screened.
- Wash hands and put on apron and gloves.
- If the drainage bag is on a stand it may not need removing. If it is hanging on the bed, you may need to access it by removing the bag and placing it over the jug.
- Clean the outlet port with alcohol swab and allow it to dry.
- Open the port and drain the urine into the receptacle.
- Close the port and wipe with alcohol swab.
- Reposition bag.
- Cover the container and take to sluice for disposal. Measure the urine first if a fluid balance chart is being kept.
- The container should be disinfected, or macerated if disposable.
- Remove gloves and apron and wash hands.

Box 6.9 Emptying a catheter bag: equipment and key points

---

of the bladder and the catheter and the inlet tubing secured in a downward position (Macaulay 1997). Anchoring the catheter in females has achieved some success, as movement of the catheter in the short female urethra is a way of introducing infection (Ayliffe *et al*. 1999).

Adequate fluid intake

If the patient's condition allows, encourage oral fluids. This results in a dilute urine which contains fewer nutrients and discourages the growth of bacteria in the drainage bag. In addition the larger volume of urine will maintain a constant flow through the drainage system and make it more difficult for bacteria to migrate from bag to bladder (Wilson 1997).

Catheter removal

Activity

Cross-infection tends to occur if antibiotics are widely used in a unit and there are a number of patients with in-dwelling catheters in adjacent beds or sitting together during the day (Ayliffe *et al*. 1999). Taking this into account, and other issues already discussed, when do you believe a catheter should be removed?

Since the risk of infection increases with each additional day of catheterization, the catheter should be removed as soon as possible (Wilson 1995), preferably within 5 days (Ayliffe *et al.* 1999).

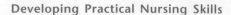

■ **Activity**   Think about how you would prepare Mrs Wilson for catheter removal.

Mrs Wilson is frightened and confused, and the support of her husband may need to be sought. A clear explanation should be given, emphasizing that the procedure is not normally painful but that there may be a feeling of discomfort. Box 6.10 outlines equipment and key points for removing a catheter. Noble *et al.* (1990) suggest that the catheter should be removed at midnight rather than the traditional time of first thing in the morning. This increases the length of time before passing urine and in turn leads to a greater initial volume and a faster return to normal voiding. This then decreases levels of anxiety. Note that it is important to ensure that urine is passed satisfactorily after catheter removal and observe for problems such as incontinence, frequency and retention. A confused client such as Mrs Wilson may well need prompting to pass urine (*see* section on promoting continence, later in this chapter). Some people, particularly men who have had prostate surgery, will need to perform pelvic floor exercises to help them to regain control (see section on pelvic floor exercises later in this chapter). In some patients, such as Sarah, who have a long-term catheter for specific medical reasons, removal of the catheter is unlikely to be an option. It will, however, need changing periodically; how often will depend on the material of the catheter and any problems Sarah is experiencing.

Summary
- Urinary catheterization is experienced by many patients/clients and may be a short-term or long-term measure.
- Catheterization is an invasive procedure and there are many complications associated with it, infection being particularly common. Therefore catheterization should only be performed if there is a clear indication, strict asepsis should be maintained, and the catheter should be removed as soon as possible, using the correct technique.
- Nurses should be aware of the different types of equipment available, and make appropriate choices in relation to types of catheter and drainage bag.
- Care should be taken to reduce physical and psychological discomfort in the catheterized patient.
  N.B. Catheterization is covered in depth by Macauley (1997), who has reviewed the literature extensively, and further reading from this source is recommended.

Equipment

Disposable gloves and apron.

A syringe of sufficient volume to remove the water from the balloon. The water capacity of the balloon is written on the catheter itself.

A disposable absorbent pad.

A receiver and a yellow waste bag.

A specimen pot, a 20 ml syringe, needle and alcohol swab, if a catheter specimen of urine is required.

Key points

- Preparation: Give explanation, ensure privacy and position the person comfortably. For a female the knees and hips should be slightly flexed and apart.
- Wash and dry hands and apply gloves and apron.
- Obtain a specimen of urine from the sampling port if indicated (*see* Box 6.3)
- Place the disposable pad under the patient's buttocks and then place the receiver between the thighs.
- Check the balloon volume, and attach an appropriately sized syringe to the balloon port of the catheter. Withdraw the water from the balloon via the syringe.
- Ask the patient to breathe in and out, and as she exhales, the catheter is gently withdrawn and placed in the receiver. If problems are encountered, stop and seek medical advice.
- Remove gloves and apron and wash hands.
- The patient should be made comfortable and because frequency may be experienced the nurse should ensure that a toilet or commode is close by. If the patient needs help with mobility, ensure a call bell is nearby.
- Document the time of catheter removal and the amount of urine in the catheter bag.
- The patient may be encouraged to increase fluid intake to 'flush' out the bladder.
- Monitor whether the person is passing urine satisfactorily. A chart may be kept so that frequency and amount can be monitored. Also ask the patient to inform a nurse if any unusual symptoms are experienced e.g. dysuria (pain when passing urine).

Box 6.10 Removal of a urethral catheter: equipment and key points

USE OF ENEMAS AND SUPPOSITORIES.

An enema is a liquid which is inserted into the rectum, while a suppository is a medicated solid formulation, usually torpedo-shaped, and is inserted into the rectum, where it will dissolve at body temperature. As will be discussed below, there are a number of indications for these procedures. However, if being given for constipation, it should be remembered that preventing constipation e.g. through diet and activity, is preferable to the use of suppositories or enemas.

Learning outcomes

By the end of this section you will be able to:

1. Identify the reasons for administering an enema or a suppository.
2. Show awareness of the precautions to be taken into account prior to administration.
3. Understand the principles to follow when administering suppositories and enemas.

Learning outcome 1:
Identify the reasons for administering an enema or suppository

Activity

An enema may be prescribed as a treatment for constipation, to prepare the bowel for investigations or surgery, or to administer medicines. When do you think an enema would be described as an evacuant enema and when as a retention enema?

Ulcerative colitis
Ulceration of the mucosa of the colon, causing offensive, watery stools with mucus and pus. Can cause haemorrhage and perforation.

If the purpose of the enema is to retain the solution for a specified period of time, this is generally referred to as a retention enema. It is primarily used for its local effect, for example a steroid enema may be administered to people with **ulcerative colitis**, for its anti-inflammatory effect. You may have identified that if the purpose of the enema is to be expelled, along with faecal matter and flatus, within a few minutes, this is called an evacuant enema. Thus this type of enema would be used for constipation or to empty the bowel prior to surgery or investigations of the gastrointestinal tract. Sarah is at risk of developing constipation due to her impaired mobility (*see* Chapter 9) and her loss of sensation is a further factor. She could, therefore, require an enema or suppository if she becomes constipated.

Suppositories are often administered for evacuant purposes too. However they are also a commonly used route to administer medication, and may be administered as a local treatment, e.g. for **haemorrhoids**.

Haemorrhoids
Dilated blood vessels in the rectal mucosa. Lay term is 'piles'.

Examples of drugs that are commonly prescribed rectally include paracetamol (for its analgesic and/or anti-pyretic effect) and anti-convulsants. What do you think are the advantages and disadvantages of this route of drug administration?

You might have thought of the following advantages:

■ An alternative route for when a person cannot take the drug orally because he is vomiting, unable to swallow (as in the unconscious person or someone who has had a cerebrovascular accident), or is nil by mouth for other reasons such as pre-operatively. An example would include a child with a high temperature who must have his temperature reduced to prevent the risk of a **febrile convulsion**, but is vomiting so cannot be given the anti-pyretic orally.

Febrile convulsion
A convulsion (fit) which can occur in a young child who has a rapid elevation of temperature.

■ The rectum is very vascular and drugs are absorbed rapidly via this route, as they avoid liver metabolism (Addison *et al.* 2000). For example, if a person is fitting, he cannot take the drug orally. Rectal absorption will be more rapid than by intramuscular injection, which could also be dangerous to administer safely to the fitting person. Note that faecal impaction can inhibit absorption of drugs via the rectal route, and therefore constipation should be prevented in the person who might require emergency use of the rectal route.

Disadvantages of both enemas and suppositories are mainly that administration is more invasive and embarrassing than oral administration, and involves some discomfort, undressing and movement, i.e. into the correct position. Schmelzer and Wright's (1996) review of the literature notes that there have been a number of traumatic and even fatal side effects of enemas reported, including, inflammation, electrolyte imbalance and perforation of the colonic mucosa. Newer pre-packaged enemas aim to prevent many of these potential problems. Nevertheless medication is only administered rectally if it is clearly indicated, and an enema would only be used if there is no alternative. Faecal impaction and diarrhoea are contraindications (Kay 2000). In addition, Kay (2000) notes that due to sexual taboos about anal penetration, there is reluctance to administer drugs rectally. She recommends that, particularly with older children and adolescents, great sensitivity should be shown.

Learning outcome 2:
Show awareness of the precautions to be taken into account prior to administration
Prior to administering an enema or suppository, the nurse should carefully assess the appropriateness of this route.

Can you think of any physical problems which might be **contraindications**?

Contraindications might include: recent colorectal or gynaecological surgery, malignancy or other pathology of the perineal area, and a low platelet count, as this would predispose to bleeding. Thus the nurse should check with both the patient and the case notes for any previous ano-rectal surgery or abnormalities. Further checks should also be made visually immediately prior to administration. The peri-anal region should be checked for abnormalities including haemorrhoids, **anal fissure** and **rectal prolapse**

Anal fissure
A painful crack in the mucous membrane of the anus, generally caused by hard faeces.

Rectal prolapse
Protrusion of rectal mucosa through the anus.

Digital rectal examinations – should they be done?

It is sometimes recommended that a digital rectal examination (DRE) is carried out to check for faecal impaction, and for abnormalities such as blood, pain or obstruction. However, there has been increasing concern about nurses doing digital rectal examinations, particularly as there have been two recent cases of professional misconduct involving the inappropriate use of DREs and manual evacuation of faeces in frail elderly people (Willis 2000). The issue has particularly concerned lack of consent to DRE by patients. Many Trusts are now developing policies and guidelines on the use of DRE, and the Royal College of Nursing has recently published a document to guide nurses (Addison *et al.* 1999). It is strongly advised that you, as a student, only carry out a DRE if it is agreed under local policy, the patient has explicitly consented to the procedure, and you are under the supervision of the registered nurse. Consent to DRE or manual evacuation of faeces (which is necessary for a small number of people with neurological disorders such as spinal injury) should be clearly documented in nursing records (Willis 2000).

Learning outcome 3:
Understand the principles to follow when administering suppositories and enemas

Choice of enemas/suppositories

This is straightforward, if you are administering prescribed medication. However when giving an enema or suppositories for evacuation purposes, there can be a choice of products. Local drug policies may vary as to whether these need to be prescribed. Often they can be administered at the registered nurse's discretion.

■ ***Activity***   Find out what types of enemas and suppositories are available to evacuate the bowel. There may be examples in the skills laboratory, or you can look at them in your practice placement.

Suppositories may be of the type that will simply soften the stools, or they may have a stimulant effect. Trounce (1997) recommends that glycerol suppositories are satisfactory, and others offer no advantage. There are microenemas available containing only 5 ml of solution which act as a colon stimulant. For more vigorous bowel cleansing (for example prior to a bowel investigation) a larger phosphate enema may be used. It is important to check the manufacturer's instructions when using these as there are a number of contraindications, and they are unsuitable for elderly or debilitated patients (Addison *et al.* 2000). They can be given for occasional constipation, but should not be given regularly. They are also not recommended in children under 3 years, and should only be given to children aged 3–12 years with medical direction.

Administration

The procedure will need careful explanation to the person, or child and family, which should include the likely effects. Addison *et al.* (2000) advises that consent must be obtained, otherwise the procedure can constitute assault and lead to legal proceedings. There are exceptions to this however, e.g. in a life-threatening situation (e.g. the unconscious fitting patient). Note that some patients may prefer to insert a suppository for themselves. If so, the nurse must carefully explain the procedure and be on hand to give assistance if required. Privacy and sensitivity when administering enemas and suppositories is very important. Kay (2000) recommends that for children, a chaperone, preferably a parent, should be present.

If the enema or suppositories are being given to evacuate the bowel, the patient/client will need to have his bowels open quite rapidly after administration. As discussed previously, if possible the person should be helped to the toilet. The more familiar environment of the toilet will be particularly helpful for a client such as Mrs Wilson, who is confused and disorientated, or for a client with learning disabilities. Otherwise, a commode is preferable to using a bedpan as it promotes a more conducive position for elimination. Safety and hygiene needs must be taken into consideration; see first section in this chapter (Assisting with elimination) for detailed discussion.

Schmelzer and Wright's (1996) study of enema administration used in-depth interviews with 24 nurses who were highly experienced in enema administration. They found that the use of interpersonal skills to gain co-operation was emphasized. The nurses suggested honesty, asking about previous experiences of enema administration, describing expected sensations, warning about discomfort, showing patients equipment, and teaching relaxation techniques. With children, the nurses used distraction, including singing and looking at colourful pictures. Schmelzer and Wright (1996) suggest that

Equipment

An absorbent under pad, tissues, lubricating gel, the enema or suppository/ies, gloves and apron.

Ensure that a good light source is available and that privacy can be maintained.

Procedure

- If the enema or suppository/ies are being given as medication they will be prescribed and therefore the checking and documenting procedures as per the local drug policy should be adhered to (*see* Chapter 11 – drug administration).

- Maintain infection control procedures throughout: hand washing, use of gloves and aprons, and correct waste disposal (*see* Chapter 3).

- Give explanations, encouragement, reassurance and feedback, and maintain privacy (Schmelzer and Wright 1996).

- Some enemas may need to be warmed before adminstration – check the manufacturer's instructions. Warming can be done by placing the enema in a jug of warm water. The temperature should be slightly greater than body temperature, feeling warm to the wrist (Schmelzer and Wright 1996).

- Position the person on his left side to allow easy flow of the fluid into the rectum by following the anatomy of the patient. Place the under-pad under the patient's buttocks, and ask him to lie at the edge of the bed with knees flexed, and covered by a blanket. This position will aid the passage of the nozzle of the enema through the anal canal. This position may need adapting for someone with a physical disability.

- Examine the perianal area.

- **Only** perform digital rectal examination if: the procedure is specifically indicated (e.g. the need to check for faecal impaction, on which suppositories would have minimal impact), if it is agreed under local policy that it can be performed by nurses, and if explicit consent has been given by the patient. A digital examination involves lubricating the index finger and gently inserting it into the rectum to check whether there is faecal impaction.

- **Enemas**: Expel any air from the enema container, because if introduced into the colon this can cause distension and discomfort. Then lubricate the nozzle of the enema. Note that some enemas have a pre-lubricated tip. Part the buttocks and gently insert into the anal canal. Squeeze the fluid gently into the rectum from the base of the container in order to prevent backflow. Some enemas include one way valves which prevent backflow. Then slowly withdraw the container nozzle to avoid reflux emptying of the rectum. Clean the perianal area and make the patient comfortable.

- **Suppositories**: Lubricate the end of the suppository with the gel. Insert the suppository blunt end foremost into the anal canal. This allows the lower edge of the contracting sphincter to close tightly around the anus. Inserting the blunt end foremost also makes it easier to retain the suppository and aids patient comfort (Abd El Maeboud *et al.* 1991). Wipe the patient's perianal area.

- If the enema or suppository/ies were given to empty the bowel, ask the patient to retain it inside for as long as possible (Schmelzer and Wright 1996). Often the patient will find it more comfortable to remain lying down. An enema, however, can be very difficult to hold onto for long as the effect is likely to be rapid. The person should be assisted to the toilet or other receptacle as necessary.
- Medication administered as a suppository should be retained by the patient. With a retention enema, the patient should remain lying down for the amount of time prescribed on the manufacturer's instructions. A call bell must be near at hand.
- Document that the enema/suppository/ies have been administered in the nursing notes or prescription chart if a medication. If the enema or suppositories were given to empty the bowel you will need to note the result.

Box 6.11 Administration of enemas and suppositories: equipment and procedure

enema technique has evolved through trial and error rather than systematic research, and their thorough review of the literature identifies much conflicting advice, and many areas which need additional research. For example, they found that most nursing texts suggest positioning patients on their left side due to the anatomy of the colon, but there are some research articles to support the right side.

Based on evidence available, principles to follow for safe administration of suppositories/enemas can be found in box 6.11.

Summary
- Suppositories or enemas may be given to administer medication or to evacuate the bowel.
- Careful assessment should precede administration as there are contraindications.
- Preparation of the patient/client should include explanation and gaining consent, correct choice of enema/suppositories and other equipment, maintenance of dignity and privacy, and correct positioning of the person to prevent damage to the wall of the rectum.
- If the enema or suppositories were given to evacuate the bowel, assistance to reach the toilet, or other receptacle if necessary, must be given.

PROMOTION OF CONTINENCE AND MANAGEMENT OF INCONTINENCE

A recent report has claimed that 70% of incontinence sufferers can be cured while the remaining 30% can benefit from proper management (Chester 1998). Incontinence is a huge topic to which whole books are devoted. This section will focus on developing understanding of the nature of incontinence and its effects, and practical issues of management, but not specialist interventions. Further reading will be indicated to enable a more in-depth exploration of the topic.

Learning outcomes

By the end of this section, you will be able to:

1. Discuss the nature of incontinence, its definition and prevalence.
2. Identify causes of urinary and faecal incontinence.
3. Show insight into the potential psycho-social and physical effects of incontinence.
4. Demonstrate understanding into how incontinence might be assessed.
5. Identify appropriate nursing interventions for the promotion of continence.
6. Discuss how incontinence can be managed.

Learning outcome 1:
Discuss the nature of incontinence, its definition and prevalence

Definitions and prevalence

Activity

You have probably encountered people with incontinence in practice placements. How prevalent do you think incontinence might be? Try to write a definition of the term incontinence.

Now compare your thoughts with the definitions and statistics below.

Continence has been described as having: 'the ability to store urine in the bladder or faeces in the bowel and to excrete voluntarily where and when it is socially appropriate' (White 1997, p. 11). Thus incontinence can be said to be any deviation from this and may be urinary or faecal. In children, incontinence is considered to be the involuntary discharge of urine or faeces in a child over 5 years. Young people and children can find incontinence particularly difficult as they may view it as a condition of the elderly, causing reluctance to seek help (Mahoney 1997).

Urinary incontinence
The International Continence Society has defined **urinary incontinence** as 'a condition in which the involuntary loss of urine is a social and hygienic

problem and is objectively demonstrable'. Urinary incontinence (UI) is a very common problem, although its actual estimated prevalence varies considerably, e.g.

- Problems with bladder control affect 23% of people over 40 years in the UK – about 6 million people (The Continence Foundation 1999).
- UI affects 3% of men under 64 years who live at home, but 40% of men and women in nursing homes (Royal College of Physicians 1995).
- The term 'enuresis' is given to nocturnal incontinence or bedwetting, which occurs most often in children but can continue into adulthood (Getliffe and Dolman 1997). This affects 10% of children aged five years and 5% of children aged ten years (Royal College of Physicians 1995).

Primary enuresis describes a state when bladder control has never been achieved, while **secondary enuresis** occurs if the child has a period of bladder control for at least a year, and then relapses.

Faecal incontinence

Faecal incontinence has been defined as 'the involuntary or inappropriate passage of faeces' (Royal College of Physicians 1995), and described as the 'last taboo' (Langford 1996). Again, incidence may vary considerably e.g.

- 1% of children aged 5–16 years.
- 0.4% of men and women under 64 years living at home.
- 15% of men and women over 85 years living at home.
- 30% of people in nursing homes (Royal College of Physicians 1995).

It may be **severe**, as when there are large volumes of stool passed involuntarily, or **mild**, when small amounts of stool stain underwear, sometimes referred to as '**staining**' (Jensen 1997). In children, the term '**encopresis**' is usually used for the passage of a normal consistency stool in a socially unacceptable place, and the term '**soiling**' is used when the stool is incomplete or loose (White 1997).

Learning outcome 2:
Identify causes of urinary and faecal incontinence

Continence is a complex skill, which relies on hormonal, muscular and neurological control, and requires elaborate interplay between the individual and the environment (Nazarko 1997). Children achieve continence by learning a complex sequence of events, and being able to co-ordinate both voluntary and involuntary actions (Stanley 1996a). Achieving bladder control depends on the child's neuromuscular and cognitive development, the manner in which potty training is undertaken, the personality of the child and the emotional environment of the family (Campbell and Glasper 1995). The age at which bladder control is achieved varies widely in different countries (Campbell and Glasper 1995). In the UK, bladder control is usually expected by the age of 4–5 years. Continence relies on being able to recognize the need to eliminate faeces and/or urine, being able to identify an appropriate place in which to eliminate and being able to wait until arriving there. When any of these fail, incontinence results.

<table>
<tr><td>Activity</td><td>Reflect back on patients/ clients that you have been in contact with. From your experience, what are the causes of urinary and faecal incontinence?</td></tr>
</table>

Causes are diverse and varied – see Table 6.3 for a summary of causes and types. Medication can also play a part in causing incontinence e.g. diuretics appear to predispose to urge incontinence (Roe and Williams 1994)

Discussion

A recent study involving nursing home residents found that they considered that urinary incontinence was an inevitable part of ageing (Robinson 2000). However, it is important to be aware that urinary incontinence is not a disease or a normal result of ageing, but a symptom of an underlying condition. According to McCreanor *et al.* (1998), stress and urge incontinence are the two main types of urinary incontinence, and may occur together – 'mixed' incontinence. Nazarko (1997) notes that the environment in a nursing home may not promote continence as the corridors can be long and confusing, and the message portrayed may be that incontinence is expected. Schnozzle *et al.* (1998) identify that in nursing homes immobility and dementia are the primary risk factors for incontinence. The problem is compounded as impaired mobility is associated with constipation, which in turn increases the risk of UTI and urge incontinence (Nazarko 1997), and constipation can also lead on to overflow faecal incontinence. For an immobile person such as Sarah, these are potential problems.

In people with a learning disability, a combination of factors may affect the learning and maintenance of continence; these include impaired brain function with possibly coexistent localized damage, as well as social and environmental factors (Stanley 1996a). Clients with learning disabilities can take time to orientate themselves to an unfamiliar environment, and incontinence can result if they don't know, or can't remember, where the toilet is. When John is admitted to hospital, the nurses will need to understand this and try to orientate him to the ward. People with a physical disability may not be able to independently reach and use the toilet, and if carers do not assist effectively, functional incontinence results. Robinson (2000) cites a nursing home resident saying 'When I have to go and I'm sitting in the wheelchair, and I'm wheeling my chair, and I can't do it fast enough, I wet my

Table 6.3 Summary of causes and types of incontinence (adapted from Colley 1996)

Causes of urinary incontinence

Type	Description	Causes
Stress	Urine leakage associated with, for example, coughing, sneezing or exercise.	Weakness of the sphincter mechanism. Most common in women, e.g. after childbirth. Can occur in men after a prostatectomy.
Urge	Leakage occurring with urgency – little or no warning of the need to void. Symptoms of frequency and nocturnal enuresis may accompany.	Detrusor instability (motor urgency) due to e.g. bladder neck obstruction, or hypersensitive detrusor muscle (sensory urgency) due to e.g. infection, bladder stones.
Overflow	Urinary leakage caused by incomplete bladder emptying.	May be due to: • Outflow obstruction: e.g. by faecal impaction • An atonic or hypotonic bladder (one which does not produce adequate detrusor contraction for micturition) e.g. in diabetic neuropathy • Detrusor-sphincter dyssynergia (lack of co-ordination between detrusor contraction and relaxation during bladder emptying) e.g. in spinal injury.
Functional	Bladder emptying when the person is unable to reach the toilet, adjust/remove clothing, and use it appropriately.	Physical impairment (e.g. lack of mobility or dexterity) or mental impairment such as confusion. An inconducive environment and unsupportive carers will also contribute.

Causes of faecal incontinence *(Jensen 1997)*

Group one	People with intact anal function e.g. CVA, diarrhoea, faecal impaction.
Group two	People with compromised anal sphincter function e.g. congenital malformation or obstetric trauma.

pants'. This is an example of probable urge incontinence, compounded by functional incontinence. A person with a learning as well as a physical disability may not be able to communicate his need to be taken to the toilet, especially if staff are not familiar with his method of communicating this need, which may be through signing or symbols.

To accurately assess the underlying cause and therefore possible management of incontinence, a thorough assessment would be necessary.

Learning outcome 3:
Show insight into the potential psychosocial and physical effects of incontinence, and the need for support

■ Activity

> Consider for a minute John (who is usually continent at home) but is now in the unfamiliar environment of a hospital ward for his operation. He knows that he needs to go to the toilet, but he does not know where it is, and cannot communicate with the nurses to ask where the toilet is. Consequently he is incontinent. How might John feel?

You probably identified both physical effects, such as discomfort, and psychological distress too.

A number of authors have highlighted the possible adverse effects of incontinence (Chiverton *et al.* 1996; Hutchinson *et al.* 1996; Norton 1996; Norton 1997; Stanley 1997; Smith 1998; Rogers 1998; Cochran 1999; Koch and Kelly 1999; Robinson 2000) (*see* Table 6.4).

Support and advice

Chester (1998) claims that incontinence is a taboo subject and that while people are willing to discuss their struggle against cancer or alcoholism, they

Table 6.4 Possible psycho-social and physical effects of incontinence

Effect	*Source*
Increase in falls	Smith (1998)
Increase in UTIs	Smith (1998)
Skin problems	Smith (1998); Robinson (2000)
Adverse effect on psychological status and socialization	Smith (1998); Robinson (2000)
Embarrassment	Cochran (1999); Koch and Kelly (1999)
Depression, isolation and adverse effects on self-esteem	Chiverton *et al.* (1996)
Distress	Koch and Kelly (1999)
Adverse effect on relationship, employment and social activities	Norton (1997)
Added workload for carers of people with learning disabilities	Stanley (1997)
Greater likelihood of admission to long-term care for clients with learning disabilities	Stanley (1997)
Social undervaluing of learning disability clients	Stanley (1997)
Adversely affects quality of life and choices on leaving school for children with learning disabilities	Rogers (1998)
Catastrophic reactions in people with early or middle-stage Alzheimer's disease	Hutchinson *et al.* (1996)

will be much less likely to talk about their incontinence. However, people with incontinence do need both support and advice, but may often be unaware of what support is available, and where it can be accessed. It is important that nurses are aware of the resources available so that they can advise clients with continence issues.

There are many local self-help support groups which can be very beneficial to participants. They give people opportunity to meet informally, and share ideas and experiences. 'Incontact' is one such organization which helps people to set up such groups. Many Disabled Living Centres (DLCs) hold the Promo-Con Continence Resource Package, which is composed of a range of products, fact sheets and other relevant information. DLCs display materials to promote continence alongside other equipment for easier living. Many organizations have developed information leaflets for people suffering from incontinence, for example the Stroke Association, Alzheimer's Disease Society, and also Help the Aged. Details about all these support services for people with incontinence are at the end of the chapter.

Activity   Try to find out about advice and support within your area. Find out where your nearest DLC is, and if possible, arrange to visit so that you can see the resources available.

Learning outcome 4:
Demonstrate understanding into how incontinence might be assessed

As discussed under learning outcome two, there are many possible underlying causes of incontinence. The key to continence promotion is an effective assessment (Nazarko 1999). Without careful assessment, people may employ inappropriate self-help strategies, such as fluid intake reduction (Robinson 2000). Temporary causes of incontinence, such as UTI, confusion, medication, faecal impaction, impaired mobility and depression, should be identified.

Activity   Assessment includes interviewing, observation and measurement. Keeping these in mind, think about how a nurse might assess incontinence. In your current or recent practice placements did you find any specific tools used for assessment of incontinence?

Table 6.5 identifies some key points, and these are expanded below.

Many practice settings will have a specific incontinence assessment tool, which will help the nurse to identify both the cause, and possible management of the individual's incontinence. Examples of these are given by Getliffe and Dolman (1997). Assessment should include a urinalysis, and sending off a urine specimen for microscopy and culture if indicated.

Nazarko (1999) suggests that the following questions will be useful when interviewing the client:

Table 6.5 Assessment of continence: some key points

Use of an assessment tool will promote a systematic approach
Referral to a continence advisor may be needed

Interviewing:
- Sensitive, empathetic approach
- Careful and appropriate use of language
- Involvement of carers

Observation
- Physical factors e.g. obstructive symptoms
- Psychological factors e.g. confusion
- Environmental factors e.g. access to toilet

Measurement
- Urinalysis
- Charting frequency and amount

- What is the patient's problem?
- What is causing the problem?
- What solutions are available?
- Who is the best person to provide those solutions?
- What outcome does the patient want?
- How can we meet the patient's needs?

Interviewing skills

When using interviewing skills to assess incontinence, approach and terminology used need careful consideration. Woodward (1996) identifies that people often see incontinence as a taboo subject and need permission from the nurse to discuss it, whilst being sensitive to the person's need for privacy and dignity. Cochran (1999) found that the term 'incontinence' was not a term used by elderly people and that it is preferable to ask 'Do you have bladder control problems?' or 'Do you leak?' Woodward (1996) also stresses the importance of terming questions clearly in understandable terms, for example the term 'frequency' may not be understood; it is preferable to ask: 'How often do you go to the toilet to pass urine during the day?' Colley (1996) emphasizes using an empathetic approach in assessment, and has developed a model for the assessment of incontinence, which is presented as a flow chart.

Cognitive impairment

For the cognitively impaired adult who may be unable to give a clear history, Thompson and Smith (1998) give useful hints for assessing incontinence, emphasizing the importance of observing for clues to indicate frequency and severity, and involving the carer in assessment. The nurse can observe the client voiding, noting signs of pain, obstructive symptoms, such as hesitancy, intermittent stream, dribbling after voiding and straining to void, urge symptoms, and functional barriers, such as being unable to undress.

Learning disability

Shaw (1998) believes that continence problems in people with a learning disability have often gone untreated, as there is an assumption that they cannot acquire the skills for continence, and an accurate assessment (including urology referral) has not been done. Accurately assessing means that signs of detrusor instability can be identified and treated with medication, prior to commencing bladder training (Shaw 1998). In a client with a physical disability and a communication difficulty, the client may know when he wants to go to the toilet, but staff are not able to recognize his need as a method of communication has not been established. Thus Stanley (1997) explains that incontinence in a client with a learning disability should be assessed by carrying out a functional analysis, considering the person, the person's situation or environment, and the significant people in the person's life. Stanley (1997) emphasizes that this individualistic approach is complex, and requires careful observation and a good knowledge about the person and his/her life; a number of structured instruments are available to help the assessment. Assessment of a child with learning disabilities must take into account developmental level, assessing motor, cognitive and language development (Rogers 1998).

Faecal incontinence

For faecal incontinence assessment, Jensen (1997) advises that history taking should address the duration of faecal leakage, current bowel management, and type, frequency, amount and duration of the faecal incontinence and how it affects lifestyle. She also suggests that physical factors (such as mobility and dexterity), environmental factors (such as access to the toilet), and psychological factors (such as motivation and cognition), should be assessed.

Referrals

In both urinary and faecal incontinence, a more specialist assessment may be needed and referral to the continence advisor should be made. Specialist investigations may sometimes be necessary, such as urodynamics.

Activity   Find out the name of the local continence advisor in your area, and how referrals are made.

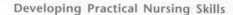
Learning outcome 5:
Identify appropriate nursing interventions for the promotion of
continence

After assessment, appropriate interventions can be planned. Complete remission may not be achievable, but at least a reduction in incontinence leading to a more controllable situation may be possible (Steeman and Defever 1998). Emphasis in this section will be on selected nursing interventions to promote continence. However it is useful to be aware that treatment for incontinence can include surgery and pharmacology (Steeman and Defever 1998), biofeedback (Jensen 1997) and intermittent catheterization.

■ **Activity**	From previous experience that you have, write down any methods that a nurse can use to promote urinary and faecal continence.

Promotion of urinary continence

How continence is promoted will obviously depend on the underlying cause and that is why an understanding of underlying causes and careful assessment is important. A holistic approach should be taken, considering contributory factors such as diet, fluids, bowels, social and physical environment as well as urinary symptoms (Lewey *et al*. 1997). Getliffe and Dolman (1997) list psychological, social and environmental adjustments which can help to promote continence, including: well sign-posted, near at hand, easily identifiable and accessible toilets, easy to remove clothing, and supportive, encouraging carers. Smith (1998) identifies that enthusiasm and commitment of staff can be very helpful in promoting continence, and also emphasizes that the nurse should refer the patient and liaise with the multidisciplinary team as appropriate. Physiotherapists can help with mobility and balance therefore enabling a quicker transfer. Occupational therapists will be able to help with making the environment and dressing and undressing easier. Two specific interventions, which you may have identified, are: **pelvic floor exercises** and **bladder re-education**.

Pelvic floor exercises

Pelvic floor exercises (PFEs) aim to strengthen the pubococcygeal muscle resulting in increased urethral closure pressure, and stronger reflex contractions, when there is a sudden rise in intra-abdominal pressure, such as when sneezing (Dolman 1997). PFEs can eradicate 70% of mild to moderate cases of stress incontinence in 3 to 6 months (Hocking 1999). Strengthening pelvic floor muscles will also improve the person's ability to hold on until reaching the toilet, and so they are useful in urge incontinence too. Dougherty's (1998) literature review on PFEs gives specific detail about all aspects of this complex subject, and Dolman (1997) also covers the topic in depth. A PFE protocol needs to be clear and specific, and address the frequency, how many to be done, the duration of each contraction, and the rest phase between repetitions (Dougherty 1998). The PFE regimen may be prescribed for a set period of weeks, followed by a maintenance plan. Clients should also be advised to squeeze these muscles if they feel the need to cough or sneeze, so that it becomes almost an automatic reaction in circumstances where stress incontinence might occur.

Bladder re-education

Bladder re-education involves re-educating the bladder to an improved pattern of voiding and has a number of variations, suitable for different client groups. When these programmes are in use for clients it is essential that all staff are fully aware, and are motivated towards them, so that they are implemented consistently.

Bladder training   Bladder training will aim to gradually extend the interval between voiding, with voiding being initiated by the clock, rather than desire to void (Anders 1999). For example, the person might initially be asked to go to the toilet every hour, and then this is gradually extended by half an hour at a time. Education of the patient and carers, use of a continence chart and continuous encouragement, are all important elements. Carers will need to praise to build up confidence and reinforce behaviour, and to be patient and understanding. There is some evidence to support its success with urge incontinence (McCreanor *et al.* 1998; Anders 1999; Roe *et al.* 1999), but it seems that more research is needed.

Timed voiding   This is often used for people with a neurogenic bladder, such as those with spinal cord lesions, and for people with a physical/mental disability. It entails voiding at fixed times, which can include techniques to trigger voiding, such as tapping over the suprapubic region, or running water.

Habit retraining   This involves developing an individualized toileting schedule (Anders 1999). Initially the person might be encouraged not to use the toilet between fixed 2-hourly intervals unless he needs to. A record of voiding and incontinent episodes is kept so that the schedule can be adjusted, with voiding intervals lengthened if the person is dry, and reduced if incontinence occurs.

Prompted voiding   Prompted voiding involves prompting the person to void at regular intervals, but only taking him to the toilet if the response is positive. This method can be very successful in promoting continence although further research is needed (Heavner 1998). Prompted voiding has been particularly used with people with learning disabilities, and with the cognitively impaired adult, where the underlying cause of incontinence is often functional and/or urge incontinence (Thompson and Smith 1998). However, this is not without difficulty, depending on the client variables: degree of confusion, physical mobility, and affective response (Hutchinson *et al.* 1996). As dementia progresses timed voiding with a toileting schedule, will be more suitable than prompted voiding (Hutchinson *et al.* 1996). Smith (1998) outlines a number of tips when using prompted voiding with clients with dementia:

- Have the word 'toilet' on the door with a picture
- Increase environmental safety e.g. hand rails
- Use simple verbal or behavioural clues
- Use pleasant distraction such as singing
- Keep to a routine and, where possible, a familiar nurse
- Use easy to remove clothes
- Stay pleasant and avoid hurrying or confrontation.

Behavioural techniques Behavioural techniques to promote continence in people with learning disabilities must include assessing the client's baseline ability, then performing a task analysis, identifying a sequence of manageable steps to be learnt, what prompts will be needed at each stage, and the necessity for reinforcement (Stanley 1997). These techniques are explained in more depth by Stanley (1996b).

Rogers (1998) gives useful suggestions in relation to toilet training in children with learning disabilities. Preparation for toilet training could include using a doll and a potty, and books. The family will need to be supported in developing a routine which fits with school and home, and any success must be praised. Day time wetting alarms (which raise the child's awareness of being wet) and star and reward charts may help to motivate. Rogers (1998) advises that lack of success should lead to abandonment of the programme, and then retrying 3 months later.

For the older child with enuresis, Dobson (1997) suggests reward schemes, alarms, medication, complementary methods e.g. hypnotherapy, and dry bed training (intensive waking schedules), all of which are tried and tested. Management of enuresis and encopresis with children, are considered in detail by Lukeman (1997).

Measures to promote faecal continence

The range of treatments for faecal incontinence is sparse – most focus on surgery and there is little nursing research into this problem (Norton 1997). However, in a recent study, biofeedback was found to have a high success rate in treating faecal incontinence with 43% regarding themselves as cured and 24% as improved (Norton and Kamm 1999). This technique can be used by specialist nurses or physiotherapists. It involves techniques used to bring under conscious control bodily processes usually considered to be beyond voluntary command (Jensen 1997). Medication, such as loperamide, may help to slow bowel transit and solidify the stool. Norton (1997) highlights that staff attitude to faecal incontinence is crucial, and that much is preventable amongst older dependent people, with proper attention to diet, fluids, mobility, medication and establishment of bowel habit.

Diet and activity

Jensen (1997) advises that mild faecal incontinence may be eliminated by changes to diet and activity level. Clients should thus be encouraged to take regular, well-timed meals, which include adequate fibre and fluids, in order to promote a soft well formed stool. Mild exercise will optimize gastrointestinal function.

Developing a pattern

People with intact sensation and normal sphincter function should be encouraged to try to establish a regular pattern for defaecation to maximize the potential benefit from the gastrocolic reflex; they should also be encouraged to respond promptly to the need to defaecate (Jensen 1997). Thus where help is needed from the nurse, such as taking the person to the toilet, the nurse should respond promptly to the person's request. When normal sensation and sphincter function is compromised (such as in spinal injured people), a programme to establish stimulation by using suppositories or enemas will be needed. Doughty (1996) reviews such programmes in detail.

Learning outcome 6:
Discuss how incontinence can be managed

Incontinence should be managed in a manner which is unobtrusive, reliable and comfortable. Thus incontinence aids should preserve hygiene, psychological and social comfort as far as possible (Steeman and Defever 1998). Urethral catheterization is rarely an appropriate means of managing urinary incontinence (except occasionally as a short-term measure), as it may lead to catheter related problems such as urinary tract infection (Vernon and Bleakly 1997) (*see* section on Catheterization), or jeopardize subsequent bladder retraining, in CVA patients for example (Hodges 1997). However for some people, such as Sarah, long-term catheterization will be the most effective solution. Generally these include people who do not completely empty the bladder due to neurological disease or injury, people with bladder outlet obstruction for whom surgical repair is not possible, and those with chronic incontinence, often with associated confusion or debility, who cannot be managed any other way (Getliffe 1997).

Activity   If you find that a patient/client has been incontinent, what would your priorities of care be?

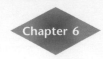

Priorities of care

The person will need to be attended to quickly, in order to prevent skin damage, relieve discomfort and restore dignity. In faecal incontinence, in particular, prompt changing of soiled pads or clothing is essential, and will help to prevent odours and skin excoriation (Norton 1997). This also applies to the soiled nappies of infants and toddlers, which should also be changed promptly. Many of the principles outlined when dealing with a person's elimination needs will also apply, in particular: approachability and communication, privacy and dignity, punctuality, prevention of cross-infection, observation, hygiene and comfort. How skin is cleaned is very important, and if incontinence cannot be prevented, then a suitable method of containment is needed, for example pads, or for a man with urinary incontinence, possibly a penile sheath.

Skin cleansing

Le Lievre (1996) has identified that nurses' skin care of incontinent patients is not always based on sound research. This may be because skin care relating to urinary incontinence has been little addressed in the literature (Vinson and Proch 1998). Box 6.12 lists some key points about skin cleansing for the incontinent person, and these are further discussed below with rationale.

- If super-absorbent, body worn pads are used, skin cleansing is not necessary at every pad change.
- Gloves and an apron should be worn for cleansing.
- Cleansing with plain water is sufficient for urinary incontinence.
- Faecal incontinence must be dealt with promptly and skin cleaned. If soap is used, rinse off thoroughly. Skin cleanser is preferable.
- Cleanse from front to back, and least soiled area to most soiled area
- Start with the labia with females, and the tip of the penis with men.
- Cleanse the anal area last.
- Dry skin carefully. Do not use talculm powder.
- Consider use of barrier creams/barrier films for particularly vulnerable skin.

Box 6.12 Skin cleansing after incontinence: a summary of key points

It is clear that nurses need to be aware of the potential skin problems which may result from incontinence. Jeter and Lutz (1996) explain that the presence of moisture from urine and sweat increases friction and shear, skin permeability and microbial load, while the frequent washings which may result, lead

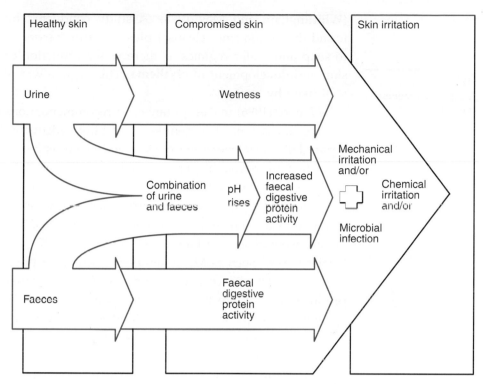

Figure 6.8 Diagram showing how incontinence affects skin. (Reproduced with permission from Paper-Pak UK Ltd)

to physical and chemical irritation. If the patient has been incontinent of both urine and faeces, their interaction can result in ammonia formation leading to a rise in pH and an increase in the activity of faecal enzymes which damage the skin (*see* Fig. 6.8). Thus Gibbons (1996) emphasizes the importance of changing a soiled product promptly in cases of faecal incontinence to prevent skin excoriation. Super-absorbent pads aim to prevent mixing of urine and faeces by keeping skin dry (*see* section on Pads, next).

Washing with soap and water can cause drying of the skin or even contact dermatitis and eczema (Spiller 1992), and after reviewing a number of studies Vinson and Proch (1998) conclude that soap and water may not provide adequate skin care. Soap, which is designed to remove dirt and grease, also removes natural skin lipids and water holding substances and weakens the epidermis. Skin is normally slightly acidic, but bars of soap are alkaline and are therefore unsuitable for use on skin assessed as at risk of breaking down, as if the skin becomes more alkaline it becomes more permeable (Jeter and Lutz 1996). If soap and water is used, it should be thoroughly rinsed with clean water, and the skin dried gently. However, the use of skin cleanser rather than soap has indicated some benefit for patient's skin

Erythema
_____

A superficial redness of
the skin.

(Whittingham and May 1998). A study conducted by Byers *et al.* (1995) found that a non-rinse cleanser plus moisture barrier cream, was preferable to soap and water regimes as there was a reduction of fluid loss from the skin and development of **erythema**. This regime was also quicker and was well liked by staff.

Le Lievre (1996) makes a number of recommendations for skin care. These include assessment of present skin condition, adequate fluid and nutritional input, daily social cleansing of skin, and use of either unscented soap which is washed off thoroughly, or preferably wash cream. When pads are changed, skin should be patted dry gently. If only urinary incontinence occurs and pads containing super-absorbents are used, then skin washing at each pad change is not necessary; however the skin should be washed as soon as possible after faecal incontinence (Le Lievre 1996). Norton (1997) recommends the use of barrier creams such as Metanium or Sudocrem for prevention and treatment of milder cases of excoriated skin due to faecal incontinence, and stoma care products to promote healing where skin is broken. These creams are also suitable for nappy wearing babies and toddlers during diarrhoeal illnesses, when there is increased risk of skin excoriation, and would thus be recommended for Toby.

Talcum powder should be avoided as it can create a warm moist environment for infection (Gibbons 1996). Cleaning with moist toilet tissue may be more comfortable for the faecally incontinent person than dry paper (Norton 1997). The anal area should always be cleaned last. There are products, such as no-sting barrier films, which can be applied to protect vulnerable skin in incontinent patients, and these have been shown to improve skin condition (Williams 1998). Skin should be cleaned and dried prior to application.

Pads

There are a vast array of incontinence pads produced by a variety of companies and all are suitable for both urinary and faecal incontinence. Pads for managing incontinence can be divided into three types: under-pads, all-in-one body worn products, and pads worn with elasticated pants (*see* Fig. 6.9).

Choice of product

While most pads used will be disposable, washable pads are also produced. Disposable pads may contain super-absorbents, which can keep the skin in a near normal state, but there are also pads containing pulp only, which encourage skin hydration and permeability. Such pads allow mixing of urine and faeces causing further enzyme activity and skin damage (Le Lievre 1996).

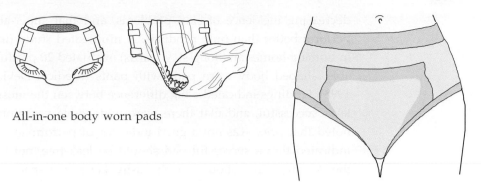

All-in-one body worn pads

Figure 6.9 Incontinence pads

Two-piece body worn pads

Gibbons (1996) suggests that faecal collectors can be used for patients who have persistent diarrhoea. Box 6.13 summarizes key points in the choice and use of incontinence pads.

A systematic review by Shirran and Brazzelli (1999) concluded that evidence available did not provide a sound basis for practice. However the review indicated that disposable pads may be more effective than non-disposable in

---

Choice of pad
- Disposable, super-absorbent pads are preferable
- Body worn pads (either all-in-ones, or pad and pants) should be used rather than under-pads.
- Choose the correct pad for the individual client, considering gender, size, and extent and frequency of incontinence.

Fitting
Always follow manufacturer's instructions for fitting, but the following general principles normally apply.
- Maintain privacy, dignity and prevention of cross-infection during pad changes
- If using pants, ensure the seams are on the outside, and pull up to mid-thigh
- Fold the pad lengthways and create a cupped shape
- Place the pad from front to back with largest area at the back
- Ensure pad is smoothed out both front and back, and fitted into the groin well.
- If using pants, pull up, or if all-in-ones, seal the tapes firmly, lower tapes should be sealed first
- Check pad is as close to the body as possible.

Box 6.13 Key points in the choice and use of incontinence pads

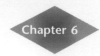

decreasing incidence of skin problems, and that super-absorbent pads may perform better than pulp products. A multi-sited study (involving 228 clients in nursing homes and long-stay wards) evaluated 20 product ranges of disposable, shaped body worn pads with pants (Medical Devices Agency (MDA) 1998). Findings indicated a big difference between the most successful and the least successful, and that there were wide price variations. However it was noted that price was not a good indicator of performance. Carers' comments indicated that a successful pad should be leak-free, not too bulky, and keep the skin dry. Pants should not rip easily, keep their shape, and not be too tight around the tops of the legs.

Choice of product should take into account comfort, easy removal for toileting, client preference and adequate protection in relation to amount of urine lost (Thompson and Smith 1998). Pads are produced for all situations, ranging from light to severe and night-time use.

■ Light would be suitable for when there is only occasional voiding of a few drops of urine.
■ Moderate for when there is frequent voiding of small to moderate amounts of urine.
■ Severe for uncontrolled daily voiding of moderate to large amounts.

Different shaped pads are available for men and women. It is important to read manufacturers' instructions for the optimal fitting of these pads as correct fitting of the product is essential to contain urine and faeces, and will reduce skin contact with excreta to the minimum (Gibbons 1996). As urine is broken down into its constituents – ammonia and urea – on contact with air, fitting the pads closely will ensure that urine and air are not mixed. Additional features, which some pads may have, are wetness indicator strips, and adhesive strips for extra security. Some pads and pants are produced which act as normal underwear. Washable pants with a built in pad can be suitable for stress or moderate incontinence. Different types to meet individuals' manual dexterity are available such as with poppers or Velcro fastenings.

Misuse of under-pads

According to Norton (1996) under-pads are one of the most misused of all items used by nurses for managing incontinence She states that one good quality body worn pad is usually more effective than using several under-pads which are costly and of little benefit to the patient. Thornburn *et al.* (1992) also emphasize the disadvantages of using under-pads rather than pads fitted to the body. Such problems include: under-pads need changing immediately to prevent urine break down and excessive skin hydration; they are not in close contact with the body so the urine rapidly becomes cold, thus waking the patient at night; and finally, they do not contain super-absorbents so excessive skin hydration results. Thus under-pads should be used only as a procedure pad when a clean (not sterile) field is needed, for extra chair/bed protection e.g. after administration of an enema, or where a body worn pad is not practical or possible e.g. with a very obese client, or for persistent diarrhoea in bed.

Additional points

When changing a pad, it should never be referred to as a 'nappy' which is demeaning. The nurse should take care not to show annoyance or embarrass the patient (*see* Chapter 2). It is important to ensure that the person has a clean pad at mealtimes and before going out anywhere. When changing the pad maintain privacy by shutting curtains, and change any wet or soiled clothing. To prevent cross-infection use of gloves, hand washing and correct waste disposal are essential (*see* Chapter 3).

Penile sheaths

Penile sheaths (*see* Fig. 6.10) are available, which channel the urine into a collection bag. These are a widely established means of managing urinary incontinence in male patients although there is a lack of research into their use (Doherty 1998). Use of sheaths avoids the disadvantages and complications of

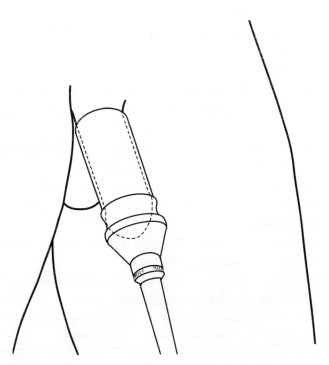

Figure 6.10 Penile sheath

long-term in-dwelling urethral catheters, and the inconvenience of pads (MDA 1995). As many people are allergic to latex (Le Lievre 1996) so use of a silicone sheath avoids this risk, and a clear sheath as opposed to an opaque one will allow observation of the penile skin. It is suggested that sheaths are most suitable for men who have a moderate to severe degree of incontinence and/or have frequency and urgency, and are not able to get to the toilet easily (MDA 1995). However the MDA identify that assessment for suitability should include assessing manual dexterity of the user (or carers), independence/availability of the carers and skin condition of the user. Sheaths may be two piece or one piece. The two-piece sheath requires application of an adhesive strip to the penis, before rolling the sheath on, while the one-piece sheath has an integral adhesive coating. The adhesive can cause skin problems in some people (Le Lievre 1996). One-piece sheaths have been rated more highly than two-piece, but acceptability of different products has been found to be highly individualized (MDA 1995). Thus men for whom a sheath might be an acceptable containment strategy, should be enabled to try out different products before deciding on one for long-term use.

Box 6.14 summarizes some important points about fitting a penile sheath but further details are given below. A clear explanation should be given to the patient about the sheath. Doherty (1998) notes that a positive attitude is necessary for successful use and that initially there may be problems but these can be overcome. Application of a urinary sheath is an intimate procedure, which may be embarrassing for both patient and nurse (Doherty 1998). The nurse should also be aware that patients with reduced or absent sensation will

---

- Assess client for suitability and give a clear explanation.
- Choose appropriate size and type of sheath. Be prepared to try out others if it is found to be unsuitable.
- Maintain principles of preventing cross-infection throughout.
- Wash and dry penis and surrounding area.
- Trim (but do not shave) pubic hair if necessary.
- If using a two-part sheath, apply adhesive strip to penile shaft in a spiral manner.
- Roll the sheath on to the penis, leaving a space between the cup of the sheath and the end of the penis.
- Gently squeeze the sheath to ensure adhesion.
- Attach to a urinary drainage bag.
- Remove by gently rolling off (preferably in the bath) every 24 hours, and wash and dry skin before reapplying

Box 6.14 Fitting a urinary sheath: key points

not be able to feel if the sheath is too tight or a sore is developing, so they and their carers will need to be observant for any such problems. In many cases the patient will be able to manage the system himself. Hands should be washed prior to application, and any cuts should be covered with a plaster. Gloves can be worn if wanted but they are not essential.

Steps to ensure effective use of urinary sheaths are outlined in some detail by Doherty (1998). These include: choice of correct size by measuring the circumference of the penis at its widest point and measuring the length – note that if it is too tight it could cause sores and discomfort, while if it is too big it will lead to leakage as urine will seep under the sheath. Doherty (1998) notes, however, that penile size can vary and that sheath measurement should allow for expansion although both latex and silicone are flexible materials. The penis and surrounding area should then be washed and dried; powder, cream or spray deodorants should not be used as they will inactivate the adhesive. If necessary, pubic hair should be trimmed but should not be shaved. A piece of paper/card, sometimes supplied by the manufacturer, can be held over the penis to keep back pubic hair while the sheath is applied.

When fitting the sheath, roll it over the penis leaving a small space between the end of the penis and the cup of the sheath, to allow for changes in the size of the penis while wearing. If the man is uncircumcised, ensure that the foreskin remains over the glans and is not retracted. Once the sheath is in place, gently squeeze it to ensure adhesion, and then attach it to a urine drainage bag. Never apply sticky tape as it is inflexible and could lead to restriction of the blood supply leading to sores or gangrene. Ensure that the tubing is not kinked, thereby allowing collection of urine and pressure on the sheath weakening the adhesive, and that the urine bag is kept lower and is well supported.

■ **Activity**   Can you think of any patients for whom this method of dealing with urinary incontinence might be particularly unsuitable?

Patients with any sore of the penis should not have a sheath applied. Patients with a small or retracted penis are not suitable (MDA 1995), unless a device such as a flange and belt is used. Patients who are confused, and do not understand what the sheath is, are likely to try to pull it off.

Summary
- Nurses within almost any setting are likely to encounter people with continence issues, and therefore an understanding of the underlying causes and the wide-ranging effects on people is important.
- Nurses should have knowledge about specialist services, e.g. the continence advisor and support organizations, so that they can advice and refer clients accordingly.

■ Promoting continence and managing incontinence requires careful assessment of each individual, and knowledge about appropriate strategies and products. Care for people with continence problems should be based on the best evidence available.

CHAPTER SUMMARY

This chapter has focused on assisting people with elimination, and has emphasized that to achieve quality care requires a sensitive and empathetic approach, effective communication skills, and a sound, evidence-based knowledge. It has also been stressed throughout that measures to prevent cross-infection whilst assisting clients with elimination are paramount. Urinalysis and specimen collection has been dealt with in some detail, as these are very common investigations which nurses assist with, but if not carried out with care, can lead to misleading results, and therefore, inappropriate treatment. Administration of suppositories and enemas is again, a relevant skill for nurses in most settings, and must be carried out with care and understanding. Urinary catheterization is invasive and potentially harmful, but is nevertheless often necessary as a short or long-term measure. An understanding of this procedure, and particularly how potential complications can be reduced, is also important. As stated, continence is a huge topic, and may require specialist involvement. Here, the practical skills in dealing with continence have been explored, and it is expected that students wishing to extend their knowledge will access the referenced material. To conclude, nurses need to value the care given in relation to patients/clients' elimination needs as, if effective, it can do much for comfort, well-being and self-esteem.

REFERENCES

Abd-el-Maeboud, K.H., el-Naggar, T., El-Hawi, E.M.M. *et al*. 1991. Rectal suppositories and mode of insertion. *The Lancet* **338**, 798, 800.

Addison, R., Ness, W., Abulafi, M. *et al*. 1999. *Digital Rectal Examination and Manual Removal of Faeces: A Guide on the Role of the Nurse.* London: Royal College of Nursing.

Addison, R., Ness, W., Abulafi, M. *et al*. 2000. How to administer enemas and suppositories. *Nursing Times NT Plus: Continence* **96** (6), 3–4.

Anders, K. 1999. Bladder retraining. *Professional Nurse* **14**, 334–36.

Ayliffe, G.A.J., Babb, J.R. and Taylor, L.J. 1999. *Hospital-Acquired Infection. Principles and Prevention*, 3rd edn. Oxford: Butterworth-Heinemann.

Ballinger, C., Pain, H., Pascoe, J. and Gore, S. 1996. Choosing a commode for the ward environment. *British Journal of Nursing* **5**, 485–6.

Bayer. 1998. *A Practical Guide to Urine Analysis.* Newbury: Bayer.

Bayer. 1997a. *Technical Information Bulletin Number 8. Urinary Tract Infection.* Newbury: Bayer.

Bayer.1997b. *Urine Analysis: The essential information*. Newbury: Bayer.

Beynon, M. 1997. Urological investigations. In: Fillingham, S. and Douglas, J. (eds.) *Urological Nursing*, 2nd edn. London: Ballière Tindall, 30–56.

Block, C., Baron, O., Bogokowoski, B. *et al*. 1990. An in-use evaluation of polypropylene versus stainless steel bedpans. *Journal of Hospital Acquired Infection* **16**, 331–38.

Brown, J., Meikle, J. and Webb, C. 1991. Collecting midstream specimens for urine – the research base. *Nursing Times* **87** (13), 49–52.

Burr, R.G. and Nuseibeh, I.M. 1997. Urinary catheter blockage depends on urine pH, calcium and rate of flow. *Spinal Cord*, **35**, 521–5.

Byers, P.P.I., Ryan, P.A. and Regan, M.B. 1995. Effects of incontinence care cleansing regimens on skin integrity. *Journal of Wound, Ostomy and Continence Nursing* **22**, 187–92.

Campbell, S. and Glasper, E.A. 1995. *Whaley and Wong's Children's Nursing*. London: Mosby.

Chester, R. 1998. *Towards Continence*. London: Counsel and Care.

Chiverton, P.A., Wells, T.J., Brink, C.A. and Mayer, R. 1996. Psychological factors associated with urinary incontinence. *Clinical Nurse Specialist* **10**, 229–33.

Cochran, A 1999. Response to urinary incontinence by older persons living in the community. *Continence* **19**, 15–24.

Colley, W. 1996. Charting new waters. *Nursing Times* **92** (24), 59–60, 62, 64.

Coyne, I.T. 1995a. Parental participation in care: a critical review of the literature. *Journal of Advanced Nursing* **21**, 716–22.

Coyne, I.T. 1995b. Partnership in care: parents' views of participation in their hospitalized child's care. *Journal of Clinical Nursing* **4**, 71–9.

Continence Foundation 1999. National Continence Awareness Campaign 1998. *Continence* **19**, 8–9.

Dobson, P. 1997. Continence. Growing Pains. *Nursing Times* **93** (30), 68, 70, 73.

Doherty, W. 1998 The clear advantage urinary incontinence sheath for men. *British Journal of Nursing* **7**, 730, 732–34.

Dolman, M. 1997. Mostly female. In: Getliffe, K. and Dolman, M. (eds.) *Promoting Continence: A Cinical and Research Resource*. London: Ballière Tindall, 68–106.

Dougherty, M. 1998. Current status of research on pelvic muscle strengthening techniques. *Journal of Wound, Ostomy, and Continence Nursing* **25**, 75–83.

Doughty, D.B. 1996. A physiologic approach to bowel training. *Journal of Wound, Ostomy and Continence Nursing* **23**, 46–56.

Edwards, C. 1997. Down and away: an overview of adult constipation and faecal incontinence. In: Getliffe, K. and Dolman, M. (eds.) *Promoting Continence: A Clinical and Research Resource*. London: Ballière Tindall, 77–226.

Emmerson, A.M., Enstone, J.E., Griffin, M. *et al*. 1996. The second national prevalence survey of infection in hospitals. *Journals of Hospital Infection*, **32**(3), 175–90.

Fader, M., Pettersson, L., Brooks, R. *et al*. 1997. A multicentre comparative evaluation of catheter valves. *British Journal of Nursing* **6**, 359, 362, 364, 366–7.

Getliffe, K. 1996. Which catheter? A guide to catheter selection *Professional Nurse* **12** (2) insert 2 pp.

Getliffe, K. 1997. Catheters and catheterization. In: Getliffe, K. and Dolman, M. (eds.) *Promoting Continence: A Clinical and Research Resource*. London: Ballière Tindall, 281–341.

Getliffe, K. and Dolman, M. 1997. Normal and abnormal bladder function. In: Getliffe, K. and Dolman, M. (eds.) *Promoting Continence: A Clinical and Research Resource*. London: Baillière Tindall, 22–67.

Gibbons, G. 1996. Skin care and incontinence. *Community Nurse* **2**, 37.

Gill, D. 1999. Stool specimen collection 2. *Nursing Times* **95** (26) insert 2 pp.

Gould, D. 1994 Controlling infection spread from excreta. *Nursing Standard* **8** (33), 29–31.

Gould, D. and Chamberlain, A. 1994. Gram-negative bacteria. The challenge of preventing cross-infection in hospital wards: a review of the literature. *Journal of Clinical Nursing* **3**, 339–45

Heavner, K. 1998. Urinary incontinence in extended care facilities: a literature review and proposal for continuous quality improvement. *Ostomy/Wound Management* **44** (12), 46–48, 50–53.

Henley, A. 1982. *Asians in Britain: Caring for Muslims and their Families: Religious Aspects of Care.* London: National Extension College.

Henley, A. 1983a: *Asians in Britain: Caring for Hindus and their Families: Religious Aspects of Care.* London: National Extension College.

Henley, A. 1983b: *Asians in Britain: caring for Sikhs and their Families: Religious Aspects of Care.* London: National Extension College.

Hocking, J. 1999. Continence problems: how to tackle reticence of patients. *Nursing Times* **95** (1), 56, 58.

Hodges, C. 1997. Continence care: choosing carefully. *Nursing Times* **93** (35), 48, 50, 52.

Hutchinson, S., Leger-Krall, S., and Skodal Wilson, H. 1996. Toileting: a biobehavioural challenge in Alzheimer's dementia care. *Journal of Gerontological Nursing.* **22** (10), 18–27.

Jensen, L.L. 1997. Faecal incontinence: evaluation and treatment. *Journal of Wound, Ostomy and Continence Nursing* **24**, 277–82.

Jeter, K.F. and Lutz, J.B. 1996. Skin care in the frail, elderly, dependent incontinent patient. *Advances in Skin Care* **9** (1), 29–34.

Johnson, A. 1989. Bedpans: disposable or reusable? *Nursing Times.* **85** (41), 72–4.

Kawik, L. 1996. Nurses' and parents' perceptions of participation and partnership in caring for a hospitalized child. *British Journal of Nursing* **5** (7), 430–4.

Kay, J. 2000. Administration of medicines. In: Huband, S. and Trigg, E. (eds.) *Practices in Children's Nursing: Guidelines for Hospital and Community.* Edinburgh: Churchill Livingstone, 29–38.

Koch, T. and Kelly, S. 1999. Identifying strategies for managing urinary incontinence with women who have multiple sclerosis. *Journal of Clinical Nursing* **8,** 550–59.

Laker, C. 1994. Urological investigations. In: Laker, C. (ed.) *Urological Nursing.* London: Scutari Press, 37–65.

Langford, R. 1996. Behind closed doors. *Nursing Times* **92** (24), 72.

Laurent, C. 1998. Preventing infection from indwelling catheters. *Nursing Times* **94** (25), 60–6.

Lewey, J., Billington, A. and O'Hara, L. 1997 Conservative treatment of urinary incontinence. *Nursing Standard* **12** (8), 45–7.

Le Lievre, S. 1996. Incontinence dermatitis. *Primary Health Care* **6** (4), 17–19, 21.

Lukeman, D. 1997. Mainly children: childhood enuresis and encopresis. In: Getliffe, K. and Dolman, M. (eds.) *Promoting Continence: A Clinical and Research Resource.* London: Ballière Tindall, 138–76.

MacQueen, S. 2000. Specimen collection. In: Huband, S. and Trigg, E. (eds.) *Practices in Children's Nursing: Guidelines for Hospital and Community.* Edinburgh: Churchill Livingstone, 261–7.

Mahoney, C. 1997. The impact of continence problems on self esteem. *Nursing Times* **93** (52), 58, 60.

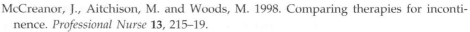

McCreanor, J., Aitchison, M. and Woods, M. 1998. Comparing therapies for incontinence. *Professional Nurse* **13**, 215–19.

McLaren, S.M. 1997. Renal function. In: Hinchliff, S.M., Montague, S.E. and Watson, R. *Physiology for Nursing practice*, 2nd edn. London: Ballière Tindall, 582–617.

McNaughton, M. and Cavanagh, S. 1998. Changing urine testing protocols through audit. *Nursing Times* **94** (1), 42–3.

Macaulay, M. 1997. Urinary drainage systems. In: Fillingham, S. and Douglas, J. (eds.) *Urological Nursing*, 2nd edn. London: Ballière Tindall, 90–130.

Mead, M. 1998a. Midstream urine testing. *Practice Nurse* **15** (7), 408.

Mead, M. 1998b. Stool culture *Practice Nurse* **16** (3), 170.

Meers, P., Sedgwick, J. and Worsley, M. 1995. *The microbiology and Epidemiology of Infection for Health Science Students*. London: Chapman Hall.

Medical Devices Agency 1995. *Penile Sheaths: An Evaluation* No. A15 Norwich: HMSO.

Medical Devices Agency 1998. *Disposable, Shaped Bodyworn Pads with Pants for Heavy Incontinence: An Evaluation*. Medical Devices Agency.

Mohammed, T.A. 2000. Urine testing and catheterization. In: Huband, S. and Trigg, E. (eds.) *Practices in Children's Nursing: Guidelines for Hospital and Community*. Edinburgh: Churchill Livingstone, 303–9.

Nazarko, L. 1995. The therapeutic uses of cranberry juice. *Nursing Standard* **9** (34), 33–5.

Nazarko, L. 1997. Continence. The whole story. *Nursing Times* **93** (43), 63–4, 66, 68.

Nazarko, L. 1999. Assess all areas. *Nursing Times* **95** (6), 68, 71, 72.

Nicol, M., Bavin, C. and Bedford-Taylor, S. *et al.* 1999. *Essential Nursing Skills*. London: Mosby.

Noble, J.G., Menzies, D., Cox, P.J. and Edwards, L. 1990. Midnight removal: an improved approach to removal of catheters. *British Journal of Urology* **65**, 615–17.

Norton, C. 1996. Faecal incontinence in adults 1: prevalence and causes. *British Journal of Nursing* **5**, 1367–74.

Norton, C. 1997. Faecal incontinence in adults 2: treatment and management. *British Journal of Nursing* **6**, 23–6.

Norton, C. and Kamm, M.A. 1999. Outcome of biofeedback for faecal incontinence. *British Journal of Surgery* **86**, 1159–63.

O'Meara, B. 1999. Hidden dangers. *Nursing Times.* **95** (31), 70–1.

Pritchard, V. and Hathaway, C. 1988. Patient handwashing practice. *Nursing Times* **84** (36), 68, 70, 72.

Robinson, J.P. 2000. Managing urinary incontinence in the nursing home: residents' perspectives. *Journal of Advanced Nursing* **31**, 68–77.

Roe, B. and Williams, K. 1994. *Clinical Handbook for Continence Care*. London: Scutari.

Roe, B., Williams, K. and Palmer, M. 1999. *Bladder Training for Urinary Incontinence (Cochrane Review)*. In: The Cochrane Library, issue 3. Oxford, Update software.

Rogers, J. 1998. RCN continuing education. Promoting continence: the child with special needs. *Nursing Standard* **12** (34), 47–55.

Rowell, D.M. 1998. Evaluation of a urine chemistry analyser. *Professional Nurse* **13**, 553–54.

Royal College of Physicians 1995. *Report of a Working Party: Incontinence – Causes, Management and Provision of Services*. London: RCP.

Schmelzer, M. and Wright, K.B. 1996. Enema administration techniques used by experienced registered nurses. *Gastroenterology Nursing* **19**, 171–75.

Schnozzle, J.F., Cruise, P.A., Alessi, C.A. *et al.* 1998. Individualising nightime incontinence care in nursing home residents. *Nursing Research* **47**, 197–204.

is available on their Incontinence Information Helpline, Monday–Friday, 9.30am–4.30pm, 020 7831 9831.

Help the Aged, St James's Walk, London EC1R OBE. Tel: 020 7253 0253. Help the Aged also have a Seniorline: a free national information service for senior citizens, their relatives, carers and friends: 0808 800 6565, Monday to Friday, 9.00am to 4.00pm. Calls are free of charge.

Incontact is an organization which supports the development of local self-help groups. It is based at St Pancras Hospital, London NW1 OPE.

Medical Devices Agency Hannibal House, Elephant and Castle, London SE 16 6TQ. Tel: 020 8268 4488. Reports of clinical trials of different products can be obtained free by health professionals.

Stroke Association Stroke House, Whitecross Street, London EC1Y 8JJ. Tel: 020 7490 7999.

Chapter

7

Monitoring vital signs

Sue Higham and Sue Maddex

This chapter discusses the measuring and recording of a person's vital signs, which are essential skills that all nurses should possess. These observations can help the nurse to establish a baseline, and to identify and monitor abnormalities, which might indicate disease or injury of a person. During any nursing observations, it is important to use effective non-verbal and verbal communication, and listening skills. This will help to ensure that the person is confident in your ability and trusts you to perform the techniques accurately. Uncertainty of your own skills may produce fear and anxiety in the person thus altering measurements of vital signs. Chapter 2 will assist you in considering your approach to the person whilst carrying out practical skills. It is also important that, when you have recorded observations, you report them to a senior member of the nursing team. This will ensure that any deficits and potential problems with the person's vital signs are addressed.

Included in this chapter are:
- ■ Measuring and recording temperature
- ■ Measuring and recording the pulse
- ■ Measuring and recording blood pressure
- ■ Neurological assessment.

Note that Chapter 8, Respiratory assessment and care, discusses the measurement and recording of a person's respiratory rate, and oxygen saturations via pulse oximetry, which are other important vital signs.

> ### Recommended biology reading
>
> The following questions will help you to focus on the biology underpinning this chapter's skills. Use your recommended text book to find out:
>
> - How is heat generated within the body?
> - How is heat lost by the body?
> - What happens if the body starts to get too hot or too cold?
> - Why do we appear flushed when too warm?
> - What are the components of the cardiovascular system?
> - Which vessels usually carry oxygenated blood?
> - Why does blood travel in one direction?
> - What are the names for the four chambers of the heart, the great vessels and valves? Draw a diagram of the heart and label these structures. Indicate the direction in which oxygenated and deoxygenated blood flows through the heart.
> - What are the layers of the heart wall and what tissue are they composed of?
> - How does the heart contract in such a co-ordinated way? Explore the route taken by impulses through the myocardium.
> - Myocardial tissue works very hard and needs its own blood supply. Where are the coronary vessels located and what would be the consequence of their blockage?
> - Compare the structure of arteries, capillaries and veins. Which vessels permit gaseous exchange and why? Which vessels contain valves?
> - When tissues are damaged, an inflammatory process is initiated to repair the damage. What are the signs of inflammation? What role does histamine play in inflammation? Why is inflammation of brain tissue potentially life-threatening?
> - What are the functions of blood? Find out the components of the blood. What roles do these components play?

PRACTICE SCENARIOS

Observation and recording of a person's vital signs is carried out for a variety of reasons. The following scenarios are used to assist you to relate your learning of these skills to patients/clients whom you might encounter in the practice setting.

■ **Adult**

Mr Ronald Atkinson is a 70-year-old man who is taken to the Accident and Emergency Unit by ambulance following a suspected **cerebrovascular**

Cerebrovascular accident (CVA)

Cerebral damage caused either by decreased blood flow or haemorrhage. Effects vary but often causes paralysis down one side of the body (hemiplegia), and speech and swallowing difficulty. Can affect level of consciousness. Commonly termed a 'stroke'

accident (CVA). He had been found on the floor at home. On his arrival, you take over his care. During his assessment you are required to observe and record his temperature, pulse and blood pressure, and perform a set of neurological observations. His family are present, and have said that he likes to be called Ron.

■ **Child**

Megan is an 11-month-old baby who has fallen down two steps of the stairs and hit her head. She is admitted to the children's ward for observation following her head injury. Megan's condition is stable but she appears drowsy at times. Megan's mother, Rebecca, says she was pale and floppy for a short while after the incident. Rebecca is resident with Megan in hospital.

■ **Learning disability**

Mr George Allen is a 60-year-old man with learning disabilities who lives in a staffed house in the community. He likes to be called George. He has epilepsy and following a prolonged fit today is just regaining consciousness. You are required to take over his care from a colleague at this point. Your colleague shows you his neurological chart and goes through how she has recorded his observations since his fit.

■ **Mental health**

Clare Woods aged 27 years is admitted to the acute mental health admission ward for opiate detoxification. The detoxification programme includes increasing doses of medication (lofexidine) to mask the effects of withdrawal from opiates. Clare's temperature, pulse and blood pressure are recorded on admission. Regular monitoring of Clare's blood pressure will be needed as lofexidine can result in hypotension (low blood pressure).

EQUIPMENT REQUIRED FOR THIS CHAPTER

Before embarking upon this chapter, find out what equipment is available locally within the skills laboratory or your practice area, for recording of vital signs. Look for:

■ **Thermometers**: may be mercury in glass, tympanic, electronic probes, and/or disposable.
■ **Sphygmomanometers**: electronic and/or manual.

Some of this equipment may be available for you to practise with, in the skills laboratory. You will also need a watch with a second hand, a pen torch, and observation charts, for temperature, pulse and blood pressure, and for neurological assessment. You may wish to work through the sections with a colleague so that you can practice this chapter's skills.

MEASURING AND RECORDING TEMPERATURE

Nurses frequently perform the measurement of temperature, as it is often important to assess whether body temperature is within the normal range. Body temperature results from a balance between heat production and heat loss (Marieb 1999). In health, various physiological and behavioural mechanisms operate to maintain the **core body temperature** (the temperature of the organs within the cranial, thoracic and abdominal cavities) within a range of 36–37.6°C (Brooker 1998). This process is called thermoregulation, and is controlled by the hypothalamus, which acts as a thermostat (Hinchliff 1996). There may be times when this process is ineffective, for a variety of reasons. Body temperature which is higher than 37°C (usually 37.2–41°C) is known as a **pyrexia**, and if a person's body temperature is lower than 35°C, this is termed **hypothermia**.

Learning outcomes

By the end of this section you will be able to:

1. Explain the rationale for monitoring temperature.
2. Identify the sites and equipment used for measuring temperature.
3. Accurately measure a person's temperature.

Learning outcome 1:
Explain the rationale for monitoring temperature

A person's body temperature is measured by a thermometer in degrees Celsius, and the reading can be used to identify disease or dysfunction.

Activity	What factors can you think of that might influence a person's body temperature?

You may have identified the following factors:

Age
The newborn's ability to regulate temperature is not fully developed as a consequence of a number of factors. A relatively thin subcutaneous fat layer, providing little insulation, and a higher ratio of surface area to body weight, combine to increase the potential for heat loss. The inability to shiver of the new born reduces their capacity to generate heat (Mohammed 2000). Once fully developed, the individual's ability to respond appropriately to temperature

changes decreases with age. Socio-economic problems or underlying disease, such as muscle weakness, arthritis or myxoedema, may exacerbate this trend (Hinchliff 1996).

Environment

If thermoregulation is impaired, the person becomes susceptible to overheating or cooling. This explains why some pre-term babies may need to be nursed in a highly regulated environment such as an incubator. Excessively high environmental temperature may lead to heat exhaustion. People with impaired cognitive function or perceptual disturbance may be unable to recognize and respond appropriately to changes in environmental temperature, for example by going out inadequately dressed in cold weather.

Level of physical activity

Brooker (1996) explains how muscular activity can produce heat energy which is used by the body to maintain the body's temperature. Intense muscular contraction, such as shivering, produces a large amount of heat (Brooker 1998), and is thus a common response to cold, being an attempt by the body to raise its temperature.

Metabolic rate

The body's metabolic processes are a source of heat production. People with an excessive metabolic rate, for example those with an overactive thyroid gland, may have a higher than normal body temperature (Edwards 1997). Likewise, low metabolic rates may cause low body temperatures.

Time of day

Body temperatures normally fall during sleep, so tend to be lowest at night, and rise during the day, peaking in the early evening (Edwards 1997).

Drugs

Alcohol diminishes perception of cold, impairs shivering and causes vasodilation, thus predisposing to a lowering of body temperature. Sedative and narcotic drugs reduce the perception of cold, reducing the likelihood of appropriate behavioural responses (Fritsch 1995).

Infection

One of the body's responses to infection is to raise body temperature above its normal value. In effect the thermostat of the hypothalamus is reset, resulting in increased heat production and inhibition of heat loss (Hinchliff 1996).

Activity Bearing in mind the above points, identify the reasons why you might record the person's temperature in each of the scenarios.

Chemical disposable thermometers
These may be used in the mouth or axilla. They are thin plastic strips that have 50 small dots of thermosensitive chemicals that change colour with increasing temperature (Torrance and Semple 1998a). As these are disposed of after use there is no risk of cross-infection.

Electronic thermometers
These consist of a probe which may be placed in the mouth, in the axilla or in the rectum, usually connected to a power supply and display unit. The purchase cost is significant, as are the ongoing costs of probe covers needed for each use. Most have a signal which operates when the maximum temperature is reached (Edwards 1997), so this should improve accuracy over mercury in glass thermometers.

Infrared light reflectance thermometers
These detect heat radiated as infrared energy from the tympanic membrane. The temperature registers within a few seconds, causing very little inconvenience or discomfort to the person (Edwards 1997). There is ongoing debate about the accuracy of these infrared devices in some circumstances. For example, in a study on a neonatal unit, Leick-Rude and Bloom (1998) found that tympanic thermometers were excessively influenced by environmental factors, such as overhead heaters. However, Schmitz et al. (1995) suggest that their use is effective in pyrexial people, and they highlight their accuracy in measuring temperatures of 38°C and above. The use of disposable probe covers prevents cross-infection, but adds to the ongoing costs in use.

Activity

Which method and site do you think is most appropriate for each of the people in the scenarios, and why?

Compare your answers with the points below:

Adult

For Ron, it would be safest to use a tympanic thermometer at this stage, due to his possible CVA. A thermometer would not be used in the mouth as Ron may have difficulty keeping this in place, due to facial weakness which may have occurred as a result of his CVA. However, a thermometer (either disposable or mercury in glass) could be used in the axilla, but he may need help to keep his arm in position for the required time. Each device would give an accurate assessment of Ron's temperature providing it is used as per manufacturer's instructions.

Child

Using an infrared thermometer and the tympanic membrane are likely to cause least distress to Megan. This method is very rapid and does not require any co-operation on her part. Care should be taken if Megan has been lying with her head on one side as this may give a higher reading in that ear, and the presence of wax in the ear canal can result in lower readings (Flo and Brown 1995). Correct positioning of the probe is essential for accuracy. Alternatively a chemical disposable thermometer or electronic probe in the axilla may be appropriate, although Megan may resist being held still for the length of time necessary. It would be dangerous to use mercury in glass because of the risk of breakage if Megan struggles. Megan is too young to understand how to co-operate when having her temperature measured by the oral route. As discussed earlier, the rectal route is not used in children except in exceptional circumstances.

Learning disability

George's temperature should be measured in the axilla using either a chemical disposable or electronic thermometer. A mercury in glass thermometer would need to be used with great care, as there is a potential risk of the glass thermometer being broken if George moves suddenly. The oral route is inappropriate as George may clench his teeth if he has a further fit or if he is confused as he regains consciousness. Alternatively an infrared tympanic thermometer could be used but as George is not in a hospital, electronic and infrared thermometers may not be available. Measuring a temperature rectally is invasive and therefore not performed unless a highly accurate reading is required, so it is unlikely that this route would be used.

Mental health

Clare's temperature could be recorded either tympanically, if an infrared thermometer is available, or orally using the mercury in glass thermometer or a disposable thermometer.

Learning outcome 3:
Accurately measure a person's temperature

Oral measurement

<table>
<tr>
<td>■ Activity</td>
<td>Find a willing volunteer with whom to practice this activity. You will need a clean mercury in glass thermometer, and a chemical disposable thermometer from the skills laboratory. Carefully work through the instructions in Box 7.1.</td>
</tr>
</table>

When recording an oral temperature there are a number of other considerations too.

<table>
<tr>
<td>■ Activity</td>
<td>List the factors that you think might affect the accuracy of oral temperature measurements.</td>
</tr>
</table>

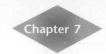
Explain the procedure to the person, including the need to keep lips closed whilst the thermometer is in position.

Using a mercury in glass thermometer

- Holding the thermometer horizontally at eye level, rotate it slightly between thumb and forefinger so that the silver column of mercury can be seen clearly.
- Check that the mercury is below the level at which the numbers start. If not, shake the thermometer in a downward direction, and check again.
- Position the thermometer (bulb first) under the person's tongue to the side; see diagram below for correct positioning.

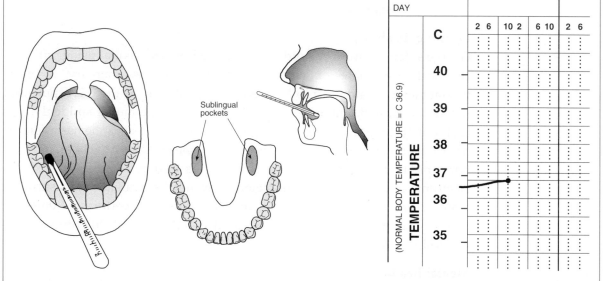

- Ask the person to hold the thermometer in place with lips closed.
- Keep the thermometer in position for a minimum of two minutes (Torrance and Semple 1998b). This should be timed with a watch, not guessed.
- Remove the thermometer and, holding it at eye level, read at the level to which the mercury has risen.
- Record the measurement on an observation chart, as per example above, of a temperature of 36.8°C. Report abnormal temperatures. Clean the thermometer thoroughly according to the local infection control policy in your practice area.

Using a disposable thermometer

- Position the plastic strip in your partner's mouth (as for the glass thermometer), with the face with the dots on (dot matrix) either way up for one minute (Torrance and Semple 1998b).
- Remove the thermometer and read the measurement by counting the number of dots that have changed colour. Dispose of the plastic strip.
- Record the measurement on an observation chart as above.

Box 7.1 Oral temperature measurement

You might have thought of the following:

- Eating or drinking hot or cold substances shortly before the procedure.
- Smoking.
- Talking.
- Breathing through the mouth.
- Incorrect positioning of the thermometer.
- Thermometer in the mouth for the incorrect time.

It is suggested that an oral temperature should not be recorded within 15 minutes of the client eating, drinking or smoking (Torrance and Semple 1998b). The time a mercury in glass thermometer should be left in place is controversial. Torrance and Semple (1998b) recommend a minimum of 2 minutes, whereas Edwards (1997) cites studies recommending times ranging from no more than 3 minutes (Pugh-Davies *et al.* 1986) to 8–9 minutes (Nichols and Kucha 1972).

Activity

If you wish to verify or challenge any of these authors for yourself, try taking your temperature with a mercury in glass thermometer at one minute intervals, from 2–7 minutes. You won't need to shake the thermometer down in between each recording, just read it and put it back in your mouth for a further minute. Does it actually make a difference to the reading? A further exercise to try, is to take your temperature just after a hot or cold drink, and see for yourself how this might affect the recording.

Axilla measurements

Activity

Now try using a chemical disposable or mercury in glass thermometer to measure a temperature in the axilla, using the instructions in Box 7.2.

You might like to compare this reading with the previous oral measurement. Generally there is 0.5 degree Celsius difference, with the axilla being the lower reading (Hinchliff 1996).

Electronic devices

For instructions for using electronic thermometers *see* Box 7.3. You may be able to practice these if they are available. Note that the tympanic temperature should not be taken with a hearing aid in place.

Activity

Whilst using a thermometer will give you an accurate measurement of temperature, can you think of other observations which could help you to assess body temperature?

You might take note of the person's colour, whether he is pale or flushed in appearance. You might also observe whether the person has cold extremities

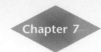
- Explain the procedure to the person, including the need to remain still whilst the thermometer is in position.
- Prepare glass thermometer as for oral temperature measurement (*see* Box 7.1).
- Raise the person's arm. Place the thermometer in the centre of the person's axilla (*see* diagram). If using a disposable thermometer, position it with the dot matrix against the torso (Torrance and Semple 1998b).
- Check to ensure that there is good contact with the skin when the arm is lowered.
- Rest the person's arm across the chest and maintain the thermometer in position for a minimum of 3 minutes for a chemical strip and 5 minutes for a mercury in glass thermometer (Torrance and Semple 1998b).
- Remove the thermometer, read and record the result as in Box 7.1. Report any abnormal readings.
- Dispose of the chemical thermometer, or clean and disinfect the glass thermometer according to local policy.

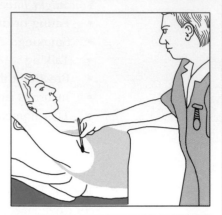

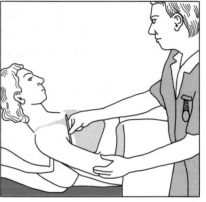

Box 7.2 Measurement of a temperature in the axilla, using a mercury in glass or a disposable thermometer

Using an electronic thermometer to record oral or axilla temperature
- The positioning of electronic probes in the mouth or the axilla is the same as for mercury in glass or chemical disposable thermometers.
- A new probe cover should be used for each person.
- Devices have either an auditory (e.g. bleeping sound) or visual (e.g. flashing) indicator when maximum temperature is reached; the probe should remain in place until this is noted.

Using an infrared tympanic membrane thermometer
- The speculum is covered with a disposable cover.
- The speculum is inserted gently into the ear canal.
- The reading is obtained within 1–2 seconds, indicated by a bleeping sound.

Box 7.3 Temperature measurement using the electronic thermometer and the tympanic thermometer

or feels hot to touch. You can observe whether the person is shivering or sweating, and ask him how he feels. It would be particularly important to use observational skills if the person is unable to communicate verbally about whether he feels cold or hot. Your observations may prompt you to record the person's temperature.

Summary

- Choice of route and method for measuring temperature should take into account individual factors such as age, and physical and mental condition, as well as the devices available in the particular practice setting.
- For each route and method, the measurement should be carried out and recorded carefully and accurately, and abnormal measurements should be reported, as action, e.g. administration of anti-pyretic medication, may be needed.

MEASURING AND RECORDING THE PULSE

Definition

The pulse is a pressure wave of blood caused by alternating expansion and recoil of elastic arteries during the cardiac cycle (Mallet and Bailey 1996). The pulse thus represents each ventricular contraction of the heart, which causes a rise in blood pressure and subsequent expansion of the arteries. In the healthy heart, one heartbeat corresponds to one pulse beat. However, disease and trauma can affect the cardiac cycle leading to a difference between the heart rate and the pulse rate. Marieb (1999) explains that the pulse rate is the number of beats of the heart in a 60-second period. The pulse is measured in time, using a watch, and is recorded as beats per minute. The rate of the person's pulse can differ with age, disease, medication and trauma.

Learning outcomes

By the end of this section you will be able to:

1. Explain the rationale for monitoring pulse rate.
2. Identify the normal values of the pulse for different age groups.
3. Locate pulses in different areas of the body, and identify which might be used in specific situations.
4. Accurately measure a person's pulse rate.

Learning outcome 1:
Explain the rationale for monitoring the pulse rate

Activity

Relook at the definition of a pulse, and then identify what feeling the pulse might actually tell you about the body.

The pulse is measured to identify the rate and strength of the ventricular contraction, and to gain information regarding the person's condition. For example, in the case of trauma and severe bleeding, the pulse rate might be weak and fast. When measuring a pulse, the following should be considered:

- **The frequency of the pulse.** This will indicate the rate of contraction of the left ventricle. This is affected by numerous factors such as age, exercise, stress, injury and disease. For example, a fever, an over-active thyroid gland and certain drugs will speed up the pulse, whilst an under-active thyroid gland, hypothermia and other drugs will slow the pulse.
- **The volume.** This indicates the strength of the ventricular contraction. For example, a weak contraction will produce a pulse which feels weak, or it may not be strong enough to produce a pulse at the periphery, such as the wrist, at all. A weak pulse may also be present when there is a lack of blood volume.
- **The rhythm.** This helps to establish if the heart is beating regularly. An irregular pulse indicates a possible abnormality in conduction of the impulse within the heart.

Note that the thickness and tension of the arteriole walls are other factors influencing the pulse. Atherosclerosis is present in many people over the age of 40 years. This degenerative process can result in structural changes in the arteries. Brooker (1996) identifies how this common disease affects the elasticity of the arteries, and this can alter the pulse rate of a person. As can be seen, then, measuring the pulse can provide very useful information about health status. As with temperature, it will be recorded on admission to hospital as a baseline, and subsequent readings may occur to monitor a person's condition.

Learning outcome 2:
Identify the normal values for the pulse for different age groups

Activity

Discuss with a colleague what might be the normal range of pulse rates for the following age groups:

- Less than 3 months
- 3 months–24 months
- 2–10 years
- Child over 10 years
- Adulthood.

The normal adult heart rate ranges from 60–100 beats per minute (Herbert and Alison 1996). For children's values, see Table 7.1. As you may have known, the younger the person, the faster the pulse rate. It is important to be aware of these expected ranges when assessing an individual's pulse rate. Note also that the heart rate diminishes by 10–20 beats per minute during sleep (Herbert and Alison 1996).

Table 7.1 Normal heart rate ranges for different age groups (Rudolph and Levene 1999, p. 33)

Age group	Beats per minute
Less than 3 months	100–180
3–24 months	80–150
2–10 years	70–110
Child over 10 years	55–90

Useful terms

- The term used for a pulse which is considered abnormally slow is **bradycardia**. In an adult this would usually be a pulse rate below 60 beats per minute.
- The term used for an abnormally fast pulse is **tachycardia**. This would usually be a pulse rate above 110 beats per minute in an adult (Wilson and Waugh 1996).

Learning outcome 3:
Locate pulses in different areas of the body, and identify which might be used in specific situations

Activity

Below is a list of pulses that can be palpated, which are illustrated in Figure 7.1. See how many you can find on yourself.

- Temporal artery, on the side of the forehead
- Facial artery, on the side of the face
- Carotid artery, located at the neck
- Brachial artery – in the antecubital fossa of the arm
- Radial artery – at the wrist
- Femoral artery – in the groin
- Popliteal artery – behind the knee
- Posterior tibial artery – at the inner side of each ankle

Note that the apex beat can be listened to with a stethoscope, and is located to the left side of the sternum over the heart.

It is important to know the sites where a pulse may be identified. A pulse can be found wherever an artery near the surface of the body is pressed against a firm surface such as a bone. The light pressure which you apply to the skin when feeling for a pulse is called **palpation**.

257

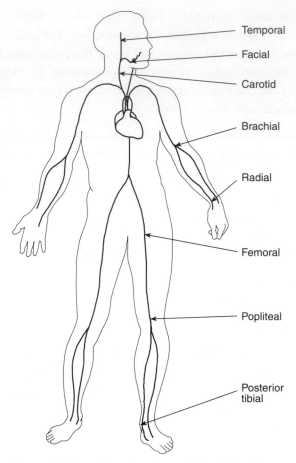

Temporal

Facial

Carotid

Brachial

Radial

Femoral

Popliteal

Posterior
tibial

Figure 7.1 Location of pulses within the body

As you will have found, some of these pulses are easier to palpate and more accessible than others, and therefore some are used more often by nurses, depending on the individual and the situation. Discussed below are the probable sites which might be used for the people in the scenarios.

Adult

Ron's pulse would probably be taken at the wrist (the radial pulse), which is where, in a non-emergency situation, the pulse is usually recorded in an adult. This is because of the ease of access to the site for the nurse and the person having his pulse recorded, and the procedure is less invasive when it is taken here. In an emergency situation, for example a collapsed person where there could be respiratory or cardiac arrest, it is often difficult to locate the peripheral pulses (e.g. the radial pulse). The carotid pulse is then used as this is closest to the person's heart and therefore, usually the last to cease. See basic life support guidelines (Webb *et al.* 1997) for further discussion regarding checking the carotid pulse in an emergency.

Child

Moules and Ramsay (1998) highlight that a child's pulse can be difficult to feel. With a young child such as Megan, who is under the age of 2 years, nurses would most likely record her apex by listening through a stethoscope. This is because young children are often reluctant to be held still for the 60 seconds required for an accurate pulse measurement. The radial pulse or brachial pulse is used for children over 2 years.

Learning disabilities

While George is unconscious, it might be easiest to feel his carotid pulse at his neck, but otherwise the radial pulse could be used.

Mental health

It will be most appropriate to take Clare's radial pulse, as she is a fully alert adult.

With all individuals, psychological state needs to be considered, and co-operation sought, prior to measuring the pulse. This would involve explaining why the pulse needs to be measured. It may be difficult to palpate some pulse sites in people with contractures. The individual must be assessed to identify which sites are the most comfortable. Note that pulses in the lower leg are usually only palpated when assessing the presence of circulation to the limb. This might be after trauma or surgery.

Learning outcome 4:
Accurately measure a person's pulse rate

Activity

You need a willing volunteer, a watch with a second hand, or a digital watch, and an observation chart from your skills laboratory. Now follow the steps in Box 7.4 to measure and record the radial pulse.

Note that when measuring the pulse rate, nurses may often count the pulse for 15 seconds and multiply by four, or for 30 seconds and multiply by two. With a regular pulse this will give a reasonably accurate measurement, but an irregular pulse should always be counted for a full minute. In children too, it is recommended that the pulse is always counted for a whole minute (Moules and Ramsay 1998). An irregular pulse rate will usually be due to an abnormality in the conduction system of the heart, and the word 'irregular' should be written by the rate.

Activity

Now ask your volunteer to jog on the spot for one minute and record the pulse again after this time. You will probably find that her/his pulse rate has risen. This is because the pulse rate rises during exercise, due to the extra oxygen demands. Can you remember any other reasons why the pulse may be faster in a healthy person?

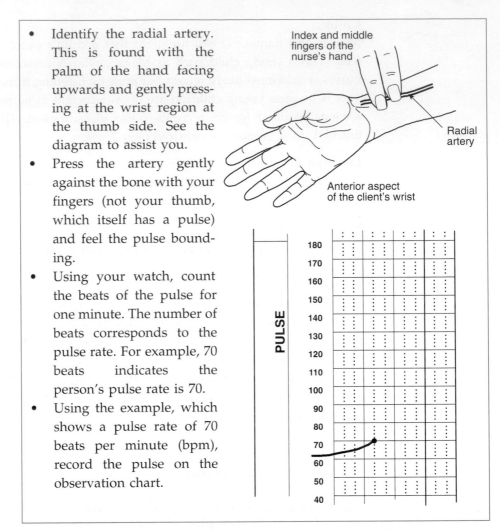

- Identify the radial artery. This is found with the palm of the hand facing upwards and gently pressing at the wrist region at the thumb side. See the diagram to assist you.
- Press the artery gently against the bone with your fingers (not your thumb, which itself has a pulse) and feel the pulse bounding.
- Using your watch, count the beats of the pulse for one minute. The number of beats corresponds to the pulse rate. For example, 70 beats indicates the person's pulse rate is 70.
- Using the example, which shows a pulse rate of 70 beats per minute (bpm), record the pulse on the observation chart.

Box 7.4 Measuring a radial pulse

Anxiety or stress will also raise the pulse rate. Thus Ron's pulse rate could be raised, due to the stress of being brought into hospital, and the anxiety about what is happening to him. Clare could be anxious as she is in a new environment and is about to undergo the detoxification process, so her pulse could be raised too. As discussed at the start of this chapter, you will need to put patients/clients at ease, thus trying to relieve some anxiety and gaining an accurate measurement.

Electronic measurement of the pulse rate

A range of equipment is available which will electronically record the pulse rate. This includes:

- The **electronic sphygmomanometer** (discussed in the next section): as well as giving a blood pressure reading, a pulse rate will usually be displayed too.
- The **pulse oximeter** (as discussed in Chapter 8): as well as measuring oxygen saturation, the pulse rate is usually displayed.
- The **cardiac monitor**: this will display the heart rate which, as we have discussed, will usually reflect the pulse rate.

Whilst all this equipment will give you a pulse measurement, it will not indicate either the volume of the pulse or its regularity. With the pulse oximeter and cardiac monitor, movement of the person can cause artefact, which leads to an inaccurate reading.

Summary

- Measuring a person's pulse is minimally invasive and uses little equipment but is a useful vital sign, giving a helpful insight into a person's health status.
- Nurses need to be able to palpate a range of pulses, and be aware of which pulse would be appropriate to measure for different age groups and in different situations.
- When measuring pulses, it is important to be aware of the normal range, and to assess the volume and regularity of the pulse as well as the rate.

MEASURING AND RECORDING BLOOD PRESSURE

Definition

Blood pressure is the force exerted by the blood on the walls of the vessels in which it is contained (Jolly 1991). The hydrostatic pressure (i.e. pressure in fluid) is measured using a manometer (i.e. an instrument for measuring pressure). In this instance, the pressure of blood is measured in the arteries using a sphygmomanometer (Marieb 1999). Blood pressure is measured in millimetres of mercury (mmHg).

Learning outcomes

By the end of this section you will be able to:
1. Identify the equipment used for blood pressure readings and the meaning of the reading obtained.
2. Identify the normal values for blood pressure, and factors affecting blood pressure readings.
3. Accurately measure a person's blood pressure using manual equipment.

Learning outcome 1:
Identify the equipment used for blood pressure readings and the meaning of the reading obtained

Activity

What sort of equipment have you seen used to measure blood pressures? If you are not familiar with the sphygmomanometer, try to access one in the skills laboratory or your practice placement, and if possible, look at electronic equipment too.

Equipment

The two main ways of measuring blood pressure are:

- Indirectly by use of electronic monitoring for example, a doppler. This is a machine which is attached to the patient's arm by means of a cuff. This is inflated automatically by the machine, which then reads the pressure within the artery. The result is displayed on the machine as two readings, the systolic and the diastolic. Some machines also display mean arterial pressure (MAP), which is the mean blood pressure during the reading.
- A more conventional method of blood pressure recording is carried out by the use of a stethoscope and mercury sphygmomanometer. Blood pressures were traditionally recorded manually this way, but in acute settings they are increasingly recorded electronically. However, nurses need to learn how to record a blood pressure manually, as electronic devices are not always available, particularly in community and non-acute settings.

As already mentioned, a blood pressure reading has two values, the systolic and the diastolic.

Systolic

This is the maximum pressure of the blood against the wall of the artery, and occurs during ventricular contraction. This is recorded as the top figure when documenting the blood pressure.

Diastolic

This is the minimum pressure of the blood against the wall of the artery, which occurs following closure of the aortic valve. This measurement, there-fore, assesses the pressure when the ventricles are at rest. This is recorded as the bottom figure when documenting a blood pressure.

Thus a recording of blood pressure recorded as 120/70, means that the systolic pressure is 120 mmHg, and the diastolic pressure is 70 mmHg.

Learning outcome 2:

Identify the normal values for blood pressure, and factors affecting blood pressure readings

Normal values

When measuring blood pressure, as with any other signs, it is important to be aware of expected normal ranges. However, O'Brien *et al.* (1997) consider that there is no such thing as a normal blood pressure as it can vary greatly between one person and another. They suggest, however, that the normal adult blood pressure ranges from 100/60 to 150/90. The two readings of diastolic and systolic should be judged as one reading to identify a person's blood pressure. The term used for a high blood pressure is **hypertension** and the term used for a low blood pressure is **hypotension**. Hypotension is often considered to be when the systolic blood pressure falls below 80–60 mmHg, while a systolic reading of over 180 mmHg, would usually be considered as hypertension. The physiological changes which occur during hypotension and hypertension are outlined by Brooker (1996) and Marieb (1999). In children the blood pressure varies with the size and age of the child. See Table 7.2. for childrens values.

Table 7.2 Typical childhood blood pressure readings in mmHg (from Hull and Johnstone, 1999, p. 357)

Age	Systolic	Diastolic
Neonate	60 85	35 57
Infant (6 months)	75–110	40–70
Toddler (2 years)	75–110	45–80
School age (7-year-old)	75–115	50–80
Adolescent (15-year-old)	100–145	60–95

Factors affecting blood pressure readings

Activity

Consider the scenarios at the start of this chapter. What factors can you identify which might affect these patients'/clients' blood pressure readings?

Physiological and genetic factors are all thought to influence the blood pressure (Montague 1996), but psychological and environmental issues also have an effect. You may have identified that both Ron and Clare have been admitted to a strange hospital environment which may induce anxiety and distress, and therefore increase their blood pressure (as well as their pulse, as discussed earlier). You may have been aware that ageing can also increase blood pressure, so men of Ron's and George's age, would be likely to have a higher blood pressure than Clare, while Megan's expected blood pressure would be lower still. You might have considered that both disease and injury (such as Ron's CVA, and Megan's head injury) could affect blood pressure, and that medication, e.g. Clare's lofexidine but many other drugs besides, could also be an influence. Some of the numerous factors which can affect blood pressure are discussed below.

■ **Blood volume**. When a patient suffers severe blood loss due to trauma or disease, blood volume drops, and consequently the blood pressure.

■ **Age**. During the ageing process, arteries often lose their elasticity and therefore an alteration in blood pressure may be found (Brooker 1996).

■ **Disease**. Elasticity of the arteries is affected directly by diseases such as atherosclerosis. Coronary artery disease will increase blood pressure (O'Brien *et al*. 1997, Brooker 1996). There are also many other diseases which may lower or higher blood pressure, ranging from heart and kidney disease, to neurological conditions, for example, a CVA, as experienced by Ron.

■ **Gravity**. A change in a person's postural position may affect the blood pressure. For example, if a person is lying down and stands up quickly, the blood pressure may fall. This is termed **orthostatic hypotension**.

■ **Drug usage**. Certain therapeutic drugs which are prescribed for the person may affect blood pressure.

■ **Environmental factors**. For example hospitalization, and its associated fear and anxiety, can all contribute to a change in blood pressure (Millar-Craig *et al*. 1978).

■ **Psychological factors, e.g. 'white coat hypertension'**. This phenomenon is associated with people feeling anxious when discussing issues with doctors and nurses, which may lead to a false reading when the blood pressure is recorded. Excitement will cause an increase in the heart rate, which in turn increases the blood pressure.

■ **Time of day**. The blood pressure is known to be lowest in the morning and then rises throughout the day reaching its peak in the afternoon, and then falls in the evening. O'Brien *et al*. (1997) highlight the importance of remembering these factors when recording the blood pressure.

■ **Weight**. An obese person's heart may have to work harder and so the blood pressure may be higher (Jolly 1991).

■ **Diet**. High salt and low calcium dietary intakes may lead to a rise in blood pressure (Millar-Craig *et al*. 1978).

Finally, faulty equipment and poor technique can affect blood pressure readings. This is discussed in Learning outcome 3.

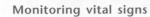
Learning outcome 3:

Accurately measure a person's blood pressure using manual equipment

Activity

Join with a colleague or work alone to identify sites for recording the blood pressure. Look back to the areas where a pulse can be found. Bearing in mind the need to attach a cuff above an artery, which arteries do you think the blood pressure could be measured from?

Any of the following arteries could be used:

- **The brachial artery.** The pulse is situated in the antecubital fossa, where the upper arm meets the lower arm at the elbow joint when the palm of the hand is uppermost. The cuff would be placed around the upper arm.
- **The radial artery.** The pulse is found where the wrist meets the palm of the hand on the side of the thumb, as already palpated in the previous section. The cuff would be placed around the lower arm.
- **The popliteal artery.** The pulse is to be found behind the knee. The cuff would be placed around the thigh.
- **The posterior tibial artery.** The pulse can be palpated where your ankle meets the inside of your foot just at your heel. The cuff would be placed around the calf or ankle.

As you have seen, blood pressure can be measured from a number of sites but in the majority of clinical situations, the brachial artery is used as it is convenient for the patient and easily accessible for the nurse. Some of the newer electronic devices measure blood pressure at the radial artery. It is advisable to avoid recording the blood pressure on an arm which is affected by disability (e.g. weakness due to a CVA), or where an intravenous infusion is *in situ*. When a person has suffered trauma or surgery which has affected both arms, the thigh may be used. In this instance, a larger cuff will be needed.

Errors in taking blood pressure

Although blood pressure recordings are frequently carried out in practice, they remain a contentious issue. O'Brien *et al.* (1997), in their British Hypertension Study, highlighted how health professionals may incorrectly record blood pressure due to faulty techniques and/or equipment. They note that controversy exists over when to record the diastolic pressure. This relates to the sounds termed Korotkoff sounds, which, when you are manually recording a blood pressure, are the sounds heard through the stethoscope (*see* Table 7.3). They are named after Nikolia Korotkoff who first identified the audible sounds of blood pressure in 1905 (Korotkoff 1905, cited by O'Brien 1997). In general, phase one is heard around 120 mmHg (systolic), and the sounds

Table 7.3 Korotkoff sounds (Kortkoff 1905, cited by O'Brien *et al.* 1997)

Phase	Sound	When they are normally heard
One	Clear tapping	Usually above 120 mmHg
Two	Blowing or whistling	Around 110 mmHg
Three	Soft thud	Around 100 mmHg
Four	Low pitched, muffled sound	Around 90 mmHg
Five	Disappearance of all sounds	Around 80 mmHg

disappear at around 80 mmHg (diastolic). However, as noted previously, these measurements vary greatly between individuals.

The main area of debate is whether the diastolic should be recorded at phase 4 or phase 5. Generally it seems preferred to measure it at phase 5. However, it is important to identify the local policy within your clinical practice area, to ensure that all recordings are done accurately and using the same approach. Note that in some individuals, there may be no phase five i.e. the beat does not disappear, so then the diastolic should be recorded at phase four. Children's blood pressure is sometimes measured at the fourth stage (Second Task Force for BP Control in Children 1987).

Accuracy in measurement is important because human or mechanical error in recording blood pressure can affect the person's future management. Shown in table 7.4 are possible problems which you may encounter and how to resolve them. Every effort must be made to reduce these errors so that blood pressure monitoring is accurate.

Table 7.4 Common problems with blood pressure measurement, and suggested solutions (O'Brien *et al.* 1997)

Problem	Solution
Incorrect blood pressure reading.	Ensure that the measurement is made to the nearest 2 mmHg.
Incorrect size and position of cuff for the patient.	Use the appropriate size of cuff for the individual. The cuff bladder (insert of cuff) should cover 80% of the arm's circumference. A too large or too small cuff will give a false reading.
Confusion about diastolic blood pressure reading.	Diastolic measurement taken at cessation of sounds.
Poorly maintained equipment causing errors in measurement.	Ensure that the manometer mercury is visible at zero and that the machine is calibrated according to the manufacturers' instructions. The tubing and all connections should be carefully checked prior to use.

1. Allow the person to sit down and relax, for 5–15 minutes if possible, prior to the recording.
2. Collect and check equipment – stethoscope and sphygmomanometer. Ensure that the tubing, bladder and cuff are intact.
3. Explain what you are going to do, to assist in allaying anxiety, and try to promote comfort and privacy.
4. Position arm on secure surface where it is in line with the person's heart (*see* diagram).
5. Locate the brachial artery with your fingers and palpate to identify the pulse.
6. Place the cuff on the arm 2.5 cm above the brachial artery.
7. Ensure that the cuff fits snugly to the arm and is secured. It is advised that the cuff bladder (the insert of the cuff, made of rubber) should cover 80% of the circumference of the upper arm. The average arm circumference is 30 cm. This needs to be considered when choosing a cuff for your client. The measurement of a cuff should be clearly visible on each cuff you use in practice. The following sizes are suggested as a guide:
   - a standard bladder 12 by 26 cm is suitable for the majority of adults.
   - an obese bladder 12 by 40 cm for obese arms.
   - a small bladder measuring 10 by 18 cm for lean adults and children.

   NB – the sizes offered are to be used as a guide only. Each person's arm measurements are different and it is important that you seek the advice of a qualified nurse to ensure the correct choice is made. The sizes indicate the size of the bladder within the velcro fastening or wrap around cuff used in practice.

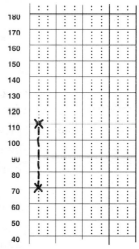

8. Whilst palpating the radial pulse, inflate the cuff until the pulse disappears. Note the level at which this occurs, as this equates to the systolic pressure.
9. Deflate the cuff fully and wait one minute.
10. Place the stethoscope over the brachial pulse.
11. Inflate the cuff, to 30 mmHg above your estimated systolic measurement, and then start to deflate slowly, listening carefully.
12. When you hear the first sound, note the measurement on the column of mercury in front of you. This is the systolic blood pressure – the top number.
13. Continue listening whilst deflating the cuff. Note the changing sounds. When the sound disappears completely, this is the diastolic blood pressure – the bottom number.
14. Record the results on your observation chart (as shown) and interpret the results. i.e. consider whether the blood pressure is high (hypertension) or low (hypotension) or within the normal range for the person.

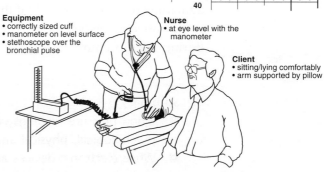

Equipment
- correctly sized cuff
- manometer on level surface
- stethoscope over the bronchial pulse

Nurse
- at eye level with the manometer

Client
- sitting/lying comfortably
- arm supported by pillow

Box 7.5 Steps in manually recording a blood pressure (adapted from O'Brien *et al*. 1997; Maslen 1995; Jolly 1991)

Steps in recording blood pressure

 Activity

If you can access manual blood pressure recording equipment – a sphygmomanometer and a stethoscope – work with a colleague, and practise taking and recording a blood pressure using the steps in taking a manual blood pressure as found in Box 7.5.

Note that in the practice setting, recording a blood pressure may be more difficult than with your healthy volunteer. Some patients may have difficulty in straightening their arms, or may have pulses which are difficult to find. Always ask for supervision when needed.

Recording children's blood pressure

The most important factor in accurate blood pressure recording in children is the cuff size (Moules and Ramsay 1998). When recording a child's blood pressure, a cuff should be used which has an inflatable bladder long enough to cover the whole length of the upper arm (Second Task Force for BP Control in Children 1987). The size of cuff used should be recorded, so that if serial readings are taken the same size cuff is used on each occasion, enabling reliable comparisons to be made.

When recording blood pressure in children, the steps in Box 7.5 will apply. However, it may be difficult to hear a young child's blood pressure with a stethoscope, and this difficulty is increased by the fact that the young child is unlikely to remain still for long (Fearon 2000a). Electronic oscillometric blood pressure devices are therefore commonly used in children. However, it should be remembered that movement may also adversely affect these readings. It is important to explain to the child what will happen during the procedure. A demonstration on a parent or carer may help the toddler or pre-school child to understand the procedure and what is expected of him/her, thus enhancing co-operation. Megan may have her blood pressure recorded once only on admission or more frequently if this reading causes concern. She may be most co-operative if she has the reassurance of sitting securely on a parent's knee during the procedure.

Summary

- Blood pressure readings can be affected by a number of factors, psychological, physical and environmental.
- While electronic devices are increasingly used for recording blood pressure, an understanding of how to accurately use manual equipment remains important for nurses.

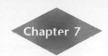

NEUROLOGICAL ASSESSMENT

Extra-dural haematoma

This is an accumulation of blood between the dura and the skull. The meningeal artery passes through the extra-dural space, and can become torn after a head injury, resulting in an arterial bleed into the extra-dural space. The brain then becomes compressed and displaced. This is a serious life-threatening condition, requiring urgent treatment.

Sub-dural haematoma

Here, blood accumulates in the sub-dural space and gradually builds up to produce a haematoma. This can lead to compression of the brain which in turn can result in loss of brain function.

Neurological observations are performed in order to assess a person's neurological status. Assessment can help to identify a neurological problem, establish what impact a neurological condition has on a person's independence or life activities, assist in establishing a baseline assessment of neurological function, determine any changes in neurological condition, and detect any life-threatening situations (Aucken and Crawford 1998). This is particularly important where there is a concern about the development of **raised intracranial pressure** (*see* Box 7.6). Being a rigid vault, the skull (cranium) cannot accommodate any swelling without impairing the function of the brain. In disease or injury, the brain tissue, blood or cerebral spinal fluid (CSF) can become increased in volume or size, causing a rise in intracranial pressure. This adversely affects cerebral blood flow (Winkelman 1995).

Neurological observation comprises an evaluation of the level of consciousness, pupil reaction, motor and sensory function and vital signs (i.e. pulse, blood pressure, temperature and respiration). This enables health-care professionals to make decisions regarding treatment, diagnosis and prognosis of the person in their care. Note that in some situations, particularly head injury, where an **extra-dural** or **sub-dural haematoma** can form rapidly, the observation of a deteriorating consciousness level is paramount, as life-saving treatment could be needed. Neurological observations should be carried out under supervision by the registered nurse, and any concerns reported immediately.

- Level of consciousness: Decrease in arousal and awareness. This is the most sensitive indicator of neurological function.
- Increasing headache.
- Pupils: enlargement, asymmetry, oval shape, decreased reaction. A new unilateral, dilated fixed pupil is a medical emergency.
- Slowing of the pulse rate: this is a late sign.
- Respirations: Abnormal or irregular pattern.
- Raised systolic blood pressure.
- Limb movements: variable responses.

If any of the above changes occur it is extremely important that you report these immediately to a qualified nurse or doctor.

Box 7.6 Signs of raised intracranial pressure (Winkelman 1995)

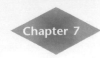

Learning outcomes:

By the end of this section you will be able to:

1. Have an understanding of when a neurological assessment would be needed, and what instruments are used.
2. Accurately perform and record an assessment of an adult's neurological status.
3. Show awareness of how neurological assessment can be carried out with children, and the special considerations which are necessary.

Learning outcome 1:
Have an understanding of when a neurological assessment would be needed, and what instruments are used

When a neurological assessment is needed

Activity

When might nurses perform a neurological assessment? Consideration of the practice scenarios will help you.

Meningitis
Inflammation of the meninges (the membranes surrounding the brain and spinal cord), usually due to infection.

A neurological assessment would be appropriate whenever there is impaired consciousness, a history of loss of consciousness, or a risk that the level of consciousness might deteriorate. The scenarios give you examples here: Megan has a head injury, Ron has had a suspected cerebrovascular accident, and George has had a fit. Other examples would include meningitis and poisoning.

Instruments used to assess neurological status

The Glasgow coma score (GCS) (Jennet and Teasdale 1974) is one of several neurological assessment tools available. It is widely used and recognized, and is often incorporated into the trauma assessment chart; Skinner *et al.* (1992) demonstrate this application in their trauma guidelines. Hudak and Gallo (1994) state that the GCS is a quick guide for evaluation of the acutely ill. There are, however, other scales available, e.g. Lowry (1998) describes an alternative instrument for observation in people with actual or suspected neurological dysfunction. *See* later section on Neurological assessment of children for details of the coma scales used with children.

Activity

If possible, find out what neurological observation scale is used in your local practice area.

As the GCS is currently the most widely used neurological assessment tool, this will now be focused on.

The GCS is used to assist the nurse in providing a consistent and standard measurement of the person's neurological state. It was developed by Jennet and Teasdale in 1974 and has become recognised for its value in adult assessment (Hudak and Gallo 1994). Scoring using the GCS is done in the form of a graph in three sections. These are eye opening, motor response and verbal response (*see* Fig. 7.2). Each activity is given a score and the best patient response equals 15 and the poorest response equals 3. The severity of a head injury can be indicated by the score attained (Jennet and Teasdale 1974). A score of less than 8 indicates a severe head injury where the person is in a coma. More than 8 indicates that the person is conscious. People with a minor head injury might have a score of 13 15. The GCS's use in people with head injuries is well documented, but it can be used for anyone who requires a neurological assessment, regardless of the underlying cause.

	Time				
Eyes open	Spontaneously	4			
	To speech	3			
	To pain	2			
	None	1			
Verbal response	Orientated, converses	5			
	Disorientated, converses	4			
	Inappropriate words	3			
	Incomprehensible sounds	2			
	No response	1			
Best motor response	Obey commands	6			
	Localizes pain	5			
	Withdraws from pain	4			
	Abnormal flexion	3			
	Abnormal extension	2			
	None	1			
	GCS score				

Figure 7.2 The Glasgow Coma Scale

Learning outcome 2:
Accurately perform and record an assessment of an adult's neurological status

Remember that priorities when assessing any person in your care must first lie with checking response, airway, breathing and circulation (Webb *et al.*

1997), and either maintaining or establishing these, before moving on to assess the person neurologically.

History

During the examination and assessment, it is important to quickly establish if the person lost consciousness at any stage and appears to be deteriorating. Hickey (1997) highlights the importance of finding out such information in an accident situation, as this will help you to determine if the person has suffered a head injury. It is useful to identify what the person recalls about the incident, and any bystanders' accounts can be helpful. Note that, after a head injury, the person may well recall some events differently from that of the bystander. Walsh *et al.* (1999) support the value of using a bystander to assist with collecting information regarding the head injury, fit or collapse. After taking a history, the person's neurological status can be assessed using the Glasgow Coma Scale (GCS). As discussed, this assessment provides a quantitative score for assessing the person's eye opening, verbal response and motor response.

Equipment required

To carry out the full neurological assessment you need a watch, a thermometer, a sphygmomanometer and a pen torch. Access a neurological observation chart incorporating the GCS if possible.

Activity

Try to find a willing volunteer to enable you to work through a neurological assessment.

- If you have accessed a neurological observation chart, you should find that it has several sections. These include the GCS, pupil reactions and limb movements, but also includes a section for charting temperature, pulse and blood pressure. If you have followed the chapter through with its activities you will be familiar with how to do these, and can practise them again now. Neurological observation charts also include respiration measurement, which is explained in Chapter 8.
- Now look at the section relating to level of consciousness (*see also* Fig. 7.2). Consider how you might assess whether your volunteer's GCS was 15/15 – the best response.

Note that the person with a GCS of 15/15 would have airway, breathing and circulation which is present and normal, would speak to you and answer any questions appropriately. In brief, a talking, breathing, alert, coherent and orientated person would normally have a GCS of 15, the maximum score. Hopefully this applies to your volunteer! Your volunteer should have scored:

- Eye opening: Spontaneous = 4
- Verbal response: Orientated = 5
- Motor response: Obeys commands = 6.

This therefore totals a GCS of 15.

Each section of the scale, and how it can be assessed, will now be explained in more detail. This will be related to the neurological assessment of Ron, who has had a suspected CVA.

Eye opening

The scores allocated to eye opening are shown in the brackets:

(4) Spontaneously.
(3) To speech
(2) To pain
(1) None

- Assessment of Ron's eye opening response indicates the arousal mechanisms found within his brain stem. If he opens his eyes or already has his eyes open and you speak to him or touch him, you should notice that his eyes follow you appropriately. It is important that you differentiate between a person sleeping and being unresponsive. This can be done by asking a simple question like *'can you open your eyes?'* Remember also, that some people with a head injury, might have difficulty opening their eyes due to swelling of the eyelids, particularly if there is an accompanying facial injury.

- When observing Ron's eye opening response, gently touch his arm when you ask a question. Touch is a very important way of communicating non-verbally and is particularly important for people with hearing and visual deficits.

- If Ron had not opened his eyes to speech, you would need to see whether he will respond to pain. How could you inflict pain? You may only use appropriate touch to centrally stimulate a person, and must take care not to cause damage e.g. bruising. One way would be by squeezing the trapezius muscle. Use your thumb and two fingers and place them at the person's shoulder where the neck meets the shoulder. Gently squeeze this muscle here. Alternatively, you can apply gentle pressure above the person's eyes. This is done by applying two fingers over the eye socket where the eye meets the skull at the eyebrow level. Finally, you could apply gentle pressure to Ron's sternum by gently rubbing his chest over the ribs where they meet his sternum. However, it must be remembered that underlying injuries must be taken into account when applying direct touch. For example, do not press over the sternum if you know the person has fractured ribs or rub over the eye if there is a sub-orbital haematoma. There are no conclusive studies which suggest these actions should not be done, but it is important not to cause more pain to the person. There is anecdotal evidence regarding the value and constraints of such

273

practices. You will need to discuss with your supervising practitioner the accepted manner within your area.

Causing pain in children is controversial. Ferguson-Clark and Williams (1998) suggest the same sites used in adults are appropriate for children. However, Fearon (2000b) advises against supraorbital pressure, and cites Frawley (1990)'s suggested alternative, which is to hold a pen at right angles to the child's extended finger and gently press the pen against the side of the finger.

Best verbal response

The scores allocated in the GCS are shown below:

(5) Orientated – converses.
(4) Disorientated – converses
(3) Inappropriate words
(2) Incomprehensible sounds
(1) None

Thus this category ranges from 'orientated' to 'no verbal response'. It is used to assess and record the person's awareness to his surroundings. Note that if a person is not able to maintain his own airway, and is intubated, he would be unable to talk. It is important then to record that the person is intubated, in the best verbal response column by recording an **I**. In some incidents of head injury, the person can become confused and disorientated to time and place. The verbal response of the person should be compared to his normal communication, and it is therefore important to be aware of how the person would communicate normally. George's neurological status is being assessed by staff who know his usual response and how he communicates, which should lead to a more accurate assessment. However, the staff in A and E who are assessing Ron have never met him before. This is where relatives' input can be particularly helpful, as they would know his usual verbal response.

Assessment of each of these categories will now be explored:

- **Orientated**. For Ron to be assessed as being orientated he should be able to tell you where he is and answer your questions appropriately. For example, he should be able to tell you his date of birth and his name.
- **Disorientated**. In this case, Ron may be able to discuss something with you but may not give you accurate answers, particularly about where he is. For example, when asked 'Where are you?' he may respond: 'I am in the garden'. Note that after a CVA, speech difficulties may result.

Sometimes a person who has had a CVA may not be confused but cannot find the right words for the context.

- **Inappropriate words.** The person may appear agitated and at times aggressive when you ask questions. He may answer the questions you ask inappropriately. He may swear at you but ask you to help him.

- **Incomprehensible sounds.** The person appears unaware of his surroundings, and he may look as though he is staring at the wall when you walk near him. He will not answer any questions nor will he initiate any conversation. He may mumble or make other verbal sounds.

- **No response.** The person will not respond to any spoken word. He will not recognize visitors nor make any verbal sounds at all.

Best motor response

This is assessed to identify the person's awareness of his environment.

The scores shown below are allocated:

(6) Obeys commands.
(5) Localizes pain
(4) Withdraws from pain
(3) Abnormal flexion
(2) Abnormal extension
(1) None

- **Obeys commands.** When you are assessing Ron, you are observing whether he can co-ordinate his actions to your requests This can easily be observed whilst you are carrying out Ron's other observations. For example, you might ask Ron to roll up his sleeve to assist you in recording his blood pressure. Note that you must consider physical ability to carry out your request. Ron is likely to have motor impairment on one side as he has a suspected CVA so other requests e.g. 'Can you close/open your eyes' may be easier for him to carry out. If Ron is unable to obey commands, you would next apply painful stimuli (as discussed previously), and note his motor response to this. If Ron, due to his CVA, has obvious flaccidity on one side, it would be better to assess motor response on the unimpaired side.

- **Localizes pain.** Here you are assessing the person's central brain responses to pain. When you have applied painful stimuli you might see Ron moving a limb towards the pain to attempt to move you away. This is termed localizing to pain, and will score a 5.

- **Withdraws from pain.** If Ron is subjected to painful stimuli and does not appear to attempt to move you away but, moves a finger or a toe away from the pain, then this is recorded as a 4. This is because this is a peripheral response rather than a central response to pain.

- **Abnormal flexion**. Here the person may move towards the painful stimulus. This inappropriate response indicates the severity of the injury to the brain as the brain is not demonstrating a response centrally.
- **Abnormal extension**. When a painful stimulus is applied to the person, the response to pain is inappropriate. The person fails to move away from the stimulus but instead extends (straightens) the limb. This indicates severe brain damage.
- **None**. The person at this stage is unresponsive to any painful stimulus. The prognosis and survival chances of this person may be poor.

■ *Activity*	When assessing a person's GCS, what issues could affect the accuracy of the assessment?

You may have considered the following:
- **Hearing loss**. If the person has impaired hearing it may be difficult to verbally communicate with the person, and this could affect the accuracy of the result in all three categories. Sign language could be used or a communication board, providing that this is appropriate to the person's level of consciousness, and that the person's vision is not impaired. The patient may well lip read and therefore be able to communicate effectively with you, and written responses are also valuable in this situation.
- **Language barrier**. A language barrier between the nurse and patient may cause communication problems too, e.g. whether the person can understand or speak English. Again a communication board may help, or interpretation via a relative or interpreter.
- **Speech difficulties and physical impairment**, as discussed in relation to Ron, can also affect an accurate assessment.
- **Alcohol**. If the person has ingested alcohol, and has a suspected head injury, it will be difficult to assess accurately. However, the nurse should always err on the side of caution. **A person's neurological assessment should never be assumed to be due to alcohol, until other causes, e.g. head injury, have been ruled out**.

It is important that both the nurse and the patient understand what is expected from them during the neurological assessment. Involvement by relatives who know the person's usual level of response is invaluable.

Pupil reaction

Recording of pupil reactions will usually form part of a neurological observation chart, as alteration in pupil sizes and reaction could indicate a rise in intracranial pressure. Take note, now, of the pupil sizes shown in Figure 7.3. You will see that they are shown in varying sizes in millimetres, ranging from

1 to 8 mm. When recording pupil reactions, it is important that the person is examined in dim light as bright lights affect the pupil reactions to your torch light.

When recording pupil reactions, the size and reaction of each eye is checked and recorded individually, L denoting the left eye and R denoting the right eye. A light beam (usually from a pen torch) is directed into the eye to assess the reaction to the light and the size of the pupil against the chart.

It is important to look at both eyes and ask yourself:

- Are they equal?
- Do they look between 2 and 5 mm?
- Do they look round?
- What reactions do you see when you shine a light into them?
    - Are they brisk? If so record B
    - Are they sluggish? If so record SL
    - Is there no reaction? If so, record – (Aucken and Crawford 1998).

You should also note at this stage whether a person is wearing contact lenses or has a false eye as these will obviously affect your recordings. In the chart in Figure 7.3, you will see that both the left and right pupils have been

Pupil sizes

- 1
- 2
- 3
- 4
- 5
- 6
- 7
- 8

Pupil scale (mm)

Recording reactions:

B = brisk reaction
SL = sluggish reaction
– = no reaction
C = closed

PUPILS	left	Size	4				
		Reaction	B				
	right	Size	4				
		Reaction	B				

Figure 7.3 Pupil sizes and recording reactions

277

recorded as 4, B, meaning that the pupils are approximately 4 mm in size and react to light briskly.

> **Activity** Now assess the size and reaction of your volunteer's pupils.

Note that people with visual impairment may have defects to their eyes which alter their pupil reactions. It is then important to try to establish what is normal for this patient. If you found that Ron had unequal pupils it would be sensible to ask him, or his relatives, whether he has any eye problems, e.g. previous eye surgery, or whether he applies eye drops. For example the person with **glaucoma** may insert drops which constrict the pupil.

Glaucoma

This is characterized by an increase in the intraocular pressure of the eye, which causes a reduction of vision in the affected eye.

Limb movements

A neurological chart will also contain a section for recording limb movements. This assessment aims to identify the effects of the neurological condition on the person's limb movements. Verbal commands are used to examine these movements. For example the nurse may ask the person to push and pull against her, with each limb. The responses are recorded for arms and legs separately. If there is a difference between the limbs, they will be recorded separately. An example is shown in Box 7.7.

Here the assessment indicates normal power in both legs, a mild weakness in the left arm, and normal power in the right arm. Normal power is recorded when the person responds appropriately to commands and shows

L I M B	M O V E M E N T	A R M S	Normal power	R		
			Mild weakness	L		
			Severe weakness			
			Spastic flexion			
			Extension			
			No response			
		L E G S	Normal power	R/L		
			Mild weakness			
			Severe weakness			
			Extension			
			No response			

Box 7.7 Recording limb movements

normal function and strength of the limb. The arm weakness recorded may be due to a CVA, as in the case of Ron. Mild weakness implies that the limb can be moved but with reduced power. 'Spastic flexion' is recorded when the limb is bent slowly, and held stiffly against the body with the lower part appearing rigid. 'Extension' is recorded when the person's elbow or knee straightens when a painful stimulus is used, for example, running your hand up the sole of the person's foot. 'No response' is recorded when no stimulus (as used in best motor response) obtains any motor response from the person.

Activity

Practise all the skills included in this chapter by recording a full set of neurological observations with your willing volunteer, which will thus include vital signs as well as level of consciousness, pupil reactions, and limb movements.

The complexity and importance of neurological observations

The neurological assessment of a person is complex and requires practice in the clinical setting. The first set of neurological observations forms the base line for future assessment. Ingram (1994) has warned that people perform neurological observations differently, thus leading to unreliable results. However, Juarez and Lyons (1995) discuss how the GCS score can provide an accurate and reliable assessment of a person's conscious level. It is recommended that a demonstration of the assessment is carried out by the previous nurse, before you take over the care of the person and his neurological observations. It is important that you firstly observe a qualified nurse recording a neurological assessment and then take part under supervision.

Learning outcome 3:
Show awareness of how neurological assessment can be carried out with children, and the special considerations which are necessary

Activity

It has already been identified that the Glasgow Coma Scale was developed for use with adults. What difficulties might there be in using this scale for children and in particular, Megan?

You may have identified the following:
- **Motor response**: the infant or young child may be yet to develop the motor control required to co-operate, so even when fully conscious and orientated, Megan would be unable to achieve a score of 6 in this category on the adult Glasgow Coma Scale. A slightly older child may have the motor ability, yet not understand what he is being asked to do.
- **Verbal response**: the child may not yet have developed the language skills required to answer questions. Also it is common for a young child in an unfamiliar environment to refuse to speak to strangers, particularly if she

CHAPTER SUMMARY

This chapter has aimed to begin to assist you in developing your skills in assessing vital signs within the practice setting. Important points which have been emphasized are:

- It is important that vital signs are assessed and recorded accurately, using the appropriate equipment in the recommended manner.
- Ensure that, as well as writing down these observations, you report them, and seek help in interpreting the results. Leaving observations unreported may result in the person being put in danger. Be vigilant and report all your findings.
- Note that some observations can change quickly along with the person's level of consciousness. Ensure that you carry out the recordings at the required frequency.
- Remember that it may take considerable practice with a range of people in a variety of settings to become really confident and competent in these skills.

REFERENCES

Aucken, S. and Crawford, B. 1998. Neurological assessment. In: Guerrero, D. (ed.) *Neuro Oncology for Nurses*. London: Whurr Publishers.

Brooker C 1996. *Nursing Applications in Clinical Practice: Human Structure and Function*, 2nd edn. London: Mosby.

Brooker, C. 1998. *Human Structure and Function*, 2nd edn. London: Mosby.

Campbell, S. and Glasper, E.A. 1995. *Whaley and Wong's Children's Nursing*. London: Mosby.

Edwards, S. 1997. Measuring temperature. *Professional Nurse*. **13** (2), s5–7.

Fearon, J. 2000a. Assessment. In: Huband, S. and Trigg, E. (eds.) *Practices in Children's Nursing: Guidelines for Hospital and Community*. Edinburgh: Churchill Livingstone, 45–54.

Fearon, J. 2000b. Neurological observations and coma scales. In: Huband, S. and Trigg, E. (eds.) *Practices in Children's Nursing: Guidelines for Hospital and Community*. Edinburgh: Churchill Livingstone, 171–8.

Ferguson-Clark, L. and Williams, C.1998. Neurological assessment in children. *Paediatric Nursing* **10** (4), 29–33.

Flo, G. and Brown, M. 1995. Comparing three methods of temperature taking: oral mercury in glass, oral dietek, and tympanic first temp. *Nursing Research* **44**, 120–2.

Fritsch, D.E. 1995. Hypothermia in the trauma patient. *American Association of Critical Care Nurses Clinical Issues* **6** (2), 196–211.

Herbert, R.A. and Alison, J.A. 1996. Cardiovascular function. In: Hinchliff, S.M., Montague, S.E. and Watson, R. (eds.) *Physiology for Nursing Practice*, 2nd edn. London: Ballière Tindall, 374–451.

Hickey, J.V. 1997. *The Clinical Practice of Neurological and Neurosurgical Nursing*, 4th edn. New York: Lippincott.

Hinchliff, S. 1996. Innate defences. In: Hinchliff, S.M., Montague, S.E. and Watson, R. *Physiology for Nursing Practice*, 2nd edn. London: Ballière Tindall, 621–53.

Hudak, C.M. and Gallo, B.M. 1994. *Critical Care Nursing: A Holistic Approach*. Philadelphia: Lippincott.

Hull, D. and Johnstone, D.I. 1999. *Essential Paediatrics*, 4th edn. Edinburgh: Churchill Livingstone.

Ingram, N. 1994. Knowledge and level of consciousness: application to nursing practice. *Journal of Advanced Nursing* **20**, 881–84.

Jennet, B. and Teasdale, G. 1974. Assessment of the coma and impaired consciousness *Lancet* **2**, 81–84.

Jolly, A. 1991. Taking blood pressure. *Nursing Times* **87** (15), 40–3.

Juarez, V. and Lyons, M. 1995. Interrater reliability of the Glasgow Coma Score. *Journal of Neuroscience Nursing* **27** (5), 283–86.

Leick-Rude, M. and Bloom, L. 1998. A comparison of temperature taking methods in neonates *Neonatal Network* **17** (5), 21–37.

Lowry, M. 1998. Emergency nursing and the Glasgow Coma Score. *Accident and Emergency Nursing* **6**, 143–48.

Luddwig-Beymer, P., Huethers, S. and Schoessler. M. 1994. Pain, temperature regulation, sleep and sensory function. In: McCance, K. and Hether, S. (eds.) *Pathophysiology: The Biologic Basis for Disease in Adults and Children*, 2nd edn. London: Mosby, 437–76.

Mallet, J. and Bailey, C. 1996. *Manual of Clinical Nursing Procedures*, 4th edn. Oxford: Blackwell Science.

Marieb, E. 1999. *Human Anatomy and Physiology*, 4th edn. California: Addison Wesley.

Maslen, B. 1995. The skills of assessment. In: Basford, L. and Slevin, O. (eds) *Theory and Practice of Nursing: An Integrated Approach to Patient Care.* Edinburgh: Campion Press, 506–30.

Millar-Craig, M.W., Bishop, C.N. and Raftery, E.B. 1978. Circardian variation in blood pressure *Lancet* **1** (8086), 795–7.

Mohammed, T.A. 2000. Incubator care. In: Huband, S. and Trigg, E. (eds.) *Practices in Children's Nursing: Guidelines for Hospital and Community*. Edinburgh: Churchill Livingstone 139–42.

Montague, S.E. 1996. The blood. In: Hinchliff, S.M. and Watson, R. (eds.) *Physiology For Nursing Practice*, 2nd edn. London: Baillière Tindall, 323–451.

Moules, T. and Ramsey, J. 1998. *The Textbook of Children's Nursing* Cheltenham: Stanley Thornes.

O'Brien, E., Petrie, J., Littler,W. *et al.* 1997. *Blood Pressure Recommendations of the British Hypertension Society*. London: British Medical Journal Publication.

O'Toole, S. 1998. Temperature measurement devices. *Professional Nurse* **13**, 779–86.

Rogers, M. 1992a. Temperature recording in infants and children *Paediatric Nursing* **4** (3), 23–6.

Rogers, M. 1992b. A viable alternative to the glass/mercury thermometer. *Paediatric Nursing* **4** (9), 8–11.

Rudolph, M. and Levene, M. 1999. *Paediatrics and Child Health*. Oxford: Blackwell Science.

Second Task Force for Blood Pressure Control in Children 1987. Report. *Journal of Paediatrics* **111** (3), 397–99.

Schmitz, T., Bair, N., Falk, N. and Levine, C. 1995. A comparison of five methods of temperature measurement devices in febrile intensive care patients. *American Journal of Critical Care* **4**, 286–96.

Skinner, D., Driscoll, P. and Earlam, P. 1992. *ABC of Trauma* London: British Medical Journal Publication.

Torrance, C. and Semple, M.C. 1998a. Recording temperature. *Nursing Times* **94** (2), Practical Procedures for Nurses Suppl.

Torrance, C. and Semple, M.C. 1998b. Recording temperature. *Nursing Times* **94** (3), Practical Procedures for Nurses Suppl.

Walsh, M., Crumbie, A. and Reveley, S. 1999. *Nurse Practitioners: Clinical Skills and Professional Issues*. Oxford: Butterworth-Heinemann.

Webb, M., Bond, M. and Beale, P. 1997. *First Aid Manual: The Authorized Manual of St John Ambulance, St Andrews Ambulance Association and the Red Cross*, 7th edn. London: Dorling Kindersley.

Winkelman, C. 1995. Increased intracranial pressure. In: Urban, N.A., Greenlee, K.K., Krumberger, J.M. and Winkelman, C. (eds.) *Guidelines for Critical Care Nursing*. St Louis: Mosby, 3–11.

Wilson, J.W. and Waugh, A. 1996. *Ross and Wilson Anatomy and Physiology in Health and Illlness*, 8th edn. London: Churchill Livingstone.

Chapter

8

Respiratory care: assessment and interventions

Lesley Baillie, Veronica Corben and Sue Higham

Nurses may care for people in many settings who require assessment and monitoring of their respiratory status, and interventions to relieve or prevent respiratory symptoms. The aim of this chapter is to help you to develop practical skills involved in respiratory care.

Included in this chapter are:
- Measuring and recording respirations
- Measuring and recording peak expiratory flow rate
- Pulse oximetry
- Observation of sputum and collection of sputum specimens
- Oxygen therapy
- Administering inhaled medication
- Managing nebulized therapy

Recommended biology reading

These questions will help you to focus on the biology underpinning this chapter's skills. Use your recommended textbook to find out:

- What are the components of the respiratory system (e.g. airways, respiratory muscles, control mechanisms) and what are their functions?
- Where does gaseous exchange occur? Which gases are being exchanged? Why does this exchange occur? What may affect this exchange?
- How does inspiration occur? What is the stimulus for us to breathe?
- What are the proportions of gases in atmospheric, alveolar and expired air?

- How does the respiratory system protect itself from infection? Where are cilia found?
- Where is bronchial smooth muscle located?
- Where are the pleural membranes? What functions do they have?
- What is surfactant? How does it prevent lung collapse?
- How can lung function be assessed? What factors could affect lung function?
- What are the functions of blood? Find out the components of the blood. What roles do these components play?

Chronic obstructive pulmonary disease
Chronic respiratory disease including conditions such as emphysema, chronic bronchitis and chronic asthma. Causes debilitating breathlessness which affects day to day living.

Asthma
A respiratory disorder characterized by recurrent episodes of difficulty in breathing, wheezing on expiration, coughing and viscous mucoid bronchial secretions.

Bronchodilator
A drug that relaxes the smooth muscle of the bronchioles to improve ventilation to the lungs. Commonly used examples are salbutamol (ventolin) and terbutaline (bricanyl).

Corticosteroid
Inhaled corticosteroids such as becotide are used for asthmatics as a preventative treatment. They appear to reduce bronchial mucosal inflammation, and thus reduce oedema and secretion of mucus in the airway.

PRACTICE SCENARIOS

The following scenarios illustrate when respiratory assessment and care may be needed, and will be referred to throughout this chapter.

■ Adult

Mr Walter Collins is an 80-year-old man who lives alone and was found by his daily carer to be unwell. He has a past medical history of **chronic obstructive pulmonary disease** (COPD). His GP referred him to the Accident and Emergency (A and E) Department to be seen by the medical team. On arrival Mr Collins' breathing is difficult and rapid, and he is coughing and trying to expectorate sputum. Oxygen therapy is being delivered.

■ Child

Michael Rawlings, aged 6 years, has had a diagnosis of **asthma** for 3 years. He has had several acute admissions to hospital with this condition, where he has needed oxygen therapy, nebulizers and sometimes intravenous medication. At home he takes **bronchodilators** and becotide (a **corticosteroid**) via an inhaler with a spacer device, and also an oral bronchodilator. It has now been decided that home monitoring of Michael's peak expiratory flow rate would help to monitor and control his asthma, and his family are keen to learn about this.

■ Learning disability

Clara Wright is a 43-year-old woman with a learning disability who lives in a small staffed unit. She has epilepsy and, this morning, had a prolonged fit for which a rectal muscle relaxant (diazepam) was administered. She is now very drowsy and unresponsive and you have been advised that her respirations need to be monitored carefully.

■ Mental health

Richard Bryant is a 28-year-old man, who has been admitted to the acute admissions ward of the mental health in-patient services, for emergency

Pabrinex

Vitamins B and C in parenteral form for the rapid correction of severe deficiency, which can occur in chronic alcoholism. Potentially serious allergic reactions may occur during or shortly after administration of this drug.

Anaphylaxis

A type of immediate hypersensitivity that is triggered when allergen molecules cross link to IgE antibodies attached to mast cells or basophils causing the release of inflammatory substances. The potential serious results of this include coma, respiratory or cardiac arrest, and swelling due to peripheral vasodilation.

alcohol detoxification. As part of his treatment, Richard was administered an intramuscular injection of **pabrinex** and shortly afterwards, he collapsed. He was unresponsive but breathing, so staff turned him into the recovery position to maintain his airway, and called the doctor urgently. As pabrinex can cause an **anaphylactic** reaction, staff were asked to observe Richard carefully and monitor his respirations.

MEASURING AND RECORDING RESPIRATIONS

Definition

The major function of the respiratory system is to supply the body with oxygen and remove carbon dioxide. When the respiratory rate is measured, it is the act of ventilation which is observed. One respiration consists of one inspiration (breathing in), and one expiration (breathing out).

Learning outcomes

By the end of this section you will be able to.

1. Discuss when and why observation of respiration is performed.
2. State normal respiratory rates for different age groups and genders.
3. Discuss what other aspects of breathing the nurse would observe when measuring the respiratory rate.
4. Accurately measure and record the respiratory rate.
5. Define terms commonly used for breathing abnormalities.

Equipment required

■   A watch with a second hand.
■   An observation chart.

Learning outcome 1:
Discuss when and why observation of respiration is performed.

Activity Why would a person's respiration be observed by a nurse? The practice scenarios will give you some clues. List possible reasons.

You may have identified the following:

•   Admission to hospital or pre-operatively, providing a baseline for future comparison.
•   When a person (in hospital or in the community) is unwell or injured, for example, loss of consciousness, chest injury, difficulty with breathing, chest pain.

- To monitor a patient's condition, for example after surgery, or during treatment, such as a morphine infusion.
- To monitor the patient's response to treatments or medication which affect the respiratory system.

Learning outcome 2:
State the normal respiratory rates for different age groups
When assessing respiratory rate you will need to know the expected normal rate for the person's age group, and if a baseline reading is available, you can make a comparison with this.

Activity

- What do you think the normal respiratory rate would be for Mr Collins, as an adult, and for a child of Michael's age?
- In health, when would respirations be slower or faster, and why?

There is considerable individual variation in respiratory rates (Stocks 1996). The respiratory rate varies according to age, size and gender, and can also fluctuate in well people, e.g. due to change in metabolic demands. The normal adult respiratory rate is about 10–15 breaths per minute (Stocks 1996). For children's respiratory rates see Table 8.1. Exercise, stress and fear will all increase the respiratory rate; this is a normal bodily response. Thus when Michael is running around kicking a football you would expect his respiratory rate to be increased as his body requires more oxygen. If a person's respiratory rate is counted when he has just arrived for admission to hospital, the anxiety and stress of the situation may lead to a raised respiratory rate which would not be an accurate baseline. In deep (stage 4) sleep, respiratory rate drops to its lowest normal level. Knowledge of normal biological functioning will help you to recognize abnormalities, and causes for concern.

An increased respiratory rate is termed **tachypnoea**. Mr Collins is likely to be tachypnoeic on admission to A and E, and even when he is at home his respiratory rate will probably be raised due to his chronic compromised respiratory status. When Michael has an acute asthma attack he is also likely

Table 8.1 Normal range for respiratory rates in children (Hull and Johnstone 1999)

Age in years	Respiratory rate (breaths per minute)
Under 1 year	25–35
1–5 years	20–30
5–12 years	20–25
Over 12 years	15–25

to be tachypnoeic. A decreased respiratory rate is termed **bradypnoea**. After a sedatory drug such as diazepam, as administered to Clara Wright, decreased respirations would be the most likely abnormality to occur.

In healthy people, the relationship of pulse and respiration is fairly constant, being a ratio of one respiration to every four or five heart beats. Very rapid respirations, such as over 40 per minute in an adult (in the absence of exercise) or very slow respirations, such as 8 per minute, are cause for alarm and should be reported promptly.

Learning outcome 3:
Discuss what other aspects of breathing the nurse would observe when measuring the respiratory rate

Activity

When you are counting the respiratory rates of the people in the scenarios, what else about their respiration would you be observing?

You should be observing:

Difficulty

Respirations are normally effortless, and you should therefore observe whether breathing is difficult or laboured (termed **dyspnoea**). Dyspnoeic patients, such as Mr Collins, may use accessory muscles of respiration such as their neck and abdominal muscles. However babies and, to a lesser extent, children up to 6 years, rely predominantly on diaphragmatic movement to breathe, resulting in greater abdominal movements during normal breathing than adults (Carter 1995). Signs of dyspnoea in babies and younger children include recession (sinking in of the soft tissues during inspiration) below the sternum and under and between the ribs, and flaring of the nostrils (Campbell and Glasper 1995). When Michael was admitted with acute asthma it would have been important for nurses to observe for these signs of laboured breathing, which can be tiring for a child.

People with dyspnoea often mouth breathe, as there is less resistance to airflow through the mouth than the nose, and this can cause drying of the oral mucosa (Stocks 1996). Oral hygiene (*see* Chapter 5) is therefore essential. The person with dyspnoea needs to be sitting up, either in an arm chair, or in bed well supported by pillows, to optimize ventilation (*see* Fig. 8.1). The baby or young child can be held in this position by the parent. **Orthopnoea** is the term used when a person cannot breathe unless he is upright. It is very likely that Mr Collins will be orthopnoeic as will Michael when he is having an acute asthma attack. Note that dyspnoea is frightening and psychological support is essential.

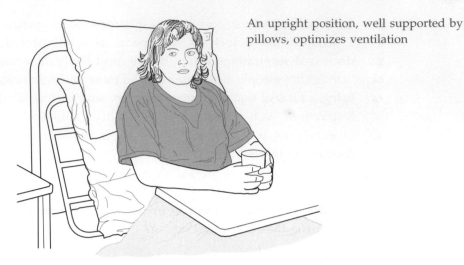

An upright position, well supported by pillows, optimizes ventilation

Figure 8.1 Correct position for the breathless person

Sound

You should also observe the sound of breathing, which is normally quiet. You may hear a variety of abnormal breath sounds, such as a wheeze or a stridor. A wheeze is a high-pitched sound which occurs when air is forced through narrowed respiratory passages. This is often heard in asthmatics, like Michael. A stridor is a harsh, high-pitched sound that is heard during respiration when the larynx is obstructed.

Depth

Depth of breathing should also be observed. This relates to the volume of air moving in and out of the respiratory tract with each breath, and is referred to as tidal volume. The term **hyperventilation** is used to describe prolonged, rapid and deep ventilations. This can occur in someone who is having an anxiety attack and can cause dizziness and faintness as the resulting low carbon dioxide level causes cerebral vasoconstriction. If you encountered this in someone, you can help by being calm and asking the person to breathe more slowly in and out of a paper bag. This enables rebreathing of expired air, which is rich in carbon dioxide, thus restoring normal levels. **Hypoventilation** is the term used for slow and shallow breathing. As Clara Wright has had a sedative administered (which could cause respiratory depression), it will be particularly important to observe for hypoventilation, which would lead to inadequate gaseous exchange. Richard, too, is particularly at risk of hypoventilation, as he is unresponsive. You should also observe whether the chest expands equally on both sides, particularly if there is a history of chest injury.

Pattern

The pattern of breathing should also be observed. Terms are given to certain abnormalities.

- **Apnoea**: is a period without breathing. This could occur during hypoventilation, with another breath only taking place when arterial carbon dioxide levels rise and stimulate breathing.
- **Cheyne–Stokes respirations**: are when there is a gradual increase in the depth of respirations leading to an episode of hyperventilation, followed by a gradual decrease in the depth of respirations, and then a period of apnoea lasting about 15–20 seconds
- Note: that it is common for infants to have an irregular breathing pattern, with alternating short (a few seconds) periods of apnoea and rapid breathing.

Learning outcome 4:
Accurately measure and record the respiratory rate

For this activity you need another person. If a colleague is not available, another friend or family member may oblige!

Activity

Measure the respiratory rate, using the instructions below:

- Observe the rise and fall of the chest. Note that in practice you should do this when the person is unaware that he is being observed, as otherwise he may alter his breathing pattern. However in an unresponsive person, for example, Clara Wright or Richard, this precaution is not relevant. In the alert individual, the respiratory rate may be counted directly after the pulse, while still outwardly counting the pulse.
- With infants and young children you should observe for abdominal movements. This may be done by placing the hand gently against the lower part of the child's chest to feel movement while continuing to hold the wrist as if taking the pulse. However if the child resists his wrist being held, this should be discontinued. In some cases it may be necessary to listen for the sounds of inspiration with a stethoscope placed on the chest in order to record a baby's respiratory rate.
- Note the placement of the second hand of your watch. Count each rise and fall of the chest.
- If respirations are regular, even and unlaboured, count the number that occur over half a minute, and multiply by two to obtain the rate for one minute. If the respirations are abnormal in any way, count them for one minute. You should not count for only 10 or 15 seconds as with numbers as small as respiratory rates, there is too much room for error. The irregular

breathing pattern of infants means it is essential for accuracy that respirations are counted for a full minute in babies aged less than one year (Wong *et al.* 1999).

Respiratory rates, particularly on admission assessment sheets, may be recorded simply as a number (the number of respirations per minute). However if the person's respiratory rate is to be recorded regularly over a period of time a graph sheet may be used. How often recordings are made varies considerably according to the person's condition. This may be quarter hourly (for the patient with acute breathing difficulties), hourly, 4-hourly, or daily. For example, it is likely that Mr Collins' respirations will be recorded quarter hourly initially, and then reduced to hourly and then 4-hourly as he stabilizes.

Activity   Ask the other person to spend a couple of minutes exercising (e.g. running up and down stairs), and then count the respiratory rate again. Using the example in Figure 8.2 as a guide, note how you would record the two respiratory rates which you have taken, on an observation chart.

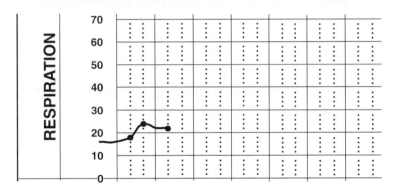

Figure 8.2 Observation chart, showing how respirations could be recorded

Learning outcome 5:
Define terms commonly used for abnormalities

Throughout this section a number of terms have been used which you may commonly hear used in relation to breathing abnormalities. For example, with application to the scenarios, Mr Collins is orthopnoeic and dyspnoeic. You will be observing Clara Wright in case she hypoventilates or becomes bradypnoeic or apnoeic.

Activity   Can you remember what the following terms mean?
- Dyspnoea
- Hyperventilation
- Tachypnoea
- Orthopnoea
- Hypoventilation
- Bradypnoea
- Apnoea.

All the terms in the list can be found in this section. Check the answers if you are unsure.

Summary

■ Measurement of respirations is performed as part of an acutely ill person's assessment, as a baseline for future comparison, and to monitor and evaluate a person's condition and response to treatment.

■ It is important to be aware of normal respiratory rates, and of possible abnormalities of respiration that can occur.

MEASURING AND RECORDING PEAK EXPIRATORY FLOW RATE

Definition

In brief, a peak flow meter measures an individual's ability to exhale. The peak flow is a measure, in litres per minute, of the maximum flow rate that an individual can achieve on forced expiration, when starting at full inspiration (Leach 1994). The more accurate term to use is 'peak expiratory flow rate' (PEFR). The measurement will help to determine lung volume, and is one of the most accurate clinical measures of the person's current respiratory status. Peak flow measurement is relatively convenient and inexpensive, and can play a key role in identifying acute exacerbations of asthma (Donohue 1996). It is therefore important that you understand how to measure and record the peak flow rate, and understand its implications.

Learning outcomes

On completion of this section you will be able to:

1. Discuss for which individuals peak flow measurement may be useful.
2. Accurately measure and record peak flow rate.
3. Show awareness of how normal peak flow measurements may differ for individuals.
4. Show insight into how peak flow measurements can be used for monitoring by patients in self-management.

Equipment required

Try to access from the skills laboratory or a clinical practice placement:

- A peak flow meter and mouth piece.
- An observation chart.

2. If a low reading was obtained, you first need to check that the patient's position and technique are correct. Then, as with any other observation, you need to report abnormal measurements to the qualified nurse, who is accountable for the patient's care. Little can usually be deduced from a single peak flow reading as a series of readings are required to produce a comprehensive picture. However a single low reading may need a quick response. Obviously the patient's general condition and other observations will be taken into account too.

3. On most adult wards peak flow will be recorded simply as a figure at the bottom of the observation chart. There are special charts available, particularly for when there needs to be ongoing monitoring, and these are often used for children, and for home monitoring of peak flow (*see* Figure 8.4).

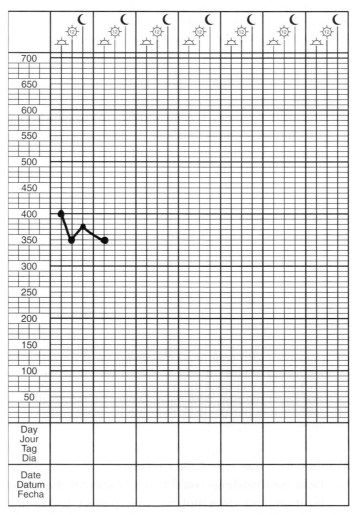

Figure 8.4 Example of a chart to monitor peak flow (reproduced with kind permission of Clement Clarke International Ltd)

4. Generally twice daily (morning and early evening) measurements are sufficient, except during acute episodes. Donohue (1996) recommends that measuring a morning pre-bronchodilator peak flow is one of the best ways of monitoring asthma. In mild cases of asthma, once or twice weekly measurements may be enough. Often it is necessary to monitor effects of medication, e.g. inhaled bronchodilators. Peak flows will then be measured before and 30 minutes after medication (when the medication is having the maximum effect) (Brewin and Hughes 1995). These pre- and post-medication measurements need recording clearly. Many wards will use different coloured pens.

Learning outcome 3:
Show awareness of normal peak flow measurements for different individuals

The normal peak flow reading varies according to a person's age, height and gender. Generally an adult should achieve 400–600 litres per minute, but males will achieve a higher figure than females, and greater height will increase the peak flow reading. A smaller measurement would obviously be expected of a child, and there are charts available on paediatric wards which can help to calculate the expected peak flow. A child of 9 years could be expected to achieve 175 litres per minute, but again this will vary according to height. Therefore accurate height measurement is essential prior to peak flow measurement in children. Even in individuals without asthma there will be variations in the measurement, with the morning figure being lower, and the highest being achieved in early evening. This tendency is likely to be exaggerated in asthmatics.

Activity   Compare your peak flow measurement with the information above. Does it fulfil what would be expected for you?

Learning outcome 4:
Show insight into how peak flow measurements can be used for monitoring by patients in self-management

Peak flow meters are increasingly being used by asthmatics to monitor and manage their condition. They have been available on prescription since 1990. The patient will normally be advised about his baseline peak flow, according to his age, height and sex. The same peak flow meter should be used for a particular individual to ensure consistency.

Activity   Reflect on why teaching patients (or families) to measure peak flow could be useful in managing asthma.

Points which you may have identified include:
- To find out how well their asthma is controlled.
- Doing regular readings may reveal a gradual (and possibly asymptomatic) deterioration, which will require action (e.g. change of medication) to

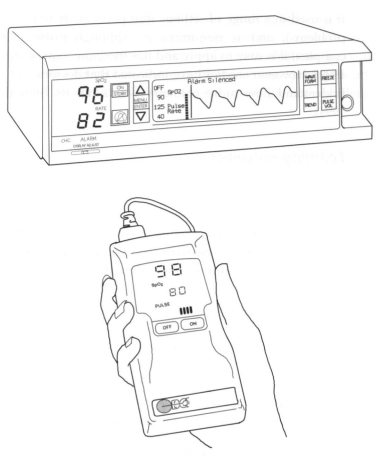

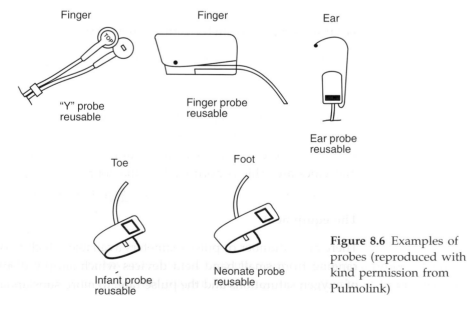

Figure 8.5 Examples of pulse oximeters (reproduced with kind permission from Pulmolink)

Finger

"Y" probe reusable

Finger

Finger probe reusable

Ear

Ear probe reusable

Toe

Infant probe reusable

Foot

Neonate probe reusable

Figure 8.6 Examples of probes (reproduced with kind permission from Pulmolink)

devices, which may also show the pulsatile waveform (*see* Fig. 8.5). Cowan (1997) summarizes the key features of a number of different devices. The box will always have a wire leading to the sensor or probe. The probe may be in the form of a clip which can be attached to a finger, toe or earlobe, or it may be in a form which can be taped to the skin or wrapped round an infant's foot or a palm. Probes can be disposable or re-usable, and are available in different sizes. Figure 8.6 shows a selection of probes.

How the equipment works

On one side of the sensor is the light source, which consists of two light emitting diodes, one giving red light (of a short wave length) and one giving infrared light (of a longer wavelength). On the other side of the sensor is a photodetector, which detects the light which passes through the area of the body to which it is attached. As the oxyhaemoglobin (HbO_2) absorbs more of the infrared light, the microprocessor can calculate the oxyhaemoglobin saturation (SpO_2), and this is displayed on the screen, along with the pulse rate. The diagram in Figure 8.7 portrays how the sensor works.

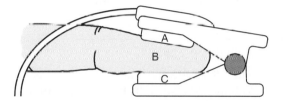

A Light emitting diodes

B Finger through which the red and infrared light passes

C Photodetector

Figure 8.7 Diagram showing how a pulse oximeter works

The pulse oximeter works on the premise that anything which pulses and absorbs red and infrared light between the light source and the light detector must be arterial blood (Lowton 1999). Pulse oximeters therefore only monitor light absorption from tissue with a pulsatile flow, so preventing false readings from fat, bone, connective tissue and venous blood. A good arterial blood flow is therefore needed for a reliable reading (Carroll 1997a).

■ *Activity*   If you have access to a pulse oximeter in your practice placement, attach the probe to your finger, and see what your SpO_2 reading is.

The normal value of oxygen saturation is **95–100%**, so hopefully your reading should have fallen within this range! This figure refers to the percentage of haemoglobin molecules fully saturated with oxygen. **SpO_2 readings below 90% will give cause for concern** (Place 1998), **and must be reported**. Nursing measures such as repositioning the person to a more upright position, if not contraindicated, may provide significant improvement (*see* Fig. 8.1). Pulse oximeters have alarm systems, which will sound if the measurement falls below a normal level. Most manufacturers claim that their devices are accurate to + or − 2%, at oxygen saturations of 70–99%. However as **hypoxaemia** (insufficient oxygenation of blood) rises, pulse oximetry does become less accurate, and at 80–85% a more detailed assessment is necessary. At any stage if there is any doubt about the accuracy of pulse oximetry, blood gas analysis, which involves analysis of a sample of blood obtained from an artery, should be performed. This is usually a medical procedure.

Learning outcome 2:

Discuss how a pulse oximeter should be used in practice

Activity

If you have seen a pulse oximeter used in practice, were you given any advice about obtaining an accurate measurement? Can you think of anything which might interfere with the detection of light by the photodetector?

There are a number of factors that can interfere with obtaining an accurate measurement and these are listed in Box 8.1. Discussion about some of these factors and possible solutions will now follow.

Incorrect positioning of probe
Use of pierced ear for probe
Probe applied to hand of arm with blood pressure cuff attached
Incorrect size probe
Tape applied too tightly
Dark nail varnish
Bright light: sunlight or artificial light
Movement
Interference from other equipment or cellular telephones
Poor peripheral perfusion

Box 8.1 Factors which can cause inaccurate pulse oximeter measurements

Positioning

The sensor must always be placed correctly, with the diodes and detector positioned directly opposite each other. If inaccurately positioned, the light may pass directly from the light emitting diode to the photodetector without passing through the vascular bed (Carroll 1997a). If the ear lobe is used, the appropriate sensor will be needed. However, a pierced earlobe should not be used as the light emitting diodes will reach the photodetector without passing through the vascular bed. Fingers should be fully inserted into the finger probes and flexible sensors should be applied correctly (Cowan 1997). Always ensure that the sensor is not applied to the finger of an arm with a blood pressure cuff attached, which would lead to inaccurate or absent readings when the cuff is inflated.

■ Activity   If you can access a pulse oximeter, attach the probe to your finger, and rather than removing it as soon as a reading appears, keep it on for 5 minutes. Is it uncomfortable? Can you imagine how you would feel if you had to wear it for several hours? How would a child or a person with confusion respond to this?

Note that the oximeter probe can lead to skin damage due to pressure, particularly if the person has poor peripheral perfusion, (as in heart failure) or has sensitive skin (such as with elderly people or children). The probe site should be checked frequently in people with continuous pulse oximetry (Le Grand and Peters 1999), and should be changed every 4–8 hours in pre-term infants (Wong *et al.* 1999). Often it is preferable with babies and children to take frequent readings, removing the probe after each reading, rather than continually monitoring.

Correct size probes and use of tape

With babies and children accuracy and safety will only be achieved if the correct size probe for the size of the child is used in the correct manner (Moyle 1999). There are special probes available for neonates, babies and small children, which will usually work through the palm, foot or arm; the manufacturer's instructions should be strictly adhered to (Moyle 1999). Figure 8.8 shows how probes might be applied. Stoddart *et al.* (1997) highlight that if an adult probe is used on the small fingers of infants and children, the pulse oximeter may under-read or over-read due to there being a different path length of tissue for each of the wavelengths. Wong *et al.* (1999) suggest that for the infant, the sensor can be taped around the big toe, and the wire taped to the sole of the foot. A sock can then be put over the foot. For the child Wong *et al.* (1999) suggest taping the sensor securely to the index finger and taping the wire to the back of the hand. Moyle (1999) warns that though it is tempting to apply extra adhesive tape around the probe, this will both affect accuracy and can cause pressure or thermal damage to the extremity. Also if a finger probe is taped too tightly venous pulsation may occur leading to measurement error (Le Grand and Peters 1999).

Nails

Accurate pulse oximetry is reliant on the translucence of the body part to which the probe is attached. A study by Peters (1997) found that unpolished acrylic nails do not affect pulse oximetry measurements of oxygen saturation

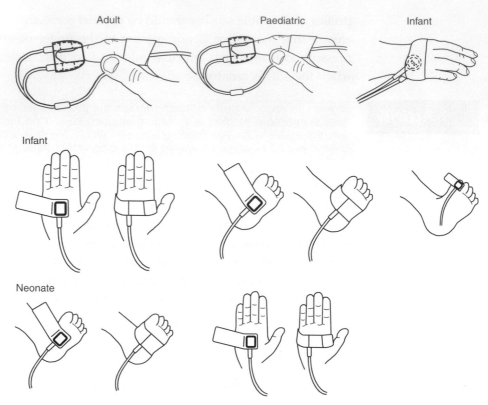

Figure 8.8 Examples of how probes might be applied (reproduced from Pumolink with kind permission)

and therefore patients do not need to remove them. However nail varnish can affect SpO_2 readings; the darker the polish the more problematic – blue, black and green are the worst. If it is not possible to remove the nail polish, or place the sensor on an unaffected area, the sensor can be placed sideways on the finger rather than across the nailbed, but it may be necessary to tape the sensor in place to prevent movement (Carroll 1997a).

Bright light

Bright lights can also interfere with measurements, and thus if phototherapy is being used (such as with a jaundiced baby) the probe will need to be covered to protect it from light (Stoddart *et al.* 1997). In bright sunlight or when a bright artificial light is being used, the sensor should also be covered with something opaque (Carroll 1997a).

Movement

Activity

When you next have access to a pulse oximeter, attach the probe to your finger, and then try moving your finger around. What happens to the reading?

Moving or partially dislodging the sensor affects the ability of the light to travel from the light emitting diodes to the photodetector (Carroll 1997a), and the accuracy of the reading may be affected. However, the technology of newer devices, has been designed to prevent movement interfering with readings. When pulse oximeters do detect excessive movement they will usually alarm as a malfunction, so this is a safe limitation of pulse oximetry as it is obvious. Carroll (1997a) notes that rhythmic movements such as **Parkinsonian tremors** or seizures, shivering, exercise and vibrations caused by transport, can all make it difficult for the pulse oximeter to identify which tissue is pulsatile. If possible the sensor should be attached to a part of the body which the patient is most likely to keep still, and if digits are used, they should be kept supported rather than held in the air (Cowan 1997). If a finger type sensor is used on a continuous basis the cable can be secured to the back of the hand. Carroll (1997a) recommends that using the ear will often reduce problems of movement. With small children, the foot or hand may have to be held still for the duration of the reading. A child who is reluctant to co-operate may be encouraged to do so by a parent.

Parkinsonian tremors
A tremor or shaking that occurs in a neurological condition called Parkinson's disease.

Poor peripheral perfusion

For a pulsatile flow to be detected there must be sufficient perfusion in the monitored area (Carroll 1997a). Any condition which reduces pulsatile blood flow to body extremities will lead to poor peripheral perfusion. Causes include **hypotension, hypovolaemia**, cardiac arrest, or hypothermia. Vasoconstricting drugs, smoking and **peripheral oedema** can also cause poor perfusion, which will adversely affect the pulse oximeter signal. If the peripheral pulse is weak or absent pulse oximetry readings will not be precise (Carroll 1997a). Cardiac arrythmias such as slow **atrial fibrillation**, can interfere with capture of the pulsatile signal, and thus reduce the technique's accuracy. If there is a pulse wave displayed on the oximeter, check that it is not dampened as this could indicate a decrease in arterial flow (Carroll 1997a).

Hypotension
Low blood pressure

Hypovolaemia
Low blood volume

Peripheral oedema
Swollen periphery of the body due to excess extracellular fluid

Atrial fibrillation
An abnormal heart rhythm whereby the atria fibrillate rather than contract, leading to a highly irregular heart rate.

Checking the pulse oximeter's accuracy

To check accuracy you can compare a palpated pulse against the displayed pulse; if they do not correlate then it is likely that the oximeter is not picking up each arteriole pulsation and thus the readings are likely to be inaccurate (Carroll 1997a). The sensor can be moved to an area of higher perfusion, e.g. the ear lobe, or the skin can be warmed. As with any technology, pulse oximeters are not immune to failure. You can attach the sensor to your own finger and if you don't obtain a normal reading then you can assume that the oximeter is faulty. Readings can also be checked against arterial blood gas measurement.

Learning outcome 3:
Identify when pulse oximetry would be used and its advantages

Pulse oximetry has widespread applications, and is recommended whenever there is risk of hypoxaemia (Grap 1998). Assessing hypoxaemia through observation is notoriously inaccurate and unreliable (Le Grand and Peters 1999; Sinex 1999) but it can rapidly lead to tissue damage. As the brain is so sensitive to oxygen depletion visual and cognitive changes can occur when oxygen saturation falls to 80–85% and other signs of hypoxaemia include restlessness, agitation, hypotension and tachycardia. However, all these signs can be missed or wrongly interpreted.

Cyanosis is the visible sign of hypoxaemia, but is only detected at a saturation of about 75% in normally perfused patients (Hanning and Alexander-Williams 1995). Moyle (1996), in identifying reasons why pulse oximetry has become so commonly used, notes that pulse oximetry can detect hypoxaemia early. Overall, pulse oximetry should be a more accurate and objective measure of hypoxaemia, alerting health professionals at an early stage. It is cheap, non-invasive and can be easily measured during transfer of a patient.

Cyanosis
A bluish, greyish or purple discolouration of the skin due to presence of abnormal amounts of reduced haemoglobin in the blood.

Activity   Have you seen pulse oximetry used in practice? If so, what care situations was it used in?

You may have thought of the following situations:

Acute illness
Pulse oximetry is used with people who are acutely ill, particularly during initial assessment and management as in the A and E Department. It is particularly useful when assessing those with dyspnoea or tachypnoea (Le Grand and Peters 1999). Thus Walter Collin's oxygen saturations will definitely need to be monitored while he is acutely breathless. When Michael was admitted with acute asthma, pulse oximetry would have been necessary. A study by Summers *et al.* (1998) found that incorporating pulse oximetry into emergency assessment did identify a small, but statistically significant group whose **hypoxia** (decreased available oxygen to the tissues to allow normal function) would otherwise have been missed. Currently pulse oximeters are not widely available outside acute hospital settings so it is unlikely that either Clare's or Richard's oxygen saturations would be monitored, although if available, it would give the nurses caring for them a useful indication of their oxygenation adequacy.

During investigations and surgery
Pulse oximetry will also be used during and after procedures involving general anaesthesia, or sedation, such as during a bronchoscopy.

In-patients with respiratory and circulatory problems

Patients with respiratory disease, particularly if receiving oxygen therapy, will have SpO_2 monitoring and indeed the amount of oxygen administered may be adjusted according to the SpO_2. Any patients who are at risk of hypoxaemia, such as those with pneumonia, congestive heart failure, COPD exacerbation, acute lung injury and babies with **bronchiolitis**, may have continuous SpO_2 monitoring via a pulse oximeter (Rodriguez and Light 1998). Patients whose cardiorespiratory status is unstable, and are undergoing transfer, will often have pulse oximetry *in situ*.

In the community

Pulse oximetry can also be used in the community with people who are at risk of hypoxaemia, for example with chronically ill patients such as those with **cystic fibrosis**. Carroll (1997b) notes the increasing use of pulse oximetry by community nurses and discusses implications. Babies discharged from neonatal units with **bronchopulmonary dysplasia** may receive oxygen therapy at home, and be monitored by pulse oximetry periodically by the community paediatric team; parents may be asked to monitor SpO_2 overnight to determine oxygen requirements and sleep patterns with and without oxygen (Stoddart *et al.* 1997).

Other advantages

Pulse oximetry can prevent or reduce the need for arterial blood gas sampling which is invasive and painful, requiring a skilled practitioner and access to a blood gas analyser. A study involving 152 patients found that use of pulse oximetry led to a significant reduction in unnecessary arterial blood gas analysis (Le Bourdelles *et al.* 1998). Pulse oximetry also provides a continuous measurement rather than intermittent as in arterial blood gas monitoring (Le Grand and Peters 1999), and thus the effectiveness of interventions, such as oxygen therapy and medication, can be evaluated. The impact of mobilization, physiotherapy and exercise can be assessed (Place 1998) and pulse oximetry may identify whether oxygen therapy is required during these procedures.

Learning outcome 4:
Show understanding of the limitations of pulse oximetry

Pulse oximetry complements measurement of other vital signs but it does not replace them (Lowton 1999); oxygen saturations are only a single physiological variable and should not be over-relied upon. Carroll (1997b) advises that the measurement obtained from the pulse oximeter must be interpreted in the light of the whole clinical picture. It has been argued that below 70% the accuracy of pulse oximetry is reduced (Schnapp and Cohen 1990). Stoddart *et al.* (1997) emphasize the importance of recognizing the limitations of pulse

Bronchiolitis
Infection of the bronchioles which affects mainly babies.

Cystic fibrosis
A genetic disease causing oversecretion of a viscous mucus predisposing to respiratory infections.

Bronchopulmonary dysplasia
A chronic lung disease that can develop in pre-term babies who have had a prolonged period of intensive therapy.

oximetry as well as its advantages. Moyle (1996) notes that there are safe limitations of pulse oximetry (where the nurse will be immediately aware that the device is not functioning properly) and unsafe where the equipment appears to be functioning but the reading is in fact false. It is important to acknowledge the limitations of pulse oximetry, which are summarised in Box 8.2 and discussed below.

Inaccurate at below 70% saturation

Does not measure adequacy of carbon dioxide elimination.

Does not measure oxygen delivery to the tissues

Does not measure lung function

Does not detect hyperoxia

Cannot distinguish between oxyhaemoglobin, and abnormal haemoglobins

Does not measure haemoglobin

Cannot differentiate between venous and arteriole pulsation

Box 8.2 Limitations of pulse oximetry

Stoddart *et al*. (1997) notes that it is the quality of oxygen delivery to the tissues which is of most importance and this depends on cardiac output, tissue perfusion and haemoglobin concentration, not just oxygen saturation of arterial blood. Oxyhaemoglobin saturation could be 99%, but this is of no value if the heart cannot deliver it to the tissues.

Activity Can you think of what signs and symptoms might indicate a lack of oxygen to the tissues (hypoxia)?

Signs which you could observe for include the warmth of peripheral areas of the body, colour of skin and tongue, urine output, and mental state (Place 1998).

Cowan (1997) identifies that oxygen therapy may lead to normal readings even though lung function is still impaired. It is also important to remember that pulse oximeters do not measure adequacy of carbon dioxide elimination.

The pulse oximeter cannot differentiate between arteriolar and venous pulsation and so in babies with certain cardiac conditions (such as tricuspid valve disease) the pulse oximeter can mistake venous saturation for arterial and give a falsely low reading (Stoddart *et al*. 1997). A further danger with using pulse oximetry in neonates is that hyperoxia, which is dangerous to neonates, retinas, and could affect sight, is not detected by pulse oximetry (Stoddart *et al*. 1997). Therefore, in practice, an upper SpO_2 limit will be established for neonates receiving oxygen therapy. If readings exceed this level, the alarm sounds indicating that the amount of oxygen needs to be reduced.

Pulse oximeters are unable to differentiate between different forms of saturated haemoglobin (Carroll 1997a). With inhalation of carbon monoxide, carboxyhaemoglobin (COHb) is formed and will be absorbed and registered as oxyhaemoglobin, leading to over-estimation of oxygen saturation. Thus for people who have been involved in accidents where there is smoke, or who are affected by carbonmonoxide poisoning, pulse oximetry is not recommended, and COHb readings are also high in tobacco smokers (Moyle 1996).

Cowan (1997) suggests that people with a low haemoglobin may have normal readings even though they may not have enough arterial oxygen to satisfy their needs. This is because the haemoglobin which they do have, even though abnormally low, may be saturated with oxygen, giving a normal but misleading SpO_2. In addition people with respiratory disease may develop high haemoglobin levels to compensate for their lack of oxygen although the haemoglobin may not be properly saturated with oxygen (Pfister 1995 cited by Cowan 1997). In some types of congenital heart disease there is mixing of oxygenated and deoxygenated blood leading to low SpO_2 readings, although the child is not in fact hypoxic.

Summary

- Pulse oximetry has become increasingly used and has many applications.
- It is non-invasive, easy to apply and provides a continuous measurement.
- It is important to understand the limitations of pulse oximetry and to be aware of its role as complementary to the overall clinical picture.

OBSERVATION OF SPUTUM AND COLLECTION OF SPUTUM SPECIMENS

Normally about 100 ml of mucus is produced in the lungs daily, but it goes unnoticed as it is usually swallowed (Rutishauser 1994). However, in a number of diseases excess mucus is produced and smoking also stimulates excessive mucus production; this excess mucus which is then expectorated from the lungs is termed sputum (Stocks 1996). When sputum is being produced, especially in suspected respiratory disease, a specimen will often be required for laboratory examination. Mr Collins, who has COPD, will be producing a large amount of sputum, and encouraging expectoration, observing his sputum, and sending a sputum specimen for analysis, will all be necessary in his care.

Learning outcomes

By the end of this section you will be able to:

1. Understand how expectoration of sputum can be encouraged, what sputum should be observed for and why.
2. Know how to collect a sputum specimen.

Learning outcome 1:
Understand how expectoration of sputum can be encouraged, what sputum should be observed for and why

Activity

It is important to encourage expectoration to prevent accumulation of secretions in the lungs (Stocks 1996). However, Dettenmeier (1992) notes that people will often deny that they are producing sputum, and some, particularly women, may feel embarrassed to expectorate, and are more likely to swallow their sputum. How could you encourage expectoration?

You can help the person to be in a well-supported, upright position which will make coughing easier (*see* Fig. 8.1), and a sputum pot and tissues should be provided. Ensuring that the person is well hydrated will render the sputum less thick and therefore easier to cough up. A dry mouth will also make expectoration difficult, and infected sputum may taste unpleasant, so you will need to provide mouth-care. Privacy should be given if there is embarrassment, and the nurse should ensure that no distaste is shown (Stocks 1996).

Activity

How would you describe normal sputum? What do you think might cause sputum to look abnormal?

Normal sputum (or mucus) of healthy individuals is odourless, clear and thin, and is similar in colour and consistency to saliva (Dettenmeier 1992). However, people with chronic respiratory disease, such as Mr Collins, will not have the normal sputum of a healthy individual but will have their own baseline which will probably be thicker than usual, and it is likely to be grey, tan or cream rather than clear (Dettenmeier 1992). It is therefore important to be aware of the individual's normal sputum when assessing for abnormalities. Signs of infection may be that the sputum is green, yellow or rust coloured, and it may also be odourous (Dettenmeier 1992). A pseudomonas infection produces thick, green sputum with a particularly characteristic odour.

A stringy mucoid specimen often occurs with bronchial asthma (Wilkins *et al.* 1995). If blood is present the sputum will be rust coloured or red, and will be termed **haemoptysis**. This may be a sign of infection but can also be present in cancer, heart failure and pulmonary embolus. It is important to check that it has actually come from the lungs and has not been vomited (**haemetemesis**) or come from the nose (**epistaxis**). Haemoptysis will be worsened by vigorous coughing, chest trauma, chest physiotherapy, anticoagulant therapy and activity.

With young children, you will need to ask parents if any sputum has been produced and if so, what it was like in colour and consistency (Woodhams *et al.* 1996). When assessing the amount being produced it is often best to ask in terms of teaspoons, tablespoons or cups. Patients may comment on the taste of the sputum which may be unpleasant if infected, or salty with cystic fibrosis.

Learning outcome 2:
Know how to collect a sputum specimen

The goal of sputum collection is to obtain fresh, uncontaminated secretions from the tracheo-bronchial tree (Wilkins *et al.* 1995). The lower part of the respiratory tract is usually sterile, but the upper respiratory tract, mouth and nose, are colonized by large numbers of different bacteria (Wilson 1995).

Activity   Why do you think a sputum specimen might need to be sent to the laboratory?

A sputum specimen may be sent for microbiological examination if infection, including tuberculosis (TB), is suspected, and may also be sent for cytology – examination for abnormal, e.g. cancerous, cells. Box 8.3 outlines the equipment needed and procedure and additional points are discussed below.

It is essential that when a sputum specimen is collected, it has actually come from the lower airways, and has not been cleared from the throat nor is in fact saliva. This will need to be explained carefully to the person, taking into

---

Equipment needed: A sterile specimen container with a leak proof lid or cap, and tissues.

Key points:
- An early morning specimen is best as bacteria counts are probably highest.
- Careful explanation is needed.
- The mouth should be rinsed with water and teeth brushed to prevent contamination with oral microbes.
- The sputum should be expectorated directly into the labelled container and the lid reapplied immediately.

Box 8.3 Key points in collecting a sputum specimen

account developmental stage and level of understanding. You can explain that the specimen must come from the 'windpipe'. Sputum will usually be more viscous and purulent than saliva; if the specimen appears to be saliva, it should be discarded (Wilkins *et al.* 1995). A physiotherapist can help the person who is having difficulty expectorating.

Woodhams *et al.* (1996) advise that children of 4–5 years upwards (particularly if they have cystic fibrosis which results in excess secretions being produced) should be able to provide a sputum specimen, if this is explained to them. However obtaining a sputum specimen from younger children will be more difficult and may require help from a physiotherapist. Occasionally suction will be needed, possibly using a mucus trap, but this is traumatic for the child so would only be used if there is no alternative (Woodhams *et al.* 1996).

When sputum is being sent for testing for TB, the specimen should be at least 10 ml (Wilkins *et al.* 1995). Three early morning specimens taken on different days will be required as the mycobacterium tuberculosis which causes TB may only be present in small numbers, particularly in the early stages of the disease (Thomlinson 1989). In small children, in whom TB is suspected, early morning gastric washings may be performed in order to collect swallowed sputum.

Testing in the laboratory involves the use of a Gram-stained smear. Most bacteria grow within 24 to 48 hours, but some bacteria, such as the mycobacterium tuberculosis, can take up to 6 weeks to grow (Wilkins *et al.* 1995). However microscopic examination of the sputum can lead to an initial tentative diagnosis. As the mycobacterium has very resistant cell walls it is stained using a special dye which cannot be removed by acid or alcohol. This method is termed 'acid-fast bacilli' or AFB (Wilson 1995).

Summary
- Nursing measures can encourage expectoration of sputum, which can then be observed for colour, consistency, amount, and odour.
- Careful explanations can help to ensure that an uncontaminated specimen of sputum can be obtained which can aid with an accurate diagnosis.

OXYGEN THERAPY

Definition

Oxygen is a colourless, odourless, tasteless gas which constitutes approximately 21% of atmospheric air at sea level (Ashurst 1995). Oxygen therapy is thus the administration of supplementary oxygen to enable a higher inspiration of oxygen than is achieved when breathing air. This may be a short term measure in acute illness (such as when Michael has been admitted with acute asthma), or it may be long-term in chronic respiratory disease, with home administration needed and, therefore, much support needed for both the individual concerned and the family.

Learning outcomes

By the end of this section you should be able to:

1. Identify reasons for oxygen therapy and for whom it will be needed.
2. Identify different devices for administering oxygen, showing insight into how different concentrations can be achieved.
3. Discuss how oxygen therapy can be administered to children and adults who may be frightened or confused.
4. Show insight into important safety aspects of oxygen administration.
5. Explain why humidification of oxygen may be needed and how this can be achieved.

Equipment required

Oxygen delivery systems: masks, nasal cannulas, headbox, and humidification equipment may all be accessible in the skills laboratory.

Learning outcome 1:
Identify reasons for oxygen therapy and for whom it will be needed

Activity

Reflect on where you may have seen oxygen therapy being used within the hospital or community and think of situations where people would benefit from receiving oxygen.

Myocardial infarction
When an interruption of blood supply to the myocardium causes death of tissue, usually resulting in severe chest pain which may radiate to the arms, jaw and/or neck, often accompanied by nausea and sweating. 'Heart attack' is the lay term for this condition.

You may have thought of the following:

- After a general anaesthetic.
- In emergency situations such as cardiac or respiratory arrest, and shock.
- In heart disease where cardiac output is reduced e.g. **myocardial infarction**.
- In chest injuries following trauma.
- In acute respiratory disease, such as an asthma attack. Michael would probably have required oxygen therapy when admitted to hospital.
- In chronic respiratory conditions (such as COPD and cystic fibrosis) where long term oxygen therapy may be needed, usually for a minimum of 15

hours per day. Two trials in the 1980s demonstrated improved survival rates in people with COPD who had long-term oxygen therapy (Dunn and Chisholm 1998). For these patients oxygen therapy can also improve quality of life as when oxygen demand is increased, such as when carrying out activities such as washing and dressing, oxygen therapy will help to reduce breathlessness, and can increase endurance by 30–50% (Rees and Dudley 1998). Mr Collins may require long-term oxygen therapy.

Learning outcome 2:
Identify devices for administering oxygen, showing insight into how different concentrations can be delivered

Oxygen supplies

In the hospital setting, the oxygen will be obtained either from a cylinder (black with white shoulders) or a wall mounted piped oxygen supply. There are a variety of flow meters in use with these, including very low flow meters to be used with infants. If cylinders are in use it is important to check them regularly as they can run out quite quickly. In the home, oxygen must be prescribed and is delivered via an oxygen company. It is usually administered from an oxygen concentrator, which uses room air, and removes nitrogen through filtration but without depleting surrounding air (Dunn and Chisholm 1998). The concentrator runs off electricity (an emergency cylinder is supplied in case of power failure), can deliver up to 4 litres per minute, and is supplied with up to 50 feet of tubing allowing considerable freedom around the home.

Delivery devices

The importance of administering oxygen using the correct mask and flow rate cannot be over-emphasized, but Bell's (1995) study found that this was achieved for only 18% of patients. Different concentrations of oxygen will be administered according to clinical need and this will affect which oxygen administration device is used. For infants and children the method of giving oxygen is selected on the basis of the concentration needed and the child's ability to co-operate with its use (Campbell and Glasper 1995). For all client groups, other than in an emergency situation, concentration of oxygen will be prescribed by the doctor according to clinical presentation or through pulse oximetry measurements or blood gas analysis. However Bell's (1995) study found that not all patients receiving oxygen therapy had a prescription for it.

Activity

Either in your clinical placement or in the skills laboratory, look at the devices for administering oxygen. How do you think different concentrations are achieved?

Oxygen therapy can be delivered at varying concentrations. These are often measured in percentages, such as 24%, 28%, 35% or 40%, which have been prescribed by the doctor according to the person's requirements. The flow of oxygen is measured in litres per minute using a flow meter. Different devices which you may have found include simple oxygen masks, Venturi masks, nasal cannulas, and non-rebreathing masks (*see* Fig. 8.9). These are disposable and packaged separately and each individual will have his own equipment. For young infants, a headbox can be used (*see* Fig. 8.10).

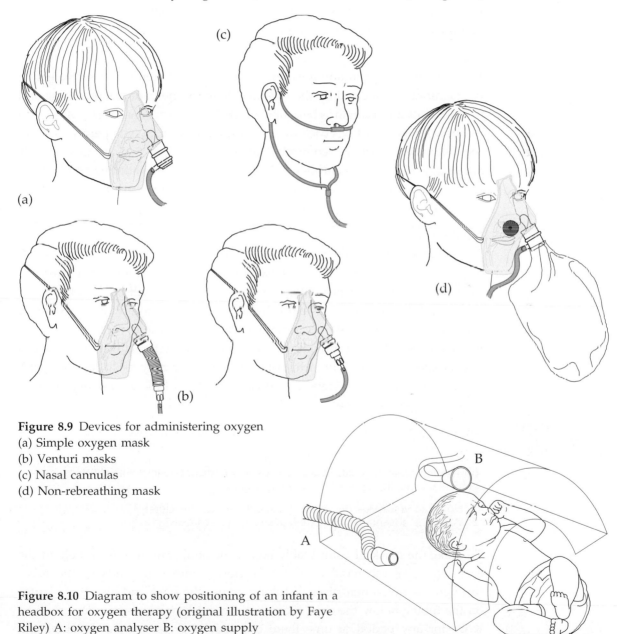

Figure 8.9 Devices for administering oxygen
(a) Simple oxygen mask
(b) Venturi masks
(c) Nasal cannulas
(d) Non-rebreathing mask

Figure 8.10 Diagram to show positioning of an infant in a headbox for oxygen therapy (original illustration by Faye Riley) A: oxygen analyser B: oxygen supply

Simple oxygen masks (such as Hudson or MC)

These masks are available in different sizes, for adults and children. The amount of oxygen delivered is adjusted only through the use of the flow meter and the exact amount delivered also depends on rate and depth of breathing (Bell 1995). However the estimated oxygen concentration achieved is 35–45% at 6–8 litres per minute (l/min), 45–55% at 8–10 l/min, and 55–65% at 10–12 l/min (Thelan *et al*. 1994). Simple oxygen masks are not suitable for administering low flow rates of 4 litres per minute or less, because with a low flow rate rebreathing of carbon dioxide may occur, as exhaled carbon dioxide accumulates within the mask (Oh 1999).

Venturi mask system

In the Venturi oxygen administration system the concentration of oxygen is not significantly affected by the rate and depth of the patient's breathing and a set concentration can thus be achieved (Bell 1995). The mask is supplied with different coloured fittings each clearly marked with an oxygen percentage and the flow rate which is required. The device ensures that oxygen flow is accurately diluted with entrained air. The nurse can thus administer the exact percentage, which has been prescribed by fitting the correct device and setting the correct flow rate.

Nasal cannulas

These administer oxygen directly into the nostrils rather than into the mouth and nose as masks do. Oxygen flow is only adjusted by use of the oxygen flow meter. Estimated percentage of oxygen inspired will be 24–28% at 1–2 l/min and 28–35% at 3–5 l/min (Thelan *et al*. 1994). Flow rates in excess of four litres per minute are not recommended due to the drying effect on the nasal mucosa. Nasal cannulas are sometimes used for chronically oxygen dependant babies, for whom high levels of oxygen may be hazardous, with special low-rate flow meters, which can deliver as little as one quarter of a litre of oxygen per minute.

■ **Activity**

For this activity you need access to oxygen administration masks and nasal cannulas either in the skills laboratory or on placement, and a colleague to use as a patient. Have a go at placing an oxygen mask on a colleague, and then try positioning nasal cannulas in place. Look at the diagrams in Figure 8.9 for guidance as to the optimal positioning. Consider:

1. How can you make the mask and nasal cannulas fit closely?
2. What the advantages/disadvantages of nasal cannulas?

To make the mask fit comfortably adjust the strap carefully to fit behind the ears. To make the nasal cannulas fit closely move the ends of the tubes through the horizontal piece of tubing across the nose and also the adaptor on the tubing below the chin. Note that if a mask or nasal cannulas are to be worn for any period of time there is a risk of pressure sore development, particularly on the bridge of the nose or behind the ears. It is important that they are a good fit and are replaced regularly. Tubing can be supported by gauze to stop sore ears (Jones 1997).

The advantages/disadvantages of nasal cannulas are analyzed by English (1994). Advantages of nasal cannulas may be that the patient can eat, drink and talk more easily and procedures, such as mouth-care, can be carried out without disrupting the oxygen administration. With babies, administering oxygen via nasal cannulas allows more freedom to the baby and care-giver, and enables feeding (including breast-feeding) to take place without disruption to oxygen therapy. Also some patients find a mask very claustrophobic. Bambridge's (1993) study found that nasal cannulas were considered comfortable by 90% of patients and were better tolerated than masks.

Administration via nasal cannulas may, however, not be very accurate, as actual intake of oxygen may vary according to whether the patient mouth breathes, and there are no concentration adjustment devices which can be fitted. With high flow rates there is likely to be discomfort and drying of the nasal mucosa (Oh 1999).

Non-rebreathing masks:
These have a large reservoir for oxygen with a series of valves to allow the patient to inhale only oxygen and prevent it mixing with expired gases. Concentration of oxygen is determined by the flow meter.

Headbox (see Fig. 8.10)
Infants best tolerate oxygen therapy when delivered via a headbox, a clear perspex box into which humidified oxygen is delivered when it is placed over the baby's head. Care must be taken to ensure that the headbox does not rest on the baby's shoulders or chin. The oxygen concentration in the headbox must be monitored continuously, using an oxygen analyzer, to ensure that the prescribed concentration is maintained.

■ **Activity**   Consider what are the advantages and disadvantages of using a headbox to administer oxygen.

You may have thought of any of these points:
Most of the baby's care can be performed without interfering with oxygen therapy. However the baby has to come out of the headbox for feeding. Observation of the baby's colour may be difficult through the headbox due to the humidity. The headbox may limit the baby's movement and older infants react vigorously to this. The headbox also represents a physical barrier between baby and family and this may be psychologically distressing for all of them. It also limits the extent to which physical comfort in the form of cuddles etc. can be offered to the baby.

Learning outcome 3:

Discuss how oxygen therapy can be administered to adults and children who may be frightened or confused

Think about how you would approach the following situations:
- A child who is frightened about oxygen therapy and reluctant to co-operate with it.
- A hypoxic adult who is confused and does not want oxygen administered.

Clear explanations are important for all age groups. With children and their families language appropriate to their level of understanding should be used. Considering level of understanding and learning ability is also particularly important in caring for a person with learning disabilities who is needing oxygen therapy. Demonstration of the mask/cannulas in position on a parent or nurse, and an explanation of the associated sensations and sounds may reassure a frightened child. Encouraging the younger child to position a mask on a doll or teddy may also help to allay fears. Treating oxygen therapy as a game or adventure may promote compliance, and distraction with toys, stories etc. may be successful in younger children. Involvement of parents in comforting their child is beneficial to all.

Mr Collins may become confused due to his hypoxia and may resist oxygen therapy. An important aspect to consider is positioning him to improve his ventilation, for example sitting him upright in a chair or in bed. With the confused adult nasal cannulas rather than a mask may be less disturbing. Again, support and explanations from a familiar relative may help.

Learning outcome 4:

Show insight into important safety factors to be considered when administering oxygen

The two main hazards are:

- Fire.
- Delivery of oxygen to people with chronic pulmonary disease, who are carbon dioxide retainers.

Fire hazard

You have probably attended fire lectures where a fire officer has outlined the 'fire triangle' necessary for a fire. Can you remember the three factors? Oxygen, fuel and heat are needed and if one of these is missing the fire cannot start or will quickly go out. Oxygen supports combustion and thus enhances the inflammable properties of other materials such as cigarettes, grease and oil (Ashurst 1995). Administration of oxygen could therefore be a fire hazard.

<table>
<tr><td>■ Activity</td><td>What precautions will be needed to reduce the risk of fire during oxygen therapy?</td></tr>
</table>

You could have thought of:
- No smoking signs.
- No toys which can spark.
- Educating patients and relatives about the risk of smoking during oxygen administration, and of using alcohol based sprays (e.g. in perfume or aftershave).
- Knowledge of fire procedure and equipment.
- Oxygen cylinders which are being used in the home will need keeping away from gas fires, naked flames and hot radiators (Jones 1997).

Carbon dioxide retainers

A further hazard is that there are certain patients for whom a high percentage of oxygen could be dangerous and actually cause the patient to develop carbon dioxide (CO_2) narcosis leading to coma (Ashurst 1995). These are patients who, due to chronic respiratory disease such as experienced by Mr Collins, continuously retain CO_2. These patients are termed CO_2 retainers. Children with cystic fibrosis are also potentially at risk from CO_2 narcosis. Normally, rising levels of CO_2 stimulate respiration. However, patients with chronic respiratory disease may continuously have a high level of CO_2 in their blood and therefore their chemoreceptors are no longer stimulated by this. For these patients, the less important hypoxic drive predominates, which means that breathing is only stimulated by lack of oxygen. Patients with chronic respiratory disease are, therefore, normally prescribed only 24–28% oxygen via a venturi mask initially and would only be prescribed a higher amount if indicated by arterial blood gas analysis (Rees and Dudley 1998). When Mr Collins is prescribed oxygen it will be important to establish whether he is a CO_2 retainer.

Learning outcome 5:
Explain why humidification of oxygen may be needed and how this can be achieved

Oxygen can be drying to the mucous membranes of the upper airway (Jones 1997), and this can lead to chest secretions being sticky and difficult to expectorate (Dunn and Chisholm 1998). Dryness to nostrils and mouth can be prevented through application of E45 cream and adequate fluid intake (Heslop and Shannon 1995). If oxygen is to be administered for more than a short period, humidification will be necessary particularly if the concentration being administered is high e.g. over 35%, or at a rate of four litres per minute or above.

Either in the skills laboratory or on your clinical placement, locate humidification equipment. What sort of water would need to be used do you think and why? What might be hazards associated with using humidification equipment?

As humidification provides a moist environment there is a risk of encouraging bacterial growth. Therefore sterile water would need to be used to minimize bacterial contamination, and the water should be changed daily. Cold water systems, where the oxygen is simply bubbled through water at room temperature, are inexpensive and easy to operate as a short-term humidification measure. These systems are noted to be fairly inefficient (Fell and Boehm 1998). In heated-water humidifiers, the oxygen is bubbled across a heated water reservoir. These systems are much more efficient, but there is a risk of mucosal over-heating or burning and excess condensation in the tubing which can reduce oxygen flow (Fell and Boehm 1998).

Any humidity supplied to young infants should be warmed as cold moist air may cause reflex bronchoconstriction (Carter 1995). However the temperature of the oxygen reaching the baby must be monitored to prevent over-heating.

Summary

■ Oxygen therapy is administered in a wide range of circumstances, to all age groups, and may be a short-term and emergency measure, or a long-term treatment.

■ A number of different devices are available for administering oxygen. The nurse must take into account age group, percentage of oxygen prescribed and tolerance when choosing a delivery system.

■ The main hazards are combustion, and administering a too high percentage to a person with chronic respiratory disease who is a CO_2 retainer. Both these hazards can be avoided by taking necessary care.

ADMINISTERING INHALED MEDICATION

The inhaled route permits medication to go directly to where it is needed in the mucous membranes of the bronchioles, providing an effective method of absorption. As less drug is required, the side effects of the drug used are less (Smith 1995). Some 39 million inhalers are prescribed in the UK each year (Myles 1999). Examples of drugs commonly inhaled are bronchodilators, and steroids for their anti-inflammatory effect. By 2002 all inhalers must be CFC free, to meet internationally agreed guidelines (Myles 1999). This is due to evidence that CFCs are destroying the ozone layer.

Learning outcomes

By the end of this section you will be able to:

1. Understand why inhalers are used.
2. Accurately explain how to use an inhaler and measure its benefit.
3. Demonstrate knowledge of various types of inhaler, and be able to adapt them in emergency situations.

Equipment required

You may be able to look at different inhalers within your practice placement. Placebo inhalers may be available in the skills laboratory.

Learning outcome 1:
Understand why inhalers are used

> ■ **Activity**
>
> For what reasons, and by whom, have you seen inhalers used?

Have you considered the following?
You may have seen inhalers used by both young children and adults. Because asthma occurs in 10–20% of children and 5–10% of adults (Hardy 1992), this will probably be the commonest reason for seeing inhalers used. It is estimated that the UK has around 3.4 million asthmatics (Myles 1999). Inhalers are also used in COPD and therefore Mr Collins might be prescribed inhalers too. Inhalers may be used as maintenance therapy as in Michael's case, as well as in emergency situations, where acute dyspnoea and cyanosis occur (do you remember what these words mean? They can all be found in the section on Measuring and recording respirations. Inhalers may also be used as prophylactic (preventative) treatment, for example before coming into contact with animal fur, grass, pollen etc, which may be **allergens** to asthmatics, or before taking strenuous activity where extra oxygen will be needed.

Allergen
A foreign substance which initiates an allergic response.

Learning outcome 2:
Accurately explain how to use an inhaler and measure its benefit

> ■ **Activity**
>
> Instructions for using an inhaler are in Box 8.4. Think about how you would actually explain this to an adult and to a child. Try to find someone who uses an inhaler, or if you have access to a skills lab, there may be a placebo inhaler, so that you can practise the explanation you have developed.

When planning your explanation you need to take developmental stage and learning ability into account. This is especially relevant if your client has a

> The person should be sitting or preferably standing, to maximize lung expansion. He should clear the respiratory tract by coughing if necessary, and then inhale and exhale deeply before commencing.
>
> 1. Check inhaler details (medication and dose) and prescription.
> 2. Remove the cap and shake the inhaler.
> 3. Place the mouthpiece into mouth and at the start of a slow deep inspiration, press the canister down, and continue to inhale deeply.
> 4. Remove the inhaler from mouth and hold breath for 10 seconds, or as long as possible (McKenzie 1994).
> 5. Wait several seconds before repeating for a second time if prescribed (note that most people are prescribed two puffs at a time).
> 6. Record administration on the prescription chart.

Box 8.4 Instructions for inhaler use

learning disability. Demonstration is a useful teaching strategy particularly with children. Devices using games (like keeping balls in the air during an inspiration) are available for a child to practise technique. Remember that inhaled medication must always be prescribed and patient details checked as per the drug policy *see* Chapter 11, Drug administration). The drug should be signed for on the drug administration sheet in the usual way.

Did you know?

One in five people do not use inhalers properly even after instruction (Asthma Training Centre 1997). Only 20% of inhaled particles reach the lungs when performed accurately and poor technique will reduce this still further.

Measuring effectiveness

What have you read in this chapter which would help you to measure the effectiveness of the inhaled therapy? You may remember that peak flow measurements can be helpful in monitoring effects of inhaled medication (*see* section on Peak flow measurement).

Learning outcome 3:
Demonstrate a knowledge of various types of inhalers and be able to use them in emergency situations

Activity

Again, thinking back to inhalers which you have seen, identify different types of inhaler currently in use.

A detailed overview of the inhaler devices available can be found in Weller (1999). Examples which you might have remembered include the volumatic, nebuhaler, diskhaler and rotohaler. With a diskhaler the inhaled particles are contained within a disk and with a rotohaler the particles are enclosed in a capsule. The disk or capsule is then inserted into the inhaler to deliver a metered amount. A volumatic inhaler ends with a large chamber, called a spacer, which contains the particles for inhalation. A nebuhaler is similar but the mouthpiece has several rings around it. These are particularly helpful for young children. The volumatic inhaler will be looked at in more detail (*see* Fig. 8.11).

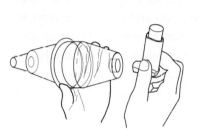
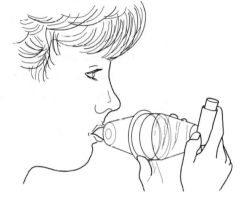

Figure 8.11 The volumatic inhaler

The volumatic inhaler

The large chamber in the spacer device slows down the speed of the drug leaving the inhaler from 70 mph to 40 mph and permits the larger particles to stick to the chamber walls (McKenzie 1994) instead of the mouth where they may cause candida infections (Hunter 1995). The smaller particles in the middle of the chamber then travel on into the trachea and bronchioles for absorption. By filling the chamber with inhaled particles of drug, the person can then breathe these in at his own rate, and the particles are less likely to be lost into the atmosphere. Using the spacer is 30% more effective (Asthma Training Centre 1997) than an ordinary inhaler. The manufacturers supply detailed instructions for using the volumatic. It is important that only one puff is squirted into the volumatic at a time.

■ Activity   Why might using a spacer be particularly useful with children (such as Michael)?

Spacers are advantageous for children as they remove the necessity to co-ordinate breathing in, with activating the canister. They can therefore be used for giving inhaled medications to very young children. Infants are unable to use the spacer's mouthpiece, but use of an inverted face mask angles the spacer so that the one way valve falls open, enabling even babies to use a spacer device (Campbell and Glasper 1995). There is a paediatric volumatic available with a soft face mask. Children may enjoy putting some favourite stickers on the volumatic. Note that spacers can also be used for elderly people if they are unable to co-ordinate breathing and using the canister.

Activity

If Michael did not have a spacer and became distressed and dyspnoeic due to his asthma, converting his inhaler into a spacer would help improve the situation in an emergency. How could you make his ordinary inhaler into a spacer device?

You will need a plastic or polystyrene cup and an inhaler. Make a slit in the base of the cup and force the mouthpiece of the inhaler through it. Michael will then need to hold the open end of the cup over his mouth and face, and you can then press the canister to release the drug into the space made by the cup. Michael should then breathe in and out slowly at least twice more before the cup is filled with a second metered dose and repeat. This is a useful first aid measure which you can use for any breathless asthmatic child or adult if a spacer is unavailable.

Summary
- Inhaled medication is frequently prescribed, particularly for asthmatics and people with chronic obstructive pulmonary disease, and a number of different devices are available.
- Inhaled medication is taken both prophylactically and as an emergency measure.
- Inhalers act directly on the respiratory tract so doses can be lower than when medication is taken systemically.
- It is very important that inhaler technique is effective so that the correct dose of medication is inhaled.

MANAGING NEBULIZED THERAPY

The nebulized route is the passage of medication to the bronchioles directly, as with inhalers, but by vaporizing the particles in a stream of air or oxygen. Nebulized particles are much smaller in diameter than inhaled particles (Critchley 1993). Medication for nebulizers is normally supplied in solution in single use plastic sealed containers called nebules. As with inhalers, the most common drugs given by nebulizer will be bronchodilators and steroids.

Learning outcomes

By the end of this section you will be able to:

1. Identify indications for nebulized rather than inhaled therapy.
2. Assemble and manage the required equipment and understand the rationale for the care of a person receiving nebulized therapy.
3. Understand how to decide whether to use oxygen or air to administer a nebulizer.

Equipment

A nebulizer with mouthpiece and mask attachments. These should be available in the skills laboratory or you might find them on placement.

Learning outcome 1:
Identify indications for nebulized rather than inhaled therapy

Activity

Can you identify the advantages of nebulized therapy over inhaled therapy?

The nebulized route enables bronchodilators to be transported more effectively than inhalers to the bronchioles because the oxygen or air in which it is converted into a vapour reduces the size of the particles, preventing them from sticking to the oral mucosa, and therefore being lost to the respiratory tract. The smaller particles can also travel more easily into the respiratory tract.

Link this information to Michael. Can you understand why in acute asthma, the nebulized route is preferred?

Activity

Think of other people who may benefit from nebulizers.

You could have thought of people who cannot manage to hold and co-ordinate a metered dose inhaler such as young children, some learning disability clients who have asthma, and unconscious patients. Nebulized medication can be delivered without a high degree of patient co-operation, for example by a mask, or holding a nebulizer mouthpiece between the lips and breathing normally. Thus nebulizers tend to be given in emergency situations, or where high doses of drug need to be administered in a situation where a person is unable to use other forms of inhaler device (Pearce 1998).

Learning outcome 2:
Assemble and manage the required equipment and understand the rationale for the care of a person receiving nebulizer therapy

Activity

Are there any special instructions you would need to give to Mr Collins and Michael if they required nebulized therapy?

The following points could all have been considered:

- Optimum position for ventilation. Can you remember this from previous sections? *See* Figure 8.1.
- Safety measures if oxygen is being used, which were discussed in the section on oxygen therapy.
- The noise of the nebulizer and the sensation within the mouth need to be explained.

The sensations associated with the nebulizer may be frightening to young children. Toddlers in particular may be unwilling to co-operate with a mask. Encouraging the child to hold the mask for himself may enhance co-operation (Campbell and Glasper 1995). A major nursing responsibility is to assess the child's tolerance of the procedure; a fighting, frightened child may become fatigued and appear worse (Campbell and Glasper 1995). The child's need for the treatment must be balanced against the distress and fatigue caused.

Activity

Can you identify any strategies which might enhance the co-operation of a small child?

You may have thought of using play strategies, or role modelling. It is not unusual to see the nebuliser without the mask being held near the child's face. However this may result in the majority of the dose being lost (Caster 1996). There are brightly coloured, child-friendly nebulizer devices available, which are aimed specifically at children, and may be more acceptable.

Activity

If you can access nebulizer equipment in the skills laboratory, try fitting the elements together. You will need to find a nebulizer unit including a mouthpiece or mask and tubing. Assemble the equipment as in Figure 8.12 or follow the manufacturer's instructions. Note that before assembling the equipment for a patient you should wash your hands, to reduce the risk of cross-infection.

Remember that nebulized medication must always be prescribed and patient details checked as per the drug policy (*see* Chapter 11, Drug administration). The drug should be signed for on the drug administration sheet in the usual way.

Activity

Before administering a nebulizer what questions would you need to ask yourself?

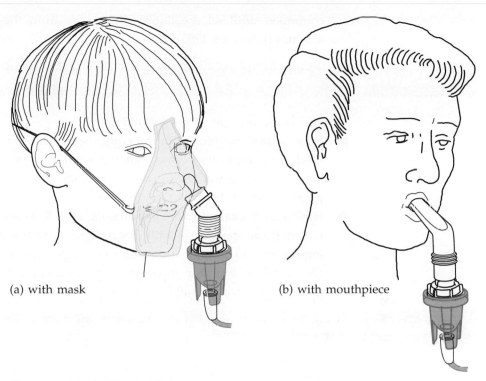

(a) with mask   (b) with mouthpiece

Figure 8.12 Nebulizer equipment

You may have considered:

■ **Does the peak flow need to be measured first?** This would serve as a baseline for comparison afterwards.

■ **Should the person use a mouthpiece or a mask?** Mouthpieces are only used where patients are physically and cognitively able to co-operate with holding it in the mouth. They should then be asked to breathe in and out of the mouth rather than the nose to gain maximum effect. A very breathless patient may find this too difficult and prefer to use a mask. However, as discussed in the section on oxygen therapy masks can be distressing to patients.

■ **Should I administer the nebulizer via air or oxygen?** See Learning outcome 3 for how you will decide on this.

■ **If using a cylinder (either air or oxygen) or piped oxygen what flow rate would be set on the flow meter?** The flow rate must be at least 6 litres per minute (Critchley 1993), else the particles will not be reduced to the appropriate size for inhalation.

■ **What instructions would I need to give to the person?** The person will need to understand that the mouthpiece or mask must be kept in place and to breathe normally. There is no need to remove to exhale. The nebulizer unit must be kept vertical throughout administration, and continued until all the liquid disappears from the unit, usually 5–10 minutes (Critchley 1993).

Activity

After administering a nebulizer, what questions might you ask yourself?

You may have thought of the following:

- **What should be done with the equipment**? The equipment can all be re-used with the same person, but the nebulizer unit and mouthpiece or mask should be washed in warm tap water and kept covered in a clean place (Critchley 1993).
- **How can I evaluate the nebulizer's effectiveness**? You can observe whether the person is still breathless, whether his/her colour has improved, and whether peak flow readings have increased. You should also consider whether there are any apparent side effects. Nebulized therapy can produce unpleasant side effects.

Activity

If you know anyone who has used nebulizers ask them to describe any side effects which they encountered.

Adverse side effects can include giddiness, tremor, palpitations, wheeziness and irritable coughing (Dodd 1996). These may be related to the drugs and then dosage may need adjustment. It is also important that the nebules are not too cold as this would cause bronchoconstriction. Mouth infections after prolonged use of certain inhaled drugs may occur too. In addition if it is a nebulized steroid which is being administered, delivery via a mask may cause irritation to the eyes and skin. Ipratropium bromide, a quite commonly prescribed bronchodilator, can also be irritating to the eyes when given via a mask. Washing the face may prevent irritation, and rinsing the mouth after inhalation of steroids may help to avoid oral candidiasis (Dodd 1996).

Learning outcome 3:
Understand how to decide whether to use oxygen or air for administering a nebulizer

Activity

Think back to the section on oxygen therapy and patients with a hypoxic drive. Do you remember what flow rate is required to administer a nebulizer? If you have seen air used rather than oxygen for administering a nebulizer, can you identify what the rationale could have been?

Remember that if a person has a hypoxic drive then it is a lack of oxygen which stimulates breathing. If oxygen is used at 6 litres per minute to administer a nebulizer, what could happen to such a person? Obviously there is a danger, as discussed earlier in this chapter, that CO_2 narcosis may result and therefore nebulizers for such patients should be administered via air, either through an air cylinder (which is grey in colour rather than the black with white shoulders oxygen cylinder), or an air compressor can be used if available. If a patient requires ongoing nebulizers at home these portable air compressor machines are much more convenient. They extract air from the atmosphere, and are available on prescription. When you are on a community placement do observe for these.

Summary

■ Nebulized therapy is widely used, particularly for people with acute respiratory disease.

■ Appropriate decisions must be made as to whether to administer a nebulizer with a mask or a mouthpiece, and via air or oxygen.

■ The nurse should be aware of side effects, and how these can be prevented or reduced.

CHAPTER SUMMARY

Respiratory problems can occur within any practice setting, and often arise very suddenly. This chapter has aimed to help you to feel confident with measurement of respiration, and other frequently used measuring skills – peak flow and pulse oximetry – were also included. These skills can appear very straightforward in nature, but it is important to understand what the measurements signify, and how accurate measurements can be obtained. Encouraging sputum expectoration can help to prevent the development of a chest infection, and nurses should be aware of the significance of how sputum may look. Oxygen therapy is administered for a range of people on both a short- and long-term basis. Nurses need to understand the potential hazards, and how it can be delivered safely. Many people with respiratory conditions use inhalers but as they are often used incorrectly, nurses need to understand how they can best be used so that they can educate clients. Nebulized medication is also often prescribed, and nurses need to understand how this can be administered safely.

There are many other specialized respiratory assessment skills and interventions, but the focus of this chapter has been to provide a foundation for how you can effectively care for someone with an actual or potential breathing problem. It is particularly important to understand the frightening nature of breathing problems, and to provide psychological support as well as competent technical care.

REFERENCES

Ashurst, S. 1995. Oxygen therapy. *British Journal of Nursing* **4**, 508–15.

Asthma Training Centre. 1997. *Asthma Training Centre Learning Package*. Stratford upon Avon.

Bambridge, A.D. 1993. Nasal catheters for oxygen administration. *British Journal of Theatre Nursing Suppl* **2** (10), S11–S16.

Bell, C. 1995. Is this what the doctor ordered? Accuracy of oxygen therapy prescribed and delivered in hospital. *Professional Nurse* **10**, 297–300.

Bellamy, D. and Bellamy, G. 1990. Peak flow monitoring. *Practice Nurse* **2**, 406–8.

Le Bourdelles, G., Estagnasie, P., Lenoir, F. *et al.* 1998. Use of a pulse oximeter in an adult emergency department. *Chest (Chicago)* **113**, 1042–7.

Brewin, A. and Hughes, J. 1995. Effect of patient education on asthma management. *British Journal of Nursing* **4**, 81–82, 99–101.

Campbell, S. and Glasper, E.A. 1995. *Whaley and Wong's Children's Nursing*. London: Mosby.

Carroll, P. 1997a. Pulse oximetry – at your fingertips. *RN* **60** (2), 22–7, 43.

Carroll, P. 1997b. Using pulse oximetry in the home. *Home Healthcare Nurse* **15**, 88–97.

Carter, B. 1995. Nursing support and care: meeting the needs of the child and family with altered respiratory function. In: Carter, B. and Dearmun, A. (eds.) *Child Health Care Nursing: Concepts, Theory and Practice.* Oxford: Blackwell Science, 274–305.

Cartridge, M. 1990. *Guidelines for Health Professionals and the Measurement of Peak Flow.* London: National Asthma Campaign.

Caster, A. 1996. Choosing nebulisers for children. *Paediatric Nursing* **8** (8), 15–16.

Cote, J., Cartier, A., Malo, J.L. *et al.* 1998. Compliance with peak expiratory flow monitoring in home management of asthma. *Chest (Chicago)* **113**, 968–72.

Cowan, T. 1997. Pulse oximeters. *Professional Nurse* **12**, 744–5, 747–8. 750.

Critchley, D. 1993. Nurses' knowledge of nebulised therapy. *Nursing Standard* **8** (10), 37–9.

Dettenmeier, P.A. 1992. *Pulmonary Nursing Care*. St Louis: Mosby.

Dodd, 1996. Nebuliser therapy: what nurses and patients need to know. *Nursing Standard* **10** (31), 39–42.

Donohue, J.F. 1996. Asthma: Indications, benefits, and pitfalls of peak flow monitoring. *Consultant* **36**, 2589–96.

Dunn, L. and Chisholm, H. 1998. Oxygen therapy. *Nursing Standard* **13** (7), 57–60.

English, I. 1994. Oxygen mask or nasal catheter – an analysis. *Nursing Standard* **8** (26), 27–30.

Fell, H. and Boehm, M. 1998. Easing the discomfort of oxygen therapy. *Nursing Times* **94** (38), 56–8.

Grap, M.J. 1998. Protocols for practice: applying research at the bedside. Pulse oximetry. *Critical Care Nurse* **18**, 94–9.

Hanning, C.D. and Alexander-Williams, J.M. 1995. Pulse oximetry: a practical review. *British Medical Journal* **311**, 367–70.

Hardy, S.G. 1992. *Nursing implications for increased asthma prevalence*. British Journal of Nursing **1**, *653–59.*

Heslop, A. and Shannon, C. 1995. Assisting patients living with long-term oxygen therapy. *British Journal of Nursing* **4**, 1123–8.

Hull, D. and Hohnstone, D. 1999. *Essential Paediatrics*, 4th edn. Edinburgh: Churchill Livingstone.

Hunter, S. 1995. The use of steroids in asthma treatment. *Nursing Standard* **9** (38), 25–7.

Jones, S. 1997. Oxygen therapy. *Community Nurse* **3**, 234.

Leach, A. 1994. Making sense of peak flow recordings of lung function. *Nursing Times* **90** (44), 34–5.

Le Grand, T.S. and Peters, J.I. 1999. Pulse oximetry: advantages and pitfalls. *Journal of Respiratory Diseases* **20**, 195–200, 206.

Lowton, K. 1999. Pulse oximeters for the detection of hypoxaemia. *Professional Nurse* **14**, 343–50.

Matthews, P. 1997. Using a peak flow meter. *Nursing* 97 **June**, 57–9.

McKenzie, S. 1994. Drugs used to control asthma. *British Journal of Nursing* **3**, 872–86.

Moyle, J. 1996. How to guides. Pulse oximetry. *Care of the Critically Ill* **12** (6), insert.

Moyle, J. 1999. Step by step guide. Pulse oximetry. *Journal of Neonatal Nursing* **5**, insert.

Myles, J. 1999. The future for asthma care is CFC-free. *Practice Nurse* **17**, 146–7.

Oh, T.E. 1999. Oxygen therapy. In: Oh, T.E. (ed.) *Intensive Care Manuel*, 4th edn. Oxford: Butterworth-Heinemann, 209–16.

Pearce, L. 1998. Know how: Asthma inhalers. *Nursing Times* **94** (9) Suppl.

Peters, S.M. 1997. The effect of acrylic nails on the measurement of oxygen saturation as determined by pulse oximetry. *Journal of the American Association of Nurse Anaethetists* **65**, 361–3.

Place, B. 1998. Pulse oximetry in adults. *Nursing Times* **94** (50), 48–9.

Rees, P.J. and Dudley, F. 1998. ABC of oxygen: oxygen therapy in chronic lung diseases. *British Medical Journal* **317**, 871–4.

Rodriguez, R.M. and Light, R.W. 1998. Pulse oximetry in the ICU: Uses, benefits, limitations. *The Journal of Critical Illness* **13**, 247–52.

Rutishauser, S. 1994. *Physiology and Anatomy: A Basis for Nursing and Health Care.* Edinburgh: Churchill Livingstone.

Schnapp, L.M. and Cohen, N.H. 1990. Pulse oximetry: uses and abuses. *Chest* **98**, 1244–50.

Seymour, J. 1995. Asthma: peak flow meters. *Nursing Times* **91** (4), 50, 52.

Sinex, J.E. 1999. Pulse oximetry: principles and limitations. *American Journal of Emergency Medicine* **17**, 59–66.

Smith, E. 1995. Guidelines for asthma treatment. RCN Nursing Update. *Nursing Standard* **9** (13), 1–8.

Stocks, J. 1996. Respiration. In: Hinchliff, S.M., Montague, S.E. and Watson, R. *Physiology for Nursing practice*, 2nd edn. London: Ballière Tindall.

Stoddart, S., Summers, L. and Platt, M.W. 1997. Pulse oximetry: what it is and how to use it. *Journal of Neonatal Nursing* **3** (4), 10, 12–14.

Stoneham, M.D., Saville, G.M. and Wilson, I.H. 1994. Knowledge about pulse oximetry among medical and nursing staff. *The Lancet* **344**, 1339–42.

Summers, R.L., Anders, R.M., Woodward, L.H. *et al.* 1998. Effect of routine pulse oximetry measurements on ED triage classification. *American Journal of Emergency Medicine* **16** (1), 5–7.

Thelan, L.A., Davie, J.K., Urden, L.D. and Lough, M.E. 1994. *Critical Care Nursing: Diagnosis and Management*, 2nd edn St Louis: Mosby.

Thomlinson, D. 1989. Laboratory intervention. In: Caddow, P. (ed.) *Applied Microbiology*. London: Scutari Press, 103–27.

Weller, T. 1999. Inhaler devices for use in asthma care. *Professional Nurse* **15**, 187–92.

Wilkins, R.L., Jones Krider, S. and Sheldon, R.L. 1995. *Clinical Assessment in Respiratory Care*, 3rd edn. St Louis: Mosby.

Wilson, J. 1995. *Infection Control in Clinical Practice*. London: Ballière Tindall.

Wong, D.L., Hockenberry-Eaton, M., Winkelstein, M.L. *et al* 1999. *Nursing Care of Infants and Children*, 6th edn. St Louis: Mosby.

Woodhams, K., Trussler, J. and Wooler, E. 1996. The Respiratory System. In: McQuaid, L., Huband, S. and Parker, E. (eds.) *Children's Nursing*. New York: Churchill Livingstone, 171–87.

Wooler, E. 1994. Asthma in children. *Paediatric Nursing* **6** (10), 29–33.

Woollons, S. 1995. Peak flow meters. *Professional Nurse* **11**, 130–2.

Chapter

9

Caring for the person with impaired mobility

Glynis Pellatt

In many settings nurses will encounter patients and clients who have impaired mobility, and are therefore at risk of a number of complications. Nurses have an important role, in actively preventing these complications, as well as seeking to promote mobility safely whenever possible. Correct moving and handling techniques will be needed when caring for the person with impaired mobility, and some principles of safe moving and handling will be referred to during this chapter. It is essential to ensure that you remain up-to-date with these techniques, and attend organized classroom sessions. As a registered nurse, you will also need yearly updates.

Included in this chapter are:
- Pressure sore risk assessment
- Pressure sore prevention
- Prevention of other complications of immobility
- Assisting with mobilization.

Recommended biology reading:
These questions will help you to focus on the biology underpinning this chapter's skills. Use your recommended text book to find out:

- What systems are involved in movement and posture?
- Which cells actually shorten and lengthen?
- What are joints?
- Find out the different types of joint.

> • Are all joints moveable?
> • What are the functions of tendons and ligaments?
> • How do we maintain flexibility?
> • What are the functions of our muscles and bones?
> • What happens to them if we are immobile?
> • What other body systems would be affected by immobility?
> • How would you feel if you were unable to move about?
>
> **Note**: that it will also be useful to revise the layers of the skin.

PRACTICE SCENARIOS

The following scenarios illustrate situations where nurses will need to assist with, and promote, mobility, and implement measures to prevent complications of immobility.

■ **Adult**

Mrs Elsie Smith is a 78-year-old woman who has been admitted to an orthopaedic ward from the Accident and Emergency Department with a fractured neck of right femur following a fall at home. She is well nourished and her general condition is good. She has been admitted into a bed with a standard hospital mattress. She will be going to theatre later today for internal fixation of the fracture. Movement is painful.

■ **Child**

Ben Chalmers aged 2 years and 2 months, has been admitted to a paediatric ward with **meningococcal septicaemia**. Movement is painful and he has a haemorrhagic rash with some exudating lesions. He is pyrexial and has an intravenous infusion in progress. He is not yet toilet trained.

Meningococcal septicaemia

Infection of the blood with meningococcus bacteria.

■ **Learning disability**

Robert Brown is a 30-year-old man with a learning disability who lives in a community unit. Due to accompanying physical disabilities he has to use a wheelchair for mobilizing. He is underweight and incontinent of urine and faeces; his skin tends to be dry. Joint deformities make it very difficult to position him comfortably in the wheelchair. He has a poor appetite and is unable to feed himself or manage his own hygiene needs. He likes to be called Bob.

■ **Mental health**

Mrs Flora Baker, who likes staff to call her Flora, is aged 80 years and lives in a community health-care trust unit for the elderly mentally ill. She has dementia and very limited mobility, needing help to walk due to

Rheumatoid arthritis
A chronic condition causing inflamed, stiff and painful joints.

rheumatoid arthritis. She is incontinent of urine and has problems communicating, and maintaining her hygiene and safety. Her general condition is fair.

PRESSURE SORE RISK ASSESSMENT

A pressure sore is a lesion that is due to:

Ischaemia
A reduction in blood flow.

■ unrelieved pressure on the skin causing ischaemia
■ sheer or friction causing mechanical stress on tissues
■ or a combination of these,

that results in underlying tissue damage. It usually occurs over a bony prominence (Simpson *et al*. 1996; Cowan and Woollons 1998; James 1998).

Learning outcomes

By the end of this section you will be able to:

1. Identify how pressure sores are formed.
2. Discuss why some people are more likely to develop pressure sores.
3. Use a pressure sore risk calculator to identify people at risk of pressure sores.
4. Discuss the importance of accurate documentation of pressure sore risk assessment.

Learning outcome 1:
Identify how pressure sores are formed

Activity

Hold a clear plastic tumbler in your hand using your fingertips. Press with your fingers and notice how your fingertips have gone very pale. Now release the pressure and look at your fingertips: they will have a red flush.

The red flush is called reactive hyperaemia.

Pressure damage occurs when skin and other tissues are compressed between bone and another surface. Body cells will die if the flow of blood in the capillary bed is not sufficient to supply oxygen, carbohydrates and amino acids for metabolism and to remove carbon dioxide and the products of catabolism (James 1998). Capillary closing pressure is the degree of external pressure required to occlude the blood vessels. It is suggested that external pressures above the mean capillary blood pressure will cause capillary closure. The average mean capillary blood pressure in healthy people is 20 mmHg, but this can be much lower in ill health (Simpson *et al*. 1996).

The time taken for irreversible changes to take place leading to tissue death varies. If pressure is relieved while the capillary and lymphatic circulation are intact, this will result in a sudden increase in blood flow to the area as the build up of metabolites acts on the arteriole sphincters. However, if the capillaries and lymphatic circulation have been irreversibly damaged the hyperaemia will be non-blanching and blistered. The reddening is caused by blood leaking from damaged capillaries. The damage will progress to deeper layers if the pressure is not relieved.

■ **_Activity_** What areas of the body will be most at risk of developing pressure sores? Use the scenarios to help you to identify these at risk areas.

You may have identified that skin over bony prominences is particularly at risk (see Fig. 9.1).

■ Sacrum, hips, heels, elbows, knees and malleoli will be a particular problem for Mrs Smith who is confined to bed until her operation. She will also be visiting X-ray and will be operated on in theatre. Lying on a trolley, X-ray table and operating theatre table will add to the risk to those vulnerable areas (Roper *et al.* 1996).

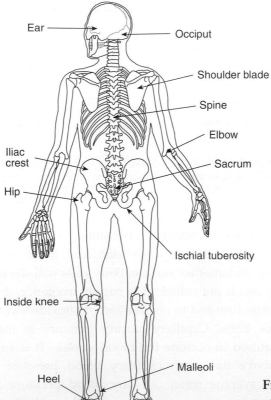

Figure 9.1 Skin areas particularly at risk of pressure sore formation

- Bob uses a wheelchair and therefore skin over his ischial tuberosities and the inner aspect of his knees is vulnerable.
- As Flora has limited and painful mobility she will probably sit in a chair quite a lot, so her at risk areas will be similar to Bob's.
- Babies and children have an uneven distribution of body weight in that their heads comprise a disproportionately high amount of the total body weight. Therefore when Ben is lying on his back his occipital region will be at risk of pressure (Olding and Patterson 1998).

You may also have identified the shoulder blades, iliac crests, sides of feet, ears and spine. However it has to be remembered that pressure sores can occur anywhere, particularly if there are tight clothes, splints or appliances that cause pressure. Areas of the body at risk of pressure sores are usually termed pressure areas.

Learning outcome 2:
Discuss why some people are more likely to develop pressure sores

Activity

Sit in a straight-backed chair. Now see how long you can sit there without moving.

Multiple sclerosis
Progressive destruction of myelin sheaths of neurones in the central nervous system. Can cause loss of movement and sensation.

Spinal cord injury
Damage to the spinal cord which causes paralysis and loss of sensation below the injury.

Cerebrovascular accident (CVA)
Cerebral damage caused either by decreased blood flow or haemorrhage. Effects vary but often causes paralysis down one side of the body (hemiplegia), and speech and swallowing difficulty. Commonly termed a 'stroke'.

How long did you manage: 5 minutes, 10 minutes or longer? What was it that made you move? You probably found that your pressure areas became very uncomfortable and eventually you had to move position. Reduced mobility is considered to be the most important factor in the development of pressure sores (Simpson *et al.* 1996). The body's defence against pressure is to shift weight frequently whether asleep or awake as a response to sensory stimulation.

Some people, however, have reduced sensation to pressure and pain neurologically induced by medical conditions such as **multiple sclerosis**, **spinal cord injury** or **cerebrovascular accident**. Some medication, such as sedatives, may cause a chemically induced reduction in sensitivity to pressure and pain. Sedation can also cause people to be too drowsy to move around. Some people, particularly if depressed, could lack the motivation to move, and others, such as those with dementia, are unable to respond to pressure stimuli and spontaneously alter their position. This, therefore, is a consideration in the care of Flora.

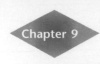

Think about factors other than reduced sensation and mobility which may make a person susceptible to pressure sores.

Factors may be extrinsic (outside the person e.g. environmental) or intrinsic (to do with the individual himself). Box 9.1 lists some of the main factors, which are discussed below.

Extrinsic	Intrinsic
Pressure	Moisture
Shearing	Acute illness: pyrexia, infection
Friction	Ageing
	Emaciation
	Obesity
	Poor nutrition
	Pain
	Poor oxygen perfusion

Box 9.1 Factors contributing to pressure sore formation

Extrinsic factors

We have already discussed the role of pressure in causing pressure sores. Shear occurs when a person begins to move or slide due to gravity but the skin under pressure, remains stationary. Tissues are then wrenched in opposite directions resulting in disruption or angulation of capillary blood vessels causing ischaemia. Shear can be very destructive to deep tissues (Simpson *et al*. 1996). Friction damage is caused by the surface of the skin sliding along the support surface when the tissue is under compression. Shear and friction could be a problem for Mrs Smith who may slide down the bed and Bob who may slide if not properly positioned in his wheelchair.

Intrinsic factors

Moisture
Moisture makes skin more vulnerable as it may stick to the support surface. Contamination by urine and faeces adds to the vulnerability. The risk of pressure sore development can increase fivefold by the presence of even small amounts of moisture (Dealey 1997). Flora and Bob are both incontinent of urine making them particularly at risk. *See* Chapter 6 (section: promotion of continence and management of incontinence) for a detailed discussion of how incontinence affects skin integrity.

Acute illness

Acutely ill patients, such as Ben, are particularly vulnerable to pressure sore formation for a number of reasons. Pyrexia increases the **metabolic rate**, particularly the demand for oxygen, which endangers ischaemic areas. Severe infection can also cause nutritional disturbances and local bacteria increase the demand on local metabolism by both their own requirements and the response of the body's defence mechanism (Simpson et al. 1996). In children a sudden rise in temperature and rapid spread of infection affects the wound healing process due to the system's inability to counteract such a significant attack. (Pickersgill 1997).

Ageing

Pressure sores are more common in people like Mrs Smith and Flora who are over 65 years old. Thinning of the dermis leads to reduced elasticity of the skin.

Body weight

Body weight is important in that emaciated patients have no protective 'padding' over bony prominences. Very obese patients may not be able to lift clear and therefore drag themselves up the bed (Russell 1998).

Poor nutrition

It has been suggested that there is a link between diet prior to admission to hospital and development of pressure sores. Lewis (1998) suggests that protein, zinc, vitamin C and iron have a role in preventing pressures sore. Older people need higher intakes of Vitamin C than young people do. In elderly patients with fractured neck of femur, such as Mrs Smith, the fracture increases metabolic requirements and reduces mobility, which may lead to pressure damage. Bob's poor nutritional intake will further his pressure sore risk.

Pain

Pain will prevent patients from repositioning themselves, particularly at night. Mrs Smith and Ben both have painful movement, and Flora may also have painful joints due to her rheumatoid arthritis.

Poor oxygen perfusion

Patients that have poor oxygen perfusion due to conditions such as heart disease, respiratory disease, **anaemia** and **diabetes** have a lower peripheral capillary pressure. Smoking exacerbates poor oxygen perfusion in all these conditions (Young 1997.

Learning outcome 3:
Use a pressure sore risk calculator to identify people at risk of pressure sores

---

Metabolic rate
The overall rate at which heat is produced in the body.

Anaemia
Reduced haemoglobin concentration in the blood, or abnormal haemoglobin, resulting in reduced oxygen carrying capacity.

Diabetes (mellitus)
A disease caused by deficient insulin release leading to inability of the body cells to use carbohydrates, and an elevated blood glucose.

Activity

Have you seen any pressure sore risk calculators used in your clinical placements? If so, which ones have you seen?

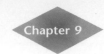
The Norton scale (Norton *et al.* 1962)

Physical condition		Mental state		Activity		Mobility		Incontinence	
Good	4	Alert	4	Ambulant	4	Full	4	Not	4
Fair	3	Apathetic	3	Walks with help	3	Slightly limited	3	Occasionally	3
Poor	2	Confused	3	Chairbound	2	Very limited	2	Usually urine	2
Very bad	1	Stuporous	1	Bedfast	1	Immobile	1	Double	1

Assessment of risk: under 14: at risk.

Waterlow pressure sore risk assessment (Waterlow 1988)

Build/weight for height		Skin type/ visual risk areas		Sex/ Age		Special risks Tissue malnutrition	
Average	0	Healthy	0	Male	1	e.g. Terminal cachexia	8
Above average	1	Tissue paper	1	Female	2	Cardiac failure	5
Obese	2	Dry	2	14–49	1	Peripheral vascular disease	5
Below average	3	Oedematous	1	50–64	2	Anaemia	2
		Clammy (temp+)	1	65–74	3	Smoking	1
		Discoloured	2	75–80	4		
		Broken/spot	3	81-plus	5		

Continence		Mobility		Appetite		Neurological deficit
Complete/ catheterized	0	Full	0	Average	0	e.g. diabetes, MS, CVA,
Occasional incontinence	1	Restricted/fidgety	1	Poor	1	Motor/sensory paraplegia 4–6
Catheter/incontinent of faeces	2	Apathetic	2	NG tube/ Fluids only	2	**Major surgery/trauma** Orthopaedic –
Double incontinence 3		Restricted	3	NBM/anorexic	3	Below waist/spinal, 5
		Inert/traction	4			on table >2 hours
		Chairbound	5			**Medication**
						Cytotoxics, High-dose
						steroids, anti-inflammatory 4

Score: 10+ At risk   15+ High risk   20+ Very high risk

The pressure sore prediction score (Lowthian 1987)

'No', 'No but' . . . etc. are how you would score to answer the questions
The questions concern the patient's state at the time the score is checked

	No	No but	Yes but	Yes
Sitting up?	0	1	2	3
Unconscious?	0	1	2	3
Poor general condition?	0	1	2	3
Incontinent?	0	1	2	3

	Yes	Yes & No	No
Lifts up?	0	1	2
Gets up and walks?	0	1	2

A total of 6 or more = danger

Box 9.2 Examples of pressure sore risk calculators

The Pattoid pressure scoring system (Olding and Patterson 1998)

Cardiovascular	1 Stable without inotropes
	2 Stable with inotropic support
	3 Inotropic support and unstable
Thermoregulation	1 Normothermic
	3 Hyperthermic/hypothermic
Respiratory	1 Self-ventilating in air
	2 Face mask/head in box oxygen
	3 Intubated
Mobility	1 Normal mobility
	2 Restricted mobility
	3 Paralysed and sedated
Nutrition	1 Unrestricted diet and fluids
	2 Fluid restriction as enteral/total parenteral nutrition only
	3 Fluid restriction
Continence	1 Fully continent
	2 Incontinent faeces only (catheterized)
	3 Incontinent of urine and faeces (that is, wearing nappies)
Skin condition	1 Intact
	2 Oedematous/clinically overloaded, discoloration/marking easily
	3 Broken/excoriated/surgical wounds/burns
Weight status	1 Average
	3 Overweight
	3 Underweight
Pressure score:	
8–14	Low risk
15–20	Medium risk
20+	High risk

Box 9.2 *Continued*

Pressure sore risk calculators are systems that have been developed to help in the identification of people at risk of developing pressure sores. There are many pressure sore risk calculators in use including:

- The Norton Score
- The Waterlow Scale
- Pressure Sore Prediction Score
- The Pattoid System.

The calculator used should be appropriate to the clinical setting and research among a similar care group should be available to support the calculator's accuracy.

We will now look at each in a little more detail. Box 9.2 displays these scales. Note that some terms used in the scales are defined in the margin.

The Norton Score (Norton *et al.* 1962)

The Norton score was developed in 1962 in a unit for the care of the elderly. It consists of five headings, each giving a numerical score. A score under 14 indicates a patient is at risk of developing a pressure sore.

Terminal cachexia
Wasting away of body tissues in the final stages of disease. Associated with malnutrition, emaciation, unhealthy skin, anaemia and general ill health.

The Waterlow Scale (Waterlow 1988)

The Waterlow risk assessment card was developed for use with general adult populations. It identifies three degrees of risk status – 'at-risk', 'high-risk' and 'very high-risk'. The aim of this tool was to provide guidelines on the selection of preventive aids and equipment and to promote the user's awareness of the causes of pressure sore development (Simpson *et al.* 1996).

Peripheral vascular disease
Disease of the blood vessels outside the heart, usually atherosclerosis. Causes insufficient blood supply to the feet.

Pressure Sore Prediction Score (Lowthian 1997)

The pressure sore prediction score was developed at the Royal National Orthopaedic Hospital for orthopaedic, trauma and spinal injured patients. The scale consists of six questions with 'yes', 'yes but', 'no', 'no but' answers.

Inotropes
Positive inotropic drugs increase the force of contraction of the myocardium.

The Pattoid System (Olding and Patterson 1998)

The Pattoid system was developed as a risk assessment tool for paediatric patients. It identifies three levels of risk – 'low-risk', 'medium-risk' and 'high-risk'.

■ Activity

Assess the people in the scenarios for pressure sore risk as follows:
- Mrs Smith using the Pressure Sore Prediction Score
- Ben using the Pattoid System
- Flora using the Norton Scale
- Bob using the Waterlow Scale.

Compare your answers with those below.

■ Mrs Smith would probably have a score of 7:
   3 in the category sitting up
   2 in the category lifts up
   2 in the category gets up and walks.

- Ben would probably have a score of 16:
  Cardiovascular 1
  Thermoregulation 3
  Respiration 1
  Mobility 2
  Nutrition 2
  Continence 3
  Skin 3
  Weight 1.

- Flora has a score of 12:
  Physical condition 3
  Mental state 2
  Activity 3
  Mobility 2
  Continence 2.

- Bob has a score of 16:
  Build/weight 3
  Continence 3
  Skin type 2
  Mobility 5
  Sex 1
  Age 1
  Appetite 1.

As you can see, there are many different scales to choose from and all our patients/clients in the scenarios are judged to be at risk of pressure sore formation on the scales used. It has been suggested that all risk calculators are based on factors that are known to predispose patients to pressure sore formation. However the variety of risk assessment scales in use today reflects the lack of consensus with regard to the relative importance of each group of predisposing factors (Pang and Wong 1998). Some calculators may over predict the risk of pressure sores, which has cost implications when pressure-relieving equipment is being provided. On the other hand if a scale under-predicts, then this has cost implications both in financial terms if a patient's stay in hospital is prolonged, as well as the human cost of pain and suffering from a pressure sore.

Simpson *et al.* (1996) offer some recommendations to optimize risk assessment tools.

1. Select a tool, which is appropriate to the patient/client group.
2. Ensure all members of the nursing team are familiar with the tool.

3. Ensure risk assessment is undertaken at appropriate times during a patient's hospital stay, especially when a major change in health status has occurred. For example, Mrs Smith should be reassessed after her surgery as her condition has changed.
4. Regularly review the cut-off point used to describe risk threshold by reviewing pressure sore incidence data in conjunction with published literature on the application of the tool.

Learning outcome 4:
Discuss the importance of accurate documentation of pressure sore risk assessment

■ Activity   Consider why it is important to record information relating to pressure sore risk in nursing documentation.

The care plan is the principle means of communication between the nurses caring for a patient. Tingle (1997) has pointed out that medico-legal problems exist in pressure sore care. There are regular cases and complaints involving poor standards of communication which include inadequate record keeping. It is vital that there is evidence of risk assessment and pressure sore prevention in patient records.

Summary
- There are many factors which can render a person vulnerable to pressure sore formation.
- Pressure sore risk calculators can help nurses to accurately identify those at risk.
- There are a range of pressure sore risk calculators available. Nurses need to choose one suitable for their patient/client group after considering available evidence.
- Documentation of pressure sore risk assessment is essential for medico-legal reasons and to promote good communication.

PRESSURE SORE PREVENTION

It is estimated that 95% of pressure sores are preventable; the 5% that are not preventable are due to pre-admission problems such as lying on the floor for a long period of time following a fall (Hampton 1998).

Learning outcomes

By the end of this section you will be able to:

1. Discuss why pressure sore prevention is an important aspect of the nurse's role.
2. Identify ways of preventing pressure sores in people at risk.

Learning outcome 1:
Discuss why pressure sore prevention is an important aspect of the nurse's role

■ **Activity**

All the four people in the scenarios have been assessed as at risk of developing pressure sores. Consider why is it important that a pressure sore prevention plan is implemented for them.

You may have thought of any of the following points:

- Pressure sores can be instrumental in a patient's death (Young 1997). Infected pressure sores have been identified as causing septicaemia and bronchopneumonia.
- Pressure sores can cause pain, loss of independence and social isolation (Arblaster 1998).
- Patients with pressure sores will remain in an acute setting 5 days longer than patients without pressure sores (Hampton 1998)
- Pressure sores are a financial drain on the National Health Service with estimates of the financial costs ranging from £60 million to £200 million annually (Kiernan 1997).
- Pressure sores have been identified as a key indicator of quality care and most provider units collate data on the number of pressure sores sustained by their patients. Purchasers use this data as a means of assessing quality of care (James 1998).

So it can be seen that there are many reasons why pressure sores must be prevented. Prevention of pressure sores has always been a nursing role; Florence Nightingale believed that good nursing care could prevent pressure sores (Russell 1998). However there is a growing opinion that a multidisciplinary approach must be taken towards the prevention of pressure sores (Dealey 1997). Nevertheless, as nurses assess, plan implement and evaluate care to meet all aspects of patients/clients' needs, they are in a key position to deliver pressure sore prevention.

Learning outcome 2:
Identify ways of preventing pressure sores in people at risk

■ **Activity**

List some methods of pressure relief that you have observed in practice placements that might be suitable for our four patients/clients.

Compare your ideas with the discussion below.

Other criteria when choosing a support system include the patient's level of risk, the size and weight of the equipment, cost implications, and ease of usage (Fletcher 1997).

Summary

■ Pressure sores can have serious consequences so when a patient/client has been identified as at risk of pressure sores, it is essential that effective measures are taken to prevent pressure sore formation.

■ Appropriate preventive measures for the individual need to be planned and should include a suitable support surface which does not impair mobility, correct moving and handling techniques, adequate nutrition, education, pain management, and skin care.

PREVENTION OF OTHER COMPLICATIONS OF IMMOBILITY

While pressure sores are an important potential problem for people with impaired mobility, unfortunately there are a number of other possible complications which they will also be at risk from. This next section considers what these complications are and how nurses can prevent them.

Learning outcomes

By the end of this section you will be able to:

1. Identify physical and psycho-social problems of immobility.
2. Identify ways in which nurses can minimize the problems of immobility.

Learning outcome 1:
Identify physical and psycho-social problems of immobility

■ **Activity** Think of patients/clients you have nursed, whose mobility was limited for some reason. They may have been confined to bed or wheelchair dependent, or physical or psychological problems may have made walking difficult. What physical and psycho-social problems did this limited mobility cause them?

Compare your answer with the list of problems in Box 9.3. These problems are now discussed below.

Circulatory and respiratory problems

■ Deep vein thrombosis can occur from pooling of venous blood in the legs. Movement of the legs normally contracts the muscles, which press upon

Deep vein thrombosis	Renal calculi
Pulmonary embolus	Incontinence
Increased cardiac workload	Muscle wasting
Orthostatic hypotension	Joint contractures
Decreased cardiac output and	Loss of self-esteem
reduced tissue perfusion	Frustration
Chest infection	Boredom
Gastro-intestinal problems	Isolation
Urinary tract infection	

Box 9.3 Physical and psycho-social problems caused by limited mobility

the veins and cause them to empty. Legs that are not mobile are unable to maintain vasoconstriction and the venous blood pools causing a deep vein thrombosis. This clot may become detached and enter the pulmonary circulation causing a pulmonary embolus (Roper et al. 1996). Mrs Smith is bed bound and could be at risk of developing a deep vein thrombosis particularly if her operation is delayed, as there can be no movement of her right leg until it has been operated on.

■ Cardiac workload increases by 20% when a healthy person lies down and 40% in people with cardiovascular impairment.

■ Orthostatic hypotension (a fall in blood pressure when moving to an upright position) can occur in chair and bed bound patients within a week of immobilization (Nazarko 1996). Robert Brown who is confined to a wheelchair may experience orthostatic hypotension, which will make him feel faint and dizzy when he is transferred from his bed to his wheelchair. Nurses should also be aware of this potential problem when getting Mrs Smith up after her surgery.

■ Decreased cardiac output and reduced tissue perfusion related to immobility may cause venous leg ulcers.

■ Impaired mobility may cause reduced ventilation of the lungs. The decreased movement and ventilation causes reduced stimulation of coughing. This leads to a build-up of secretions in the bronchi and bronchioles, which may become infected, causing a chest infection. This problem could occur in any of the people in the scenarios.

Gastro-intestinal problems

• Lack of mobility and changes in diet and fluids may cause constipation. Constipation increases the risk of urinary tract infections and urge incontinence (Nazarko 1997).

- Immobile patients may find it difficult to pour out their own drinks or feed themselves. Bob is unable to feed himself, and Mrs Smith may not be able to comfortably reach her drinks or food. Correct positioning for eating may be difficult for the immobile person.
- Lack of mobility may lead to a reduced appetite.

Urinary problems

■ Urinary stasis may be caused by reduced mobility, which can cause urinary tract infection, or renal calculi (stones). The latter occur when crystalline substances such as uric acid, calcium phosphate and oxalate which are normally excreted in the urine, crystallize out of solution (Anson 1997).

■ Immobile patients may rely on staff to take them to the toilet or provide bedpans or commodes. Impaired mobility may cause difficulties removing or adjusting clothing. Older people such as Mrs Smith do not become aware of the need to empty their bladder (voiding) until the bladder is 90% full and they are less able to 'hold on' than younger people. This may lead to incontinence, when the person is unable to get to the toilet quickly. Incontinence due to physical impairment such as immobility is termed 'functional' incontinence.

Chapter 6 'Meeting elimination needs' covers these issues in detail and will help you to develop your practical skills in relation to those who need help with elimination.

Musculo-skeletal problems

■ In immobile parts of the body muscle wasting will commence and this muscle degeneration will deplete the capacity for movement leading to further impairment. The lack of muscle activity will cause degenerative changes involving the release of calcium from the bones (osteoporosis).

■ If joints are allowed to stay in one position too long the muscle fibres around the joint shorten and the loose connective tissue within the joint transforms into dense tissue. This combined process causes a contracture (Roper et al. 1996). Bob already has some joint deformities. Joints particularly at risk are the shoulders, elbows, wrists, neck, fingers, hips, knees, ankles and toes. Contractures reduce stability and increase the risk of falls and this can restrict mobility further.

Psycho-social problems

■ Loss of mobility can cause patients to experience loss of self-esteem, and they may feel frustration at being dependent on others.

■ Children in hospital such as Ben can have difficulty playing in their usual ways, particularly when they are confined to bed, and may experience boredom, as may adults with impaired mobility.

■ Elderly people like Mrs Smith who are admitted to hospital for an acute medical episode may become functionally impaired, not only because of the disease process but also from the hospitalization process – some becoming confused and disorientated.

■ For Bob with profound learning and multiple disabilities there may be frustration at having to rely on carers to move him around, and having to make his needs and wishes known with limited communication ability.

■ Impaired mobility can also affect the ability and opportunity to socialize and communicate with others, leading to isolation.

Learning outcome 2:
Identify ways in which nurses can minimize the problems of immobility

Roper *et al.* (1996) suggest that when planning care, the objective of the plan is:

• To prevent identified potential problems from becoming actual problems.
• To solve actual problems.
• Where possible to alleviate those which cannot be solved.
• To help the person to cope positively with those problems that cannot be alleviated or solved.

Activity

We have identified a number of potential and actual problems related to impaired mobility in our four patients/clients. Consider the nursing interventions that could be implemented to solve or alleviate those problems.

A few points, which you may have considered, are discussed below

Potential problem – deep vein thrombosis/ pulmonary embolus

The signs and symptoms of deep vein thrombosis – painful, swollen calf, and of pulmonary embolus – chest pain and cough, are all part of the nursing observations. The nurse, in liaison with the physiotherapist, can help the person with active, passive and isometric exercises of the legs. Passive exercises are where another person puts the limb through a range of movement, while active exercises are when the person himself carries out the exercises. Isometric is muscle contraction with minimal muscle shortening so that there is no movement (Bronte and Gray 1995). Graduated compression stockings are another possible preventive measure. These enhance venous return and blood flow, but there are contraindications to their use, e.g. leg deformities, severe arteriosclerosis and local skin disorders (Mills 1997). When applying these stockings it is essential to measure the leg carefully so that the correct size is chosen, and to follow the manufacturers' instructions for application. Anticoagulants may also be prescribed for those at high risk.

Potential problem – orthostatic hypotension

This can be alleviated by gradually sitting Bob up in bed before he is transferred into his chair. When Mrs Smith first gets up after her surgery this precaution should also be taken.

Potential problem – chest infection

Frequent repositioning and encouragement to do deep breathing exercises can help to prevent chest infection. The optimal position for breathing can be seen in Fig. 8.1. The person can also be encouraged to cough to clear secretions and prevent them pooling in the lungs. Chapter 8 has a section on observation of sputum which includes tips on how expectoration of sputum can be encouraged.

Potential problem – alteration in diet and fluid intake leading to constipation

Mrs Smith needs to have her food and drinks positioned so that she can reach them. Her pain must be adequately managed so that she is not afraid to move to pour herself a drink. Bob would benefit from a high fibre diet. People with profound and multiple disabilities may have difficulty with feeding and the nurse's aim is to enhance the quality of the mealtime experience. The nurse should sit face to face with Bob to enable good contact making a sociable occasion of being fed. Flora will also benefit from a high fibre diet. She could have problems due to the joint deformities caused by her rheumatoid arthritis, and may need to be provided with a non-slip mat to prevent her plate moving, a plate guard to help keep the food on the plate and a non-spill feeder if a cup is not practical. Flora may need verbal prompting or assistance to ensure that she remembers to eat her meal (Oddy 1996). Chapter 4 'Assessing and meeting nutritional needs' includes more detail about these issues. Ben has an intravenous infusion but his mouth must be kept clean and moist (*see* Chapter 5) so that he will have no problems when he is well enough to eat and drink normally.

Potential elimination problems – urinary tract infection, incontinence

Patients/clients at risk of urinary tract infection should be observed for signs such as cloudy, foul smelling urine. In Chapter 6 the section on urinalysis explains how urinary tract infection might be suspected and when a specimen of urine should be sent for microscopy, culture and sensitivity (p. 183). Continence aids will be required to meet Bob's needs but consideration must be given to body image, comfort and skin care, and as to how continence can be promoted, rather than only contained. As Flora's rheumatoid arthritis will make it difficult for her to walk, she may need to be positioned within a short walking distance from the toilet. She may also need guidance to get to the toilet as she may have difficulty finding it. Making toilets easy to identify by using colour, signs and pictures can help (Nazarko 1997). Mrs Smith's requests for help with elimination should be answered promptly. These issues are all examined in detail in Chapter 6.

Problem – muscle wasting and contractures

This is a particular issue for Bob because as muscle contraction increases, this further limits joint movement. People with profound learning disabilities who are immobile are particularly at risk of developing deformities. Prevention and management will need a multi-professional approach with physiotherapy as part of his everyday activities, occupational therapy input and devices such as splints and body braces.

Problem – Psycho-social effects: Loss of self-esteem, frustration, boredom, isolation

As discussed in Chapter 1, how the nurse carries out care may affect how the patient/client feels about himself and thus reduce the psycho-social effects of impaired mobility. Chapter 2 looks at the approach of the nurse when carrying out practical skills, and emphasizes self-awareness. Family and friends have an important role in helping to reduce isolation. Family-centred care is considered in depth by Whittaker (1998). Parental participation is viewed in terms of partnership by Casey (1993), with the emphasis on the family providing care, complemented by the nurse. Ben will require considerable technical care which his parents may prefer the nurses to do (Coyne 1995). However, the presence of Ben's parents will be essential to his psychological well-being, and will relieve potential boredom and isolation. Most children's units will also have play therapists, who will have an important role with the child with restricted mobility.

Summary
- The person with restricted mobility is at risk of a number of physical and psycho-social complications.
- The nurse has an important role in identifying potential complications and implementing preventive care, thus promoting well-being.

ASSISTING WITH MOBILIZATION

This is an important role of the nurse in many settings, and will involve the nurse enabling barriers to be overcome, and working closely with other disciplines, particularly the physiotherapist and the occupational therapist.

Learning outcomes

By the end of this section you will be able to:

1. Identify barriers to mobilization.
2. Understand how you can assist patients/clients with mobilization.

Learning outcome 1:
Identify barriers to mobilization

Activity

To enable nurses to help people to mobilize there needs to be an awareness of possible barriers to mobility. What barriers can you identify that could prevent a patient or client from mobilizing?

A few possibilities are listed below but you may well have thought of others.

- Pain or fear of pain may prevent a person from maintaining or regaining their mobility. Therefore the cause of the pain must be assessed and strategies implemented to control it.
- Fear of falling is a common problem. Mrs Smith has already fallen once and fractured her femur and may have lost confidence in her ability to walk (Nazarko 1996). This fear of falling can cause a fear of going outside, and even lead to agoraphobia.
- Lack of motivation, in the person with depression or dementia, may lead to a reluctance to move around.
- Foot problems such as untrimmed toenails can impede mobility by causing pain and discomfort (Love 1995). Bunions and arthritic feet make it difficult to wear normal shoes.
- Unsuitable footwear makes mobilizing difficult and dangerous. Slip-on shoes or slippers will increase the tendency to shuffle, shiny or plastic soles will cause a frightened, small-step gait. Narrow shoes inhibit normal foot movement, reducing normal toe function and preventing normal toe 'push off' which affects gait pattern and weight transference (Finlay and Fullerton 1996).
- Arthritic knees, which Flora has, may cause instability and falls, which in turn can lead to loss of confidence.
- Shortening of one leg may occur after the surgical correction of a fractured neck of femur making it difficult for the person to put both feet on the ground together.

Learning outcome 2:
Understand how you can assist patients/clients with mobilization

■ **Activity**   Focus on the practice scenarios and identify strategies and equipment which might assist with mobilization.

You probably considered involvement of the multidisciplinary team, and will have encountered mobility aids. Helping a person to mobilize certainly requires a multidisciplinary approach. For example the orthotist will be able to supply callipers, shoes or knee braces to overcome some of the barriers to mobility. Physiotherapists will assess people for mobility aids such as crutches or walking frames, both standard or wheeled ones for those who cannot lift a standard frame. Post-operatively, physiotherapists would decide which walking aid would be most appropriate for Mrs Smith. Gutter frames can help people with arthritis such as Flora. Those unable to walk, like Bob, will be supplied with wheelchairs. Special chairs with cushions that rise slowly can be helpful for people who have difficulty getting up from a chair.

Restoring or minimizing loss of mobility in people with dementia such as Flora can be challenging but Oddy (1996) has suggested an approach that uses both communication and movement strategies (*see* Box 9.4). These strategies are used to bridge the gap that keeps the person with dementia disconnected from their environment and from those around them.

As Ben improves play therapy will be an important part of his rehabilitation to increase his mobility and enable him to maintain his normal activities.

Dressing and undressing Bob, who has severe contractures, can be very difficult and the occupational therapist can advise about suitable clothing. Splints and braces can help to maintain body and limb posture. Arm gaiters can help to minimize involuntary muscle action so that he might be able to

---

- Specific verbal strategies, involving thoughtful wording e.g. encouraging and reinforcing, using simple terms: *'Keep going'*, *'You're doing well'*.
- Non-verbal strategies, making use of cues e.g. holding out your hand towards the person, and using touch.
- Strategies to minimize the fear of falling, such as filling the empty space in front of the person with a solid object such as a chair, or ensuring that there is a rail to hold onto by the side.
- Movement strategies, where the carer interprets the environment for the person with dementia. This might entail getting the person to follow you, and copy how you are walking.

Box 9.4 Restoring, or minimizing loss of, mobility in people with dementia (Oddy 1996)

use an adapted motorized wheelchair thus increasing his independence in mobilizing.

When helping a person to mobilize the safety of both the individual and the nurse must be a major consideration. As we have already discussed, some people may be unsteady on their feet or have lost confidence. Therefore a risk assessment must be carried out before any attempt is made to assist with mobilizing. You have probably looked at risk assessment within moving and handling sessions, and will also be aware of the importance of documentation.

Risk assessment

- **Task**. What exactly is the manoeuvre to be carried out? For example the task might be to get Mrs Smith to stand for the first time since her operation.
- **Individual capability**. How much can the patient do for herself? Mrs Smith is reasonably fit and has no problems with communication and should just need support and guidance to build her confidence.
- **Load**. Is the person heavy and unable to move him or herself? Bob, although not particularly heavy, is unable to move and therefore needs a hoist to move him out of bed.
- **Environment**. Make sure that there is enough room for you and the patient to work in. Slippery floors are a danger for people learning to walk or who are unsteady on their feet.

Remember that if the person cannot move himself or herself then equipment must be used. When assisting a person to stand, you stand beside them, facing forward so you both move the same way. The use of a transfer belt around the person's waist gives you something to hold. For example, if the patient has a slight weakness on the left side, you stand at her left side in a walk stance, with your right hand holding the belt around her waist, and the patient's left hand in your left hand, using a palm to palm grip (*see* Fig. 9.2). On the command 'Ready, brace, stand', you both move forward as you transfer your weight from the back leg to the front. You can now use this hold to give the person confidence to walk. You will have the opportunity to practise these techniques under supervision in the classroom. A very important aspect is not to hurry the client, maintaining a slow steady pace.

Summary
- Building a person's confidence and self-esteem is an important aspect of mobilization and the nurse is part of a multidisciplinary approach to the care and management of people with problems of mobility.

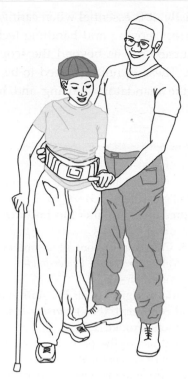

Figure 9.2 Helping a person to walk

■ The nurse should be aware of barriers to mobilization, in order that these can be addressed.
■ When assisting with mobilizing, risk assessment is essential and must be documented.
■ Appropriate mobility aids should be provided for each individual and the nurse can give encouragement and support to the person who is regaining mobility.

CHAPTER SUMMARY

The underlying reasons for impaired mobility are wide ranging, and may be temporary or permanent. However, the possible complications of impaired mobility can lead to much discomfort and further health problems, so nurses must take a proactive role to prevent these ill effects. Pressure sores were focused on in some depth within this chapter, as their incidence remains widespread even though it is well recognized that they are largely preventable. Throughout this chapter, emphasis has been placed on identifying potential problems, so that effective preventive strategies for each individual can be implemented. The promotion of mobility wherever possible is the key to preventing many of these problems, and a multidisciplinary approach to this should be taken. Finally, it is essential when caring for the person with impaired mobility, that correct moving and handling techniques are used to protect both clients and nurses. It was beyond the scope of the chapter to address this topic in depth. These techniques need to be learnt under supervision and attendance at the mandatory moving and handling sessions is essential.

REFERENCES

Anson, R. 1997. Urinary tract stones. In Fillingham, S and Douglas, J. (eds). *Urological Nursing*. 2nd ed. London: Ballière Tindall, 131–70.

Arblaster G. 1998. Reducing pressure sores after hip fractures. *Professional Nurse* **13**, 749–52.

Bronte, M. and Gray, A. 1995. Care implications of disorders of the cardiovascular system. In: Peattie, P. and Walker, S. (eds.) *Understanding Nursing Care*, 4th edn. Edinburgh: Churchill Livingstone, 385–439.

Carr, E. 1998. Experiencing and managing pain: the nurse-patient relationship. In: Hinchliff, S., Norman, S. and Schober, J. (eds.) *Nursing Practice and Health Care: A Foundation Text*, 3rd edn. London: Arnold, 337–62.

Casey, A. 1993. Development and use of the partnership model of care. In: Glasper, A. and Tucker, A. (eds.) *Recent Advances in Child Health Care*. London: Scutari, 183–93.

Coyne, I.T. 1995. Partnership in care: parents' views of participation in their hospitalized child's care. *Journal of Clinical Nursing* **4**, 71–9.

Cowan, T. and Woollons, S. 1998. Dynamic systems for pressure sore prevention. *Professional Nurse* **13**, 387–94.

Cullum, N., Deeks, J., Song, F. and Fletcher, A.W. 1999. *Beds, Mattresses and Cushions for Pressure Sore Prevention and Treatment.* (Cochrane review). In: The Cochrane Library, issue 4, Oxford: Update Software.

Dealey, C. 1997. *Managing Pressure Sore Prevention.* Salisbury: Quay Books, Mark Allen Publishing.

Dunford, C. 1998. Managing pressure sores. *Nursing Standard* **12** (24), 38–42.

Finlay, O. and Fullerton, C. 1996. Feet and footwear in older people. In: Squires J. (ed.) *Rehabilitation of Older People*, 2nd edn. London: Chapman and Hall.

Fletcher J. 1997. Pressure-relieving equipment: criteria and selection. *British Journal of Nursing* **6**, 323–8.

Hampton S.1998. Can electric beds aid pressure sore prevention in hospitals? *British Journal of Nursing* **7**, 1010–17.

James H. 1998. Classification and grading of pressure sores. *Professional Nurse* **13** (10), 6–10.

Kiernan, M. 1997. Pressure sores: adopting the principles of risk management. *British Journal of Nursing* **6**, 329–32.

Lewis, B. 1998. Nutrient intake and the risk of pressure sore development in older patients. *Journal of Wound Care* **7** (1), 31–35.

Love, C. 1995. Nursing or chiropody? Nurses' attitudes to toe nail trimming. *Professional Nurse* **10**, 241–44.

Lowthian, P. 1987. The practical assessment of pressure sore risk. *Care – Science and Practice* **5** (4), 3–7.

Lowthian, P. 1997. Notes on the pathogenesis of serious pressure sores. *British Journal of Nursing* **6**, 907–12.

Mills, C. 1997. Pulmonary embolus. *Nursing Times* 93 (51), 50–53.

Nazarko, L. 1996. Power to the people . . . rehabilitation, mobility. *Nursing Times* **92** (14), 48–9.

Nazarko, L. 1997. Continence. The whole story. *Nursing Times* **93** (43), 63–4, 66, 68.

Norton, D., Exton-Smith, A. and McLaren, R. 1962. *An Investigation of Geriatric Nursing. Problems in Hospital.* London: National Corporation for the Care of Old People.

Oddy, R. 1996. Strategies to help people keep moving. *Journal of Dementia Care* **4** (4), 22–4.

Olding, L. and Patterson, J. 1998. Growing concern. *Nursing Times* **94** (38), 76–79.

Pang, S. and Wong, T. 1998. Predicting pressure sore risk with the Norton, Braden and Waterlow scales in a Hong Kong rehabilitation hospital. *Nursing Research* **47**, 147–53.

Pickersgill, J. 1997. Taking the pressure off. *Paediatric Nursing* **7** (8), 25–7.

Roper, N., Logan, W. and Tierney, A. 1996. *The Elements of Nursing.* Edinburgh: Churchill Livingstone.

Russell L. 1998. Physiology of the skin and prevention of pressure sores. *British Journal of Nursing* **7**, 1088–100.

Simpson, A., Bowers, K. and Weir-Hughes, D. 1996. *Pressure Sore Prevention.* Gateshead: Athenaeum.

Tingle J. 1997. Pressure sores: counting the cost of nursing neglect. *British Journal of Nursing* **6**, 757–58.

Young T. 1997. Pressure sores: incidence, risk assessment and prevention. *British Journal of Nursing* **6**, 319–21.

Waterlow, J. 1988. The Waterlow card for the prevention and management of pressure sores: toward a pocket policy. *Care – Science and Practice* **6** (1), 8–12.

Waterlow, J. 1998. Pressure sores in children: risk assessment. *Paediatric Nursing* **10** (4), 22–23.

Whittaker, N. 1998. Family-centred care. In. Hinchliff, S., Norman, S. and Schober, J. (eds.) *Nursing Practice and Health Care: A Foundation Text*, 3rd edn. London: Arnold, 457–77.

A complication of diabetes mellitus, where ketones accumulates in the body due to faulty carbohydrate metabolism. If untreated, leads to coma and can be life-threatening.

Tattooing

When dirt is trapped in the dermis and epidermis, permanently discolouring the skin.

Clozapine

An atypical anti-psychotic drug which has been proved to have efficacy in treatment resistant schizophrenia and ameliorating negative schizophrenic symptoms (King 1999).

Abscess

A localized collection of pus. Pus is a thick fluid containing leucocytes, bacteria and cellular debris, and indicates infection.

unwell with the flu and collapsed at home in a **keto-acidotic coma**, lying unconscious at home in the kitchen until discovered by his sister at least 2 hours later. He was initially managed in the intensive therapy unit to stabilize his diabetic condition. He was then transferred to your ward 4 days later with a large area of black dead tissue on his sacrum, and discoloured areas on both elbows, which appear to have been caused by the period of prolonged pressure when unconscious on the kitchen floor. On exploration of his feet, sensory awareness is absent, and an **ulcer** (open sore), surrounded by hard, yellowish skin, is discovered on one of his toes. This appears infected, and has an offensive discharge. Mr Nixon is keen to get home as soon as possible. He normally smokes 30 cigarettes a day, is underweight and his appetite is poor.

■ Child

Chloe is 11 years old and fell off her bicycle, sustaining a series of abrasions and lacerations to her face. Her wounds, although superficial, contain small gravel pellets and dirt, and therefore require cleansing under general anaesthetic, to prevent 'tattooing'. Chloe received initial assessment and care in the Accident and Emergency Department, and was then transferred to your ward, to await surgery. Chloe's father is in attendance.

■ Learning disability

A week ago, Alison Jones, aged 35 years, who has Down's syndrome, slipped in the snow and broke her forearm. As the fracture was unstable, she was admitted to hospital for surgery, which involved plating of the radius and ulna bones. She has now returned to your residential unit and has a wound on her forearm with clips *in situ*. Alison is worried about the wound and its healing.

■ Mental health

Christopher Davis is 32 years old, and has been homeless and unemployed for several years. He is being treated as an in-patient in the acute mental health unit, after a deterioration in his mental health, which has further affected his self-care ability. He has a diagnosis of substance abuse and schizophrenia, which is currently being treated by **clozapine** Christopher requires careful blood monitoring, as clozapine can affect white blood cell levels. Whilst on the unit he complained of pain in his left upper buttock. A large, hot, swollen area was found, which was diagnosed as being an **abscess**. Christopher says that he has had several of these before. Incision and drainage took place in theatre and he has now returned to the unit, with a pack *in situ* in the wound. Antibiotics have been prescribed.

THE STAGES OF WOUND HEALING

A wound can be defined as 'a defect or break in the skin that results from physical, mechanical or thermal damage, or that develops as a result of the presence of an underlying physiological disorder' (Thomas 1990, p. 1). Wound healing is a very complex phenomenon, and is still incompletely understood (Dealey 1999). Different wounds do not necessarily follow the same pattern in the healing process. Doughty (1992) explains that:

■ When wounds are confined to the epidermis and dermis, they will heal by **regeneration**.
■ Wounds extending through the dermis heal by scar formation, composed of connective tissue, because deeper tissues e.g. hair follicles, subcutaneous tissue, are unable to regenerate (Cuono 1985 cited by Doughty 1992). Connective tissue is developed from cells termed fibroblasts.

To assist understanding of wound healing, we will start by exploring simpler surgical and minor traumatic wounds (which tend to heal in an orderly manner), and progress to the more complex, often long-standing wounds such as venous leg ulcers.

Learning outcomes

By the end of this section you will be able to:

1. Distinguish the phases of healing and recognize tissue appearance at each stage.
2. Be aware that healing does not in reality occur in a simple linear fashion.
3. Recognize the appearance of scar tissue, and abnormalities which can occur.

Learning outcome 1:
Distinguish the phases of healing and recognize tissue appearance at each stage

The process of wound healing is usually described in four stages, although Williams and Young (1998) point out that this is a false division, which is done in an attempt to simplify this very complex process. Some authors describe only three stages and others more, but these variations are either a compression or expansion on the four stages described. Similarly you may find that different names are used to describe the identified stages within the texts which you refer to. This chapter employs the approach that, following haemostasis (the control of bleeding by the body), there are four stages of healing:

Granulation tissue
Refers to tissue in the proliferative phase of healing. Blood vessels, collagen and ground substance – a specialist non-cellular healing material – combine to produce a defect filling material that will eventually produce a scar. Granulation tissue is very delicate and bleeds easily owing to the profuse blood supply. It requires careful protection.

- The **inflammatory phase** prepares the tissue for repair. This protective mechanism aims to minimize injury and initiate the healing response (Williams and Young 1998). The cellular aspect of this stage occurs within hours of the wound occurring (Krizek *et al.* 1997).

- The **destructive phase** breaks down damaged tissue, and involves wound cleaning of the devitalized tissue by the white cells (Williams and Young 1998).

- The **proliferative phase** rebuilds the tissue. Collagen and an elastic mesh is formed. New blood cells grow into the mesh to complete the formation of **granulation tissue**.

- Finally, the **maturation phase** involves re-moulding the tissue to form a scar. This can take a year or more (Krizek *et al.* 1997).

■ **Activity**

Prior to observing and assessing wounds, you will need some theoretical knowledge to base your approach upon. Prepare notes on the phases of healing, which are outlined briefly above, from your recommended biology textbook. Clancy and McVicar's (1997) paper explains the homeostatic responses of wound healing, so this is also a useful source. Try to focus in your reading, on the requirements for each stage of the healing process.

Your reading should have helped you to understand that:

- Wound healing is, in essence, a sequential process.
- The previous stage has to be completed before the next stage can occur.
- Certain cells are very important in each stage.
- Any stage can be prolonged, due to factors relating to the individual person.

■ **Activity**

Aim to observe a simple uncomplicated surgical wound, or a minor traumatic wound (e.g. a laceration) that is exposed or reasonably visible – this could even be on your own (or a relative's skin), if you've had a recent mishap! Compare the appearance of the wound to the described criteria for different phases of healing. Discuss with your practice assessor which stage of healing the wound has reached.

You should have noticed that at different stages of wound healing, the tissue will have a different appearance:

- When observed in the **inflammatory** phase, the wound appears swollen and red, and the surrounding tissue feels warm and can be painful. Recognizing these signs (which occur due to local vasodilation) can be difficult at first.

- In the **destructive** phase, as the wound progresses, there may be oozing through the wound edges, a dry scab, or minimal signs of either.

- In the **proliferative** phase, signs of the wound shrinking appear, small lines appear around the wound as it contracts, and some wounds may be raised and inflamed. The appearance of tiny red dots is the first sign of granulation tissue (Williams and Young 1998). At this stage the wound can be itchy, but the granulation tissue is very delicate and therefore it is essential that it is left undisturbed.

■ A surgical wound in the **maturation** phase may remain in this stage for up to 2 years after the surgery. It will appear very much smaller, and may be white and hard (scar tissue), and fixed to surrounding tissue, or similar in appearance to surrounding tissue, indicating a well healed mature wound. However, few wounds are as simple as the latter.

Casey (1999) summarizes the implications of the different colours of wounds as:

• **Black:** Necrotic (dead) tissue and therefore no healing has begun.
• **Yellow:** Slough (made up of dead cells). Occurs near the end of the inflammatory stage.
• **Red:** Granulation tissue.
• **Pink:** Epithelialization. During this stage epithelial cells, through division and migration, move across the wounded surface from the edges, to meet in the middle. This cannot take place until granulation tissue is in place, and thus epithelialization is the last stage of healing.

Activity

Now that you have some understanding of the stages of healing and the possible appearance of the wound at different stages, consider how you might prepare Alison for the wound healing process, so that you can reduce her anxiety.

Points which you might have considered are:
• Use of effective communication skills to ascertain Alison's understanding of the healing process, and her anxieties about this.
• Use of simple diagrams might be helpful.
• If you know of anybody who has a healed surgical wound, perhaps Alison could, with the person's permission, talk to him. Actually seeing a healed wound might help to allay her anxiety, if this is possible to arrange.
• You could gently encourage Alison to look at the wound and point out the signs of healing.

Learning outcome 2:
Be aware that healing does not in reality occur in a simple linear fashion

Due to a number of factors, wound healing is not always a straightforward process, and an overview of wounds caused by trauma, pressure or ulceration will illustrate this issue. These wounds are considered in further detail in the later section 'Classification of wounds and their management'.

Activity

If possible, select a patient with a wound caused by trauma, pressure or ulceration, in discussion with your practice assessor. Try to find out about the history of the wound, and its healing process to date.

Compare your investigations to the discussion below.

■ **Trauma**: Traumatic wounds vary greatly in nature. While minor wounds may heal in a straightforward manner, others involve extensive skin loss and contamination, which can affect the healing process and may require surgical intervention.

■ **Pressure sores**: Wounds such as pressure sores follow a progressive path. The impairment of the circulation to the skin for even short periods in susceptible individuals, such as the frail, elderly or malnourished, is problematic. Mr Nixon, as an elderly person who also has diabetes and had a period of immobility on a hard surface (the kitchen floor), was obviously a high-risk individual (see Chapter 9, Pressure sore risk assessment). Even in healthy people, what appears to be an area of redness on the scalp, spine, elbows, sacrum, or heels can change over a period of days to a large black necrotic wound. The discoloured areas on Mr Nixon's elbows could potentially develop into necrotic sores similar to his sacral sore. With correct management the pressure sore will change to a clean empty crater, which heals from the base upwards to produce often, over a period of months, a very pale weak scar that will easily break down if subjected to subsequent trauma. Figures 10.1, 10.2, 10.3 and 10.4 show pressure sores of differing depths.

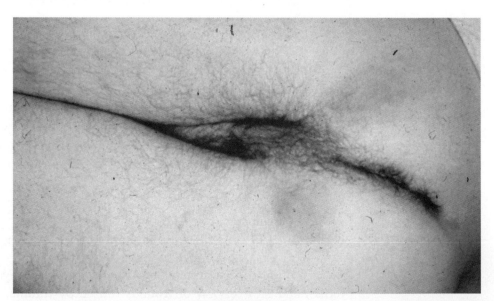

Figure 10.1 Pressure damage indicated by erythema
Caused to buttocks by prolonged pressure. The individual has been sitting on a hospital trolley without adequate pressure relief following a collapse. The damage has led to reddening of the skin. Continuing to place the individual on such damaged skin will cause skin breakdown, especially if the skin has already been sensitized by pressure.

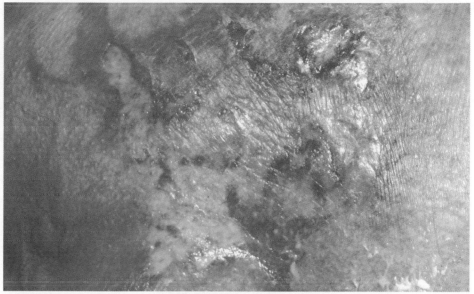

Figure 10.2 Pressure damage caused by friction
These wounds occurred in an older person who was suffering from a systemic
infection. Profuse sweating and sliding down the bed at home led to the skin being
stuck to the sheets, the resulting friction tearing at the epidermis.

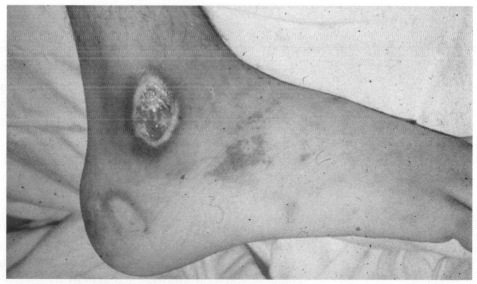

Figure 10.3 Pressure sore caused by loss of sensation
This individual, as a result of a spinal injury, has no muscle tone or sensation in the
legs. The wound is the product of the foot rubbing against the leg supports on a
wheel chair. The wound is deeper, and located on the external malleolus may be
very close to exposing bone (feel the amount of skin covering your own external
malleolus).

367

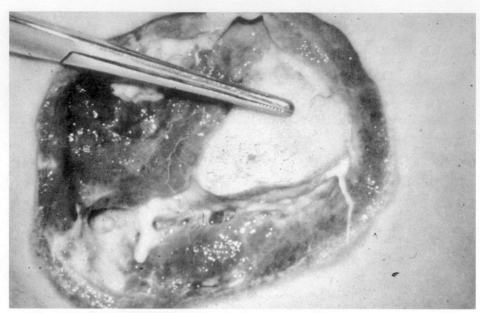

Figure 10.4 Very deep pressure sore
This wound is the result of prolonged pressure over weeks in a patient who has
suffered a stroke and is shown after remove of dead tissue above the exposed
tissue. Bone, muscle and slough are present with sinuses that track deeply into the
wound.

■ **Ulcers**: An ulcer is a secondary skin lesion involving a focal loss of epidermis and dermis (Wysocki and Bryant 1992). Leg ulcers are an increasingly
common chronic wound, and are often an extensive and long-standing
problem (Dealey 1999). There are a number of different types of leg ulcers,
each having differing distinguishing features, underlying pathology and
treatment. A useful overview of lower leg ulceration can be found in Zink
et al. (1992). There are also a number of books devoted entirely to leg ulcers
and their management (*see* Morison and Moffat,1994; Cullum and Roe,
1995; Negus 1995). Some examples of leg ulcers are:

– Venous ulcers: Hollinworth (1998) describes venous leg ulceration as a
cascade of events, with chronic venous insufficiency being the initiating factor, while a number of risk factors can be identified e.g. varicose
veins, rheumatoid arthritis. (*see* Fig. 10.5)
– Arterial ulcers: Caused by inadequate tissue perfusion. (*see* Fig. 10.6)
– Mixed ulcers: Caused by venous and arterial disease.
– Diabetic ulcers: This term is given to ulcers occurring on the feet of
diabetics; these are complex wounds by nature (*see* Fig. 10.7), and cause
unacceptably high levels of morbidity and mortality (Foster 1999).

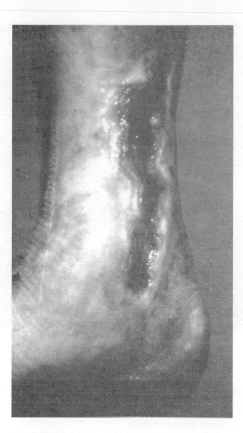

Figure 10.5 Venous leg ulcer
Venous ulcers occur in the lower leg, as a result of damage to the valves in superficial veins of the leg. Pressure builds up forcing products out of the veins into the tissue causing brown staining. The ulcers occur as a result of processes we do not fully understand. Essentially the blood supply to the skin is affected by an accumulation of white blood cells in the microcirculation and a fibrin cuff forming around the small vessels.

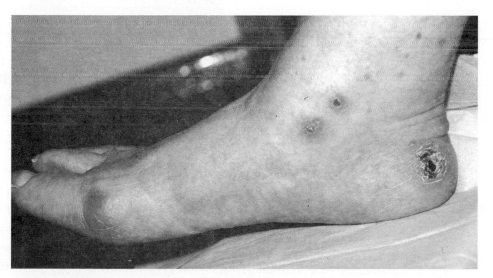

Figure 10.6 Arterial foot ulcer
The ulcers are caused by factors relating to impaired arterial blood supply to the leg. The foot will feel cold, pulses may be weak or absent. The ulcers occur as areas of blood supply to the skin become blocked. When closely examined the ulcers appear punched out. The ulcers in the picture are covered with encrustation containing dead skin and dried blood.

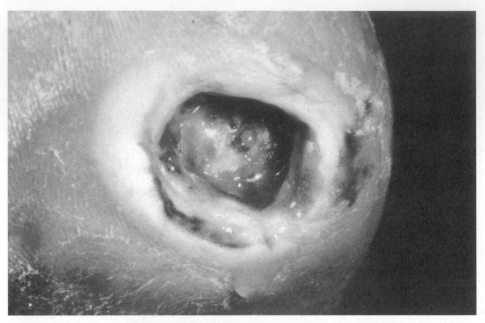

Figure 10.7 Diabetic neuropathic ulcer
This type of wound occurs usually in longstanding and poorly managed diabetic individuals. Prolonged high blood sugars (hyperglycaemia) impair nerve function. The individual is unaware of the damage. The area of white skin (hyperkeratosis) is the product of pressure and overproduction of hardened skin. The tissue is a classic feature of the diabetic neuropathic ulcer.

Attention to foot care, with the aim of preventing these lesions, is very important for the diabetic person, such as Mr Nixon, but note that his depression will affect his ability to carry out this self-care. *See* Chapter 5, Box 5.3: Foot care.

Over 70% of leg ulcers are caused by venous disease, 10% by arterial disease, and 10–15% by a combination of the two (Williams and Young 1998). Goldstein *et al.* (1998) suggest that a non-healing ulcer of the lower extremity can be multi-factoral in origin, and discusses how diagnosis can thus be made.

From reading the above you should now be aware that some wounds are caused by underlying health problems which may be difficult to resolve (if at all), and thus healing is unlikely to progress in a straightforward fashion. Some of these complex wounds necessitate a multidisciplinary team approach in diagnosing the problem affecting the individual, and its management. Investigations will be performed to ensure an accurate identification of the problem. For example, a venous ulcer is traditionally managed, if uncomplicated, by

Compression therapy
Compression therapy aims to provide graduated compression, with the highest pressure at the ankle and the lowest at the knee.

Doppler
The Doppler ultrasound (which should only be used by a suitably trained and experienced professional) records systolic pressure recordings at the foot or ankle, in order to obtain a ratio, known as the ankle brachial pressure index (ABPI). A normal reading is about 1 and if the reading is 0.8 or above it is considered safe to apply compression.

compression therapy, which ensures that blood in the lower limb is returned and does not pool in distended lower leg veins. However, an arterial ulcer is caused by reduced blood supply to the area. Therefore all patients presenting with an ulcer should be screened for arterial disease by **doppler** measurement of ankle brachial pressure index (RCN 1998), alongside a thorough clinical investigation. **Applying, in error, compression to a limb with an arterial ulcer will have catastrophic results for the ulcer and the patient, leading potentially to loss of the limb affected!**

Learning outcome 3:
Recognize the appearance of scar tissue and abnormalities which can occur

A scar is the end result of healing, but the formation of a mature scar can be a slow process. Understanding how Alison's scar is likely to develop over the coming months, will mean that you can be supportive and reassuring.

To gain understanding of scar tissue, you need to observe what appears to be a healed wound, i.e. there is no scab, open wound or discharge. So, select a client who does not have an obvious wound healing problem in the inflammatory, destructive, or proliferative phase of healing. Your practice assessor may be able to guide you towards a suitable individual, and remember to be sensitive and tactful. If the person is happy to show you the wound scar, carry out the activity below to examine its appearance and explore its stage of maturity (eventual appearance). Provided the wound is not too personal most people will provide a very good history of events, and be happy to show the scar to you. This can provide useful information relating to assessing potential problems with any surgery to be undergone, or if new wounds appear. If it is difficult to access a client with a scar in the practice setting, you yourself may have a scar which you could examine, or perhaps a friend/relative would help you with this exercise.

Activity

Remember that you need warm hands as some wounds are extremely sensitive to the cold. Do not touch unhealed wounds with bare hands – potential risk of contamination to the client and/or you! You will need paper and pen to record your findings.

For your record, aim to note:
- The appearance: Is the scar white or pink? Is it surrounded by normally coloured or discoloured tissue? Are stretch marks visible?
- The size: How big is the scar? Draw a diagram especially if large.
- The location: Where is it located? Scars located on joints and pressure points such as the sacrum or elbows, can be potential problems in future.
- Features of the scar: Is it intact, or has it signs of breakdown and repair? This will often relate to the location, as scars on joints undergo continuous stretching and contraction, and are likely to be damaged.
- The texture of the scar: Is it hard or soft, does it feel mobile or attached to surrounding tissue?

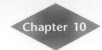
Discussion

Relate your observations to the points below.

A scar is the product of many cells. However specialist 'myo-fibroblast' cells, which possess muscle fibres, have a key role in healing, by shrinking the wound by contraction. Note that 75% of normal wound healing is by contraction which results in a smaller, less visible scar. A scar consists of tissue which initially is raised and very well vascularized – hence the red colour for several months after creation. Over a longer time period, the redness disappears, as the number of blood vessels reduces, and the colour changes to white. This is explained by alterations to the material forming the scar. Scar tissue is estimated to achieve a maximum strength of 80% of the normal tissue (Williams and Young 1998). This can mean that individuals who are susceptible to pressure sores, following e.g. a cerebrovascular accident, can have repeated skin breakdown on the same area. Thus unfortunately, Mr Nixon is at increased risk of a further sacral sore, should he be immobile on a future occasion. Careful assessment of risk using an effective pressure sore risk assessment tool (see Waterlow 1988; Bergstrom *et al.*1987 for examples), can enable appropriate preventive measures to be implemented. Chapter 9 discusses pressure sore risk assessment and prevention of pressure sores in detail.

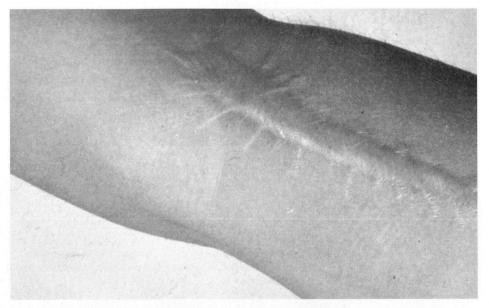

Figure 10.8 Hypertrophic scar
This is less a wound than the results of abnormal healing. This wound has over-produced collagen in the proliferation and maturation stages of healing causing a raised scar. Discuss with your practice assessor the management of such scars.

Some individuals have problems with hypertrophic scars and keloids (Figs. 10.8 and 10.9). A hypertrophic scar is a raised, healed red scar that is uncomfortable and tight. This is the result of an increased deposition of collagen within the area of the original wound (Weiss 1995). A keloid is a firm mass of scar caused by excessive collagen deposition, but it extends outside the wound boundaries (Weiss 1995). While hypertrophic scars can regress, keloid scars do not. Management of both of these problems requires specialist approaches, and a multidisciplinary approach, for both the physical and psychological problems that may accompany them.

Summary

- Wound healing is a complex process involving phases of healing, through which the wound must pass in order to adequately heal.
- The process is theoretically sequential, but in reality parts of different phases occur concurrently.
- The end result is a scar of uncertain appearance and weakened structure in comparison to surrounding undamaged tissue.

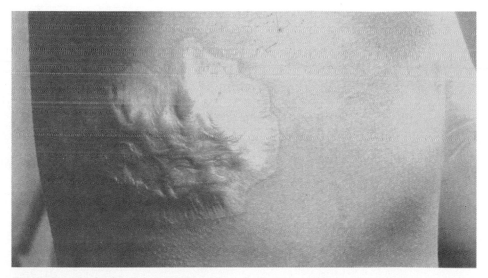

Figure 10.9 Keloid scar

This keloid scar is the result of a partial thickness scald injury some months before. The tissue has healed abnormally with an excess of abnormal collagen being deposited. The resulting hard raised scar differs from a hypertrophic scar. Firstly because it extends beyond the site of the original wound (this can be observed in the lighter patch at the border of the keloid). Secondly because it does not normally regress with time. Certain racial groups are predisposed to keloid scarring; especially individuals from the Mediterranean and North Africa.

CLASSIFICATION OF WOUNDS AND THEIR MANAGEMENT

From the exploration of healing in the previous section, you will have noticed that surgical wounds and minor trauma wounds heal relatively quickly if no complications occur. These are **acute wounds** and are called acute because of their sudden occurrence, short duration, and minimal need for external interventions. Doughty (1992) suggests that as an acute wound begins with an injury that initiates haemostasis, this triggers the wound-healing cascade, thus promoting rapid healing, especially in a healthy individual. **Chronic wounds**, she points out, are usually caused by underlying health problems so haemostasis is absent from the process, added to which, the individual's ability to heal is often impaired. As Doughty (1992) emphasizes wound healing is a systemic process and is therefore significantly affected by 'systemic conditions' (p. 42). Features of chronic wounds include their problematic and slow nature of healing, and the accompaniment of other health, social and psychological problems. In chronic wounds, the inflammatory response is continually stimulated by the underlying disease process, resulting in a prolonged and excessive inflammatory phase of wound healing (Williams and Young 1998). These wounds occur predominantly in the elderly.

Classifying wounds will enable you to appreciate issues affecting their management, and so plan more effective care. When exploring the classification of wounds, be aware that there are a variety of ways of performing this. This chapter will use a simple classification based on the cause, distinguishing between mechanical injuries, chronic ulcers, and thermal chemical injuries.

Learning outcomes:

By the end of this session you will be able to:

1. **Distinguish between acute and chronic wounds.**
2. **Discuss the principles of wound closure for different types of acute and chronic wounds.**

Learning outcome 1:
Distinguish between acute and chronic wounds

> ■ **Activity**   Table 10.1 shows a classification of wounds. Working from this, how would you classify the wounds of Mr Nixon, Alison, Christopher and Chloe?

You should have identified that Mr Nixon's sacral wound is a chronic pressure sore, and his toe wound is probably a diabetic neuropathic ulcer. Alison's is an acute surgical wound, and Chloe's wounds are acute abrasions and lacerations. How did you classify Christopher's wound? This, too, is an acute surgical

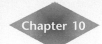

Table 10.1 Wound classification

Classification	Type of wounds	Causes and features
Acute	Penetrating wounds	Wounds penetrating the skin provide the opportunity for infection to gain access. Causative objects could include missiles (e.g. bullets, explosion debris) or hand-held objects (knives, billiard cues etc.).
Acute	Lacerations	Healing of lacerations is affected by the cause i.e. whether it is a clean wound or is contaminated by dirt/debris, age of the wound and the individual. Wounds involving the eyes and joints are priorities.
Acute	Abrasions	Abrasions tend to be caused by a part of the body being dragged against an abrasive surface, thus removing surface epithelium. They can be very painful and sensitive as nerve endings are exposed, and if they are not meticulously cleaned, 'tattooing' will result from the dirt trapped in the dermis and epidermis, which is almost impossible to remove (Evans and Jones 1996).
Acute	Bites	These are a common cause of wounds, most of which are caused by dogs, but human bites account for a substantial proportion too (Higgins *et al.* 1997). Infection is of particular concern due to the large number of micro-organisms to be found in mouths.
Acute	Surgical wounds	As these wounds are planned, risks (e.g. of infection) can be reduced to a minimum (Dealey 1999). Infection rates vary according to the type of surgery (*see* Table 10.2). Mishriki *et al.* 1990) found an overall infection rate of 7.3% but this was affected by a number of variables e.g. age, surgeon. Bremmelgaard *et al.* (1989) found infection rates ranging from 2.3% (clean wounds) to 27.1% (dirty wounds). Patients with infections stayed in hospital an average of 21.5 days longer than those without infections.
Chronic	Venous leg ulcers	Caused by damage to the venous system in the leg, especially the valves, resulting in pooling and distending of vessels. Bi-products of this process cause tissue death and ulcer formation. Venous ulcers are commonly located in the midcalf to heel area, and are usually shallow and irregularly shaped (Wysocki and Bryant 1992). Accompanying pain is usually described as a constant dull ache or pain (Williams and Young 1998)
Chronic	Arterial leg ulcers	Occur when impairment of the blood supply by a variety of causes (including atheroma, white blood cell accumulation and loss of red blood cell flexibility) causes areas of skin death, as the blood vessel supplying the area becomes occluded. They are frequently located on the feet, toes and lower leg, are usually deep lesions with distinct punched out margins. They are extremely painful although the pain can be relieved when legs are dangled as gravity improves arterial perfusion (Wysocki and Bryant 1992).

Continued

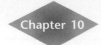
Table 10.1 *Continued*

Classification	Type of wounds	Causes and features
Chronic	Diabetic neuropathic or neuro-ischaemic leg ulcers	Chronic hyperglycaemia can cause impairment of the nerve supply to the foot and lower limb. The resulting loss of sensation can lead to pressure damage, repeated trauma and/or penetration by foreign bodies. These ulcers can be said to be neuropathic in origin. In neuro-ischaemic ulcers, the combination of neuropathy and arterial disease produces a very complex wound with a very poor outcome, soon leading to amputation.
Chronic	Pressure sores	Prolonged pressure on the skin produces obstruction of small vessels, resulting in death of skin, and sometimes deeper tissues, due to lack of blood supply. Can be accompanied by friction injury, where skin undergoes dragging against surface, and is torn off.
Chronic	Infection-induced ulcers	Tropical ulcers are one of the most common forms of these. Opportunistic organisms gain access through the skin via a small wound, and produce an ulcer.
Chronic	Ulcers caused by cancer	Most commonly seen in the elderly is the rodent ulcer: a basal cell carcinoma, which is a 99% non-proliferating local cancer.
Acute	Flame or scald induced burns	Burns can produce damage to the epidermis alone (superficial), the epidermis and dermis (partial thickness), and to deeper tissue (full thickness). Pronounced pain unusually is a good indicator of a more superficial and quicker to heal burn.
Acute	Alkali/acid burns	Need specialist treatment to neutralize the chemical.
Acute	Radiation burns	Are rare but extremely damaging. Pre-World War Two, radiotherapy was used to treat some skin cancers. The long-term effects were often radiation burns requiring specialist management.

Table 10.2 Classification of surgical wounds (Cruse and Foord 1980)

Type	Features	Infection rate
Clean	Surgery without infection present and no entry into hollow muscular organs. Appendicectomy, cholecystectomy, and hysterectomy, are also included in this category if there is no acute inflammation	1.5%
Clean contaminated	Hollow muscular organ penetrated, but minimal spillage of contents occurred	7.7%
Contaminated	Hollow muscular organ opened with gross spillage of contents, or acute inflammation but no pus found. Traumatic wounds less than 4 hours of occurrence	15.2%
Dirty	Traumatic wound over 4 hours old. Surgery where there is presence of pus or a perforated viscus	40%

wound, but while Alisons would be considered a clean surgical wound, Christopher's is a dirty wound as it contained pus. Now try using the table to classify wounds of patients/clients in the practice setting, in the following exercise.

Activity

Table 10.1 provides you with information to distinguish the majority of wounds that are met in the care environment. Within your practice setting, explore the nature and cause of wounds that you have identified. Do all the wounds clearly fit into a category type? Are there any wounds that started as acute, and have ended up as chronic? If so why?

You may have identified that wounds are not always easy to place in a category; acute surgical wounds can break down and sometimes appear similar to pressure sores, i.e. these wounds started as acute and ended as chronic (*see* Fig. 10.10). The reasons for this are not always clearly understood, but often relate to the physical health state of the individual. This could indeed happen to Christopher's wound, if his general health is poor.

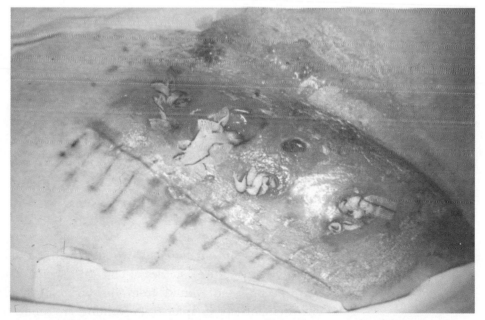

Figure 10.10 Infected abdominal wound
This wound is the product of infection, which as found its way to the surface causing the profound inflammation and breakdown of the skin barrier. This is an old picture showing how in the past wounds were packed with ribbon gauze. Ribbon gauze in a wound can result in lost cotton fibres delaying healing (see Box 10.6: criteria for the ideal dressing).

Learning outcome 2:
Discuss the principles of wound closure for different types of acute and chronic wounds

If possible you should relate this content to the practice setting which you are working within.

In a useful overview of wound closure techniques, Gottrup (1999) identifies that wounds may be closed through:

- Primary closure.
- Early (delayed primary) closure i.e. 4–6 days (performed before there is visible granulation tissue).
- Late (secondary) closure i.e. 10–14 days.
- Grafting using skin or artificial skin products.
- No closure (leaving the wound to heal by granulation).

When wounds are closed (i.e. the skin edges are brought together) the wound is said to be healing by **first intention**. Potential for infection and tissue defect is thus minimized and these wounds heal quickly, with minimal scarring, if infection and secondary breakdown are prevented (Doughty 1992). When wounds are left open, this is termed healing by **second intention**.

Activity

Try to find out how and when wounds are closed, in order to keep them protected from the surrounding environment. Observations in practice, and asking placement staff, should help you. Consider:

- The surgical wound (such as Alison's arm wound)
- The traumatic wound (such as Chloe's lacerations)
- The chronic wound (such as Mr Nixon's pressure sore).

Also find out:

- How long are closure materials (clips, staples or sutures), if present, left in the wound before removal and does the site of the wound have any effect on this?

Points which you may have identified:

The surgical wound

- Clean or clean-contaminated wounds will be managed by primary closure, using sutures, staples or clips, at the end of surgery, with the aim of protecting the wound from the bacteria circulating in a hospital environment (*see* Chapter 3, Preventing cross-infection), and promoting the best cosmetic result. Thus Alison's arm wound will have been managed by primary closure, at the end of her operation.
- With contaminated or dirty surgical wounds, delayed primary closure may be preferable, and in some cases the wound may be left open, to heal by second intention. A dirty, infected wound, such as Christopher's, will

be left open to enable continuing drainage; closing the wound would allow build up of pus, and a further abscess.

The traumatic wound

Management of traumatic wounds, such as Chloe's, depends on the degree of contamination (taking into account where and how the wound occurred), the extent of skin damage/ skin loss, the site of the wound, and how long ago the injury occurred. Gottrup (1999) advises that a clean incisional wound (e.g. caused by a knife), with little tissue damage, that occurred less than 6 hours previously, can be irrigated, debrided and managed by primary closure. However he suggests that if the injury is more than 6 hours old, or is heavily contaminated, e.g. by soil, then primary closure should be delayed.

There may sometimes be differing priorities though. Although Chloe's wounds are heavily contaminated, as they are facial wounds, after removal of the gravel and thorough cleansing and irrigation of the wounds, primary closure would be applied to the lacerations. Facial wounds do have an excellent blood supply and rarely become infected (Higgins *et al.* 1997). Incised wounds and lacerations can be closed with tapes, sutures or tissue adhesive; the decision on which to use will depend on factors such as size, depth and site. For example, tissue adhesive could be very suitable for a small, superficial scalp wound, but should not be used for lacerations of the mouth or eye (Young 1997). Where, for cosmetic reasons, extreme accuracy of alignment is essential, e.g. a lacerated nostril, lip or eyebrow, suturing is preferable (Young 1997).

If the client with a traumatic wound has delayed seeking attention, then prolonged bacterial access will have occurred. Usually the wound will be cleansed with the aim of free drainage and/or detection of infection, followed by delayed primary closure by suturing, at 4–6 days. Gottrup (1999) explains that secondary closure (at 10–14 days) has been used when a wound is heavily contaminated, and that although this leaves a broader scar than after primary (early or delayed) closure, it is still cosmetically preferable to that achieved through the healing of an open granulating wound. Note that **tetanus** prophylaxis should be ensured with any traumatic wound.

Tetanus 'lockjaw'
Tetanus is an acute infection caused by *chlostridium tetani*, an anaerobic organism which is found in substances like road dust and soil. A tetanus toxoid injection is given to produce immunity against tetanus in healthy individuals, and those at risk of developing tetanus after a dirty wound.

The chronic wound

The chronic wound is usually allowed to heal by **second intention**. Granulation tissue fills the defect, and new epidermis covers the surface. While satisfactory, this is slow and time-consuming, and as discussed, provides poor protection against risks such as repeated pressure. It can, nevertheless, provide a successful outcome. Mr Nixon's pressure sore will need to heal by second intention. When surgical excision of necrotic tissue as in a pressure sore is performed, the aim is also for healing to occur by second intention. Attempts to directly close large defects by bringing the edges of the wound together have consistently proved a disaster, since the tension on the suture line pulls the wound apart. An alternative is to use surgical techniques such as skin grafting and skin flaps; Gottrup (1999) gives a brief overview of these techniques.

When to remove skin closures

The decision on when to remove skin closures depends on a number of factors including:

- Site: The face heals faster – sutures are often removed in 5 days. The feet heal more slowly so sutures may remain *in situ* for 7–10 days.
- Factors such as ageing, steroid therapy, and diabetes, can affect the rate of healing (*see* later section 'Factors affecting wound healing').

It will be important to ensure that patients being discharged from hospital with skin closures *in situ* are informed of exactly when and where the skin closures will be removed. Alison's clips would probably be ready for removal at 7 days, and she could attend her local health centre for their removal by the practice nurse. Sometimes it may be necessary to arrange for the district nurse to visit a patient's home for skin closure removal, such as if it is difficult for the person to leave the house due to poor general condition or lack of mobility. If adhesive glue was used to close any of Chloe's lacerations, this has the advantage of not needing removal. If any sutures were inserted, being facial they can be removed at 5 days, at the health centre by the practice nurse. However, Chloe might be asked to return to a hospital clinic (e.g. the plastic surgery clinic) so that the cosmetic result can be assessed, and further follow-up arranged. Paper strips can be gently removed at 5 days too.

Summary
- Acute wounds usually heal more uneventfully and quickly, but can in certain situations become chronic.
- Different types of wounds are managed in different ways: in general, clean surgical wounds by primary direct closure, contaminated traumatic wounds by delayed primary closure, and chronic wounds by secondary intention healing.

FACTORS AFFECTING WOUND HEALING

The factors influencing wound healing are many and complex; knowledge is not yet able to explain the range of biological, psychological and sociological elements that influence the individual. Nevertheless there are some common elements that can be identified and addressed in order to achieve a successful outcome. Identifying factors which may influence wound healing for the individual is important, as a perpetuating wound will result if underlying causes are not addressed (Williams and Young 1998).

Learning outcome

On completion of this section you will be able to explore the range of factors that can affect wound healing

Miller (1995) suggests that when assessing an individual with a wound, the following two questions are necessary:

1. What factors are interfering with wound healing?
2. Which of these can be changed in order to move the healing process forward?

The following exercise is based on this framework.

Activity

With the guidance of your practice assessor, identify a patient/client (such as Mr Nixon) who has a problematic wound, and carry out this activity:

1. Look at the patient's assessment documentation. Identify factors that have been recorded which could influence wound healing, and try to provide a rationale for your identification of each factor. Remember to consider the person (biologically and psychologically) as a whole, as well as the wound itself.
2. Then ask yourself, can these factors be altered/changed? Try to think of what action could be required.

Points which you may have considered:

Table 10.3 includes factors which might have been identified for Mr Nixon, with suggested action. Compare the list you prepared for your patient with this. You may well have identified a much wider range of issues, depending on your individual patient (*see also* Miller 1999a; Mulder *et al.* 1995; Partridge 1998). Are you aware of the effect of steroids on wound healing? The anti-inflammatory response of steroids reduces the inflammatory response, and affects the function of the **macrophages** thus slowing healing (Williams and Young 1998). Chronic conditions which affect wound healing include respiratory and cardiovascular disease, due to their effect on tissue oxygenation (Williams and Young 1998).

You probably considered general health status, age, nutrition, and body-build: has the individual reserves to help use for wound repair? Did you also identify stress and anxiety as a factor? This too can have a major influence on wound healing (Partridge 1998); however employing techniques such as provision of information (Boore 1978) and therapeutic touch (Daley 1997) can contribute to healing. Christopher has a number of problems, and the discomfort associated with his wound may be a further source of stress. Alison, too, has been through a stressful experience. Now that she is back in

Macrophage

Cells that can destroy bacteria and devitalized tissue, and are therefore important in the destructive phase of wound healing.

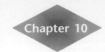

Table 10.3 Factors affecting wound healing, as applied to Mr Nixon

Factor	Rationale for identification	Can be influenced?	Action required
Lifestyle: heavy smoker	Effects of smoking on tissue function are outlined in detail by Siana and Gottrup (1992). Smoking causes a compromised blood supply to the wound, and impairs the cardiovascular system, delaying healing. It leads to inhibition of epithelialization and a reduction in wound contraction (Williams and Young 1998).	Potentially	Reduction in smoking balanced against quality of life issues.
Diabetes mellitus and high blood glucose levels	Diabetics have impaired wound healing (Davidson *et al*. 1984; Silhi 1998). Insulin needs to match bodily needs, e.g. should be increased if the body is under stress, such as in the presence of infection.	Yes	Multidisciplinary team approach to bring blood glucose nearer to normal range. Will include blood glucose monitoring, dietary considerations and balancing insulin prescription.
Depression	Depression affects ability to self-care.	Yes	Pharmacology and therapeutic approach from keyworker to moderate depression.
Poor nutritional status: low calorie intake and appetite poor	Adequate nutrients required for wound healing (*see* Table 10.4)	Yes	High calorie and protein supplements. Dietician involvement, monitoring of intake.
Ageing	The skin's ability to repair reduces with ageing (Desai 1997). In addition, the disease processes which often accompany ageing are likely to affect healing (Partridge 1998).	Indirectly by improving overall health	Multidisciplinary team and client involvement to promote health.
Stress and anxiety about being in hospital	Stress delays healing (Boore 1978; Kiecolt-Glaser *et al*. 1995).	Potentially	Develop nurse–patient relationship, listen to concerns, information giving and involvement in care.

Continued

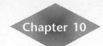

Table 10.3 *Continued*

Factor	Rationale for identification	Can be influenced?	Action required
Underweight	Bony prominences less protected, putting patient at further risk of skin breakdown	Sometimes dependent on the health status, and psychological status	Use of appropriate positioning and equipment to minimize risk of skin damage to pressure areas, particularly those already affected. Also dietician involvement and promotion of nutrition to increase weight. *See* Chapter 9 (Pressure sore prevention) and Chapter 4 (Promoting healthy eating).
Infection in toe wound	Infection compromises healing, places stress on the body, and impairs diabetes stabilization	Yes: management of infection	Medical and nursing team action, including investigations (e.g. X-ray to identify whether there is bone infection). Precription/ administration of antibiotics. Appropriate wound care.
Neuropathic ulcer to toe	Repeated trauma/ stress to the wound due to lack of sensation	Yes	Foot care (*see* Chapter 5). MDT liaison, including podiatrist, tissue viability nurse, diabetic nurse specialist.
Presence of necrotic tissue in sacral wound.	Causes a continued inflammatory response, thereby delaying wound healing	Yes	Debridement of necrotic tissue.

her own environment with familiar staff members, it will be important to be supportive and reassuring. Chloe and her father could be upset and anxious due to her trauma and emergency hospital admission. Thus the nurses' approach to them is paramount in relieving their stress and helping them to relax (*see* Chapter 2, Approach to patients/clients). Casey (1999) notes that even minor wounds can have a significant psychological impact on both the child and the parents, and that there is often associated parental guilt. Box 10.1 summarizes common fears and anxieties which parents of children with wounds can experience. Note also the effect that a wound may have on the child's body image, see Price (1993) for further discussion on this aspect.

If you worked through Chapter 4 (Assessing and meeting nutritional needs) you are probably well aware of the need for an adequate and increased nutritional intake for wound healing. However, there is evidence that many people with chronic wounds e.g. pressure sores have poor nutritional intake and risk

> - Dealing with their child's anxiety
> - Their child's pain, particularly during dressing removal
> - How to manage dressings and keep them in place
> - How to keep the child amused
> - Subsequent scarring.

Box 10.1 Sources of parental anxiety, in relation to wound care (based on Casey 1999)

factors for malnutrition, as do other community patients (Green *et al*. 1999). Williams and Young (1998) suggest that every patient with a wound should be assessed nutritionally. Table 10.4 outlines the key nutrients required for wound healing and their role in the process. McLaren (1992) extensively reviews the literature linking nutrition and wound healing.

Activity Consider Mr Nixon, Christopher, Chloe and Alison, in our scenarios at the start of this chapter. How might you ensure that their additional nutritional needs are met?

Look back to Chapter 4 if you need to check that you addressed this activity comprehensively.

Finally, you may also have identified factors to do with the condition of the wound and how it is being managed. Miller (1999a), acknowledging the

Table 10.4 Nutrients required for wound healing and their function (adapted from Williams and Young 1998, p. 26–7)

Nutrient	Function
Carbohydrate	Energy source for increased cellular activity during wound healing
Fat	An alternative energy source. Fat soluble vitamins are essential for the building of new cell membranes in wound repair
Protein	Essential for building the new wound bed, i.e. collagen formation. Patients already protein depleted before wounding are worse effected
Vitamin A	Supports epithelial proliferation and consequent migration across granulation tissue. More efficient when given prior to wounding
Vitamin B	Assists formation of collagen mesh which supports new blood vessels as they move into granulating tissue
Vitamin C	Assists formation of collagen mesh
Vitamin E	With vitamin C, attacks damaging oxygen free radicals that are present in infected wounds and during the inflammatory phase of wound healing
Minerals: zinc, copper and iron	Required for collagen formation. Zinc also has an antibacterial effect, mainly against Gram-positive bacteria.

systemic nature of wound healing, states that the wound itself is the last place practitioners should look at, when questioning why a wound is not healing. Relevant factors include:

■ Aspects to do with the wound itself e.g. the presence of necrotic (dead) tissue or infection.

■ Aspects to do with how the wound is being managed e.g. frequent and excessive exposure of the wound which causes a drop in temperature at the wound bed, inappropriate use of antiseptics or certain wound products, which might damage fragile new tissue.

All these factors could delay healing and are considered later in this chapter in the section 'Wound management'.

Summary
■ A range of factors can potentially interfere with the healing process of a wound. These factors will relate to the individual's general health status, the condition of his wound, and the care being received.
■ Some of these factors cannot be significantly altered; others very significantly.
■ The use of nursing skills has a major effect on this process.

WOUND ASSESSMENT

As discussed in the previous section, when assessing a wound you will need to consider the whole person, so that factors that could interfere with healing can be addressed wherever possible. This section now prepares you to assess the wound itself, based on your accumulated knowledge of the stages of wound healing, the ability to classify wounds, and finally the ability to be aware of the range of wider issues that affect healing. All these aspects underpin the assessment process.

Recommended reading: identifying wound assessment scales
Referring to texts relating to wound assessment tools, and considering their strengths and weaknesses, will be beneficial when working through this section. Ensure that you distinguish these from pressure sore risk assessment tools e.g. the Waterlow Scale (Waterlow 1988), and the Braden Scale (Bergstrom *et al.* 1987). The function of these is to assess the risk of the individual developing a pressure sore (see Chapter 9: Pressure sore risk assessment). Grading tools on the other hand, aim to provide information on the wound itself. Some e.g. the Stirling Scale (Reid and Morison 1994) are used to grade the type of pressure sore. The Red Yellow and Black Scale (RYB) (Cuzzell 1988)

is American, simple to use, aims to be more widely usable, and provides information on treatment; however it has had little uptake in the UK. Cooper (1992) warns that although this tool is useful, it over-simplifies wound assessment, as it considers only a single variable. Useful articles relating to wound assessment include Miller (1996; 1999b). A number of texts include wound assessment charts (e.g. Dealey 1999, p. 58; MacQueen, 2000, p. 320).

Learning outcomes

By the end of this section you will be able to:

1. Assess an individual with a wound using a recognized assessment tool.
2. Be able to record key information in a useful format, which can be used to plan appropriate interventions.

Learning outcome 1:
Assess an individual with a wound using a recognized assessment tool

Activity

Find out whether there is a wound assessment tool used in your local practice setting, and try to access this. Otherwise use one from the literature. Liaise with your practice assessor, and using the tool, assess a client's wound. You will also need a measuring instrument e.g. ruler, and good light. While carrying out this exercise, consider:

(a) Should a wound assessment tool be used for all wounds?
(b) What aspects should be included in a wound assessment tool?

Discussion points

(a) Should a wound assessment tool be used for all wounds?

■ Minor straightforward wounds do not require a formal recorded assessment. If the wound is judged by both your assessor and yourself to be healing uneventfully, a record of this in the care plan will suffice. This should be quite sufficient for Alison's straightforward surgical wound, unless problems developed.

■ Judging when to use a tool will involve issues such as a wound that is not healing as expected, possibly reverting to a previous stage, wounds with problems or where required as a legal record, for example after an assault. Mr Nixon's pressure sore, and ulcerated toe (which could, as a diabetic ulcer, deteriorate) are both chronic and problematic wounds, and as such the use of an assessment tool will be advantageous.

(b) What aspects should be included in a wound assessment tool?
Box 10.2 lists the features which might be included in a wound assessment tool, based on those found within the literature. These are discussed in fuller detail below.

- Presence of a fistula or a sinus
- Presence of a wound drain, and drain site
- Presence of dehiscence
- Anatomical location
- Size of the wound
- Wound age
- Extent of tissue involvement
- Is the wound open or closed?
- Description of tissue at the wound base
- Presence, nature and extent of exudate
- Status of the edge of the wound
- Presence of foreign bodies
- Condition of surrounding skin
- Pain.

Box 10.2 Aspects included in a wound assessment tool

■ Presence of a **fistula** (an abnormal connection between two spaces such as skin surface and bowel) or a **sinus**. A sinus is a tract that ends in a blind cavity; these are frequently found in deep pressure sores. A sinus should heal from its base, as if it heals at the surface, fluid will accumulate within, promoting an abscess which will subsequently break through to the surface.

■ Wound drain, and drain site. Wound drains are inserted into some surgical wounds to promote the removal of fluid that would otherwise accumulate and form a potential growing medium for infection, or interfere with healing.

■ A **dehisced** wound is one where tissue has become separated from deeper tissue owing to the presence of infection, a **haematoma** (collection of blood) or **seroma** (collection of serous fluid).

■ Anatomical **location**.

■ **Size** of the wound (recorded on a graph or as width by length; depth is very difficult to measure). Sometimes a tracing is made, which creates a record of shape as well as size.

■ Wound **age**: how long has the wound been present?

■ **Extent** of tissue involvement: does it involve epidermis, dermis, fat, fascia, muscle, and/or bone?

■ Is the wound **open or closed?** Remember from earlier in this chapter: an open wound is one healing by second intention, a closed wound is predominantly healing by first intention. Thus Alison's wound will be healing by first intention but Mr Nixon's sacral wound is healing by second intention.

■ **Description of tissue** at the wound base. Colour: Is there black necrotic tissue, yellow slough, or red granulation tissue? There may be elements of all three at the same time. Necrotic tissue (as is present in Mr Nixon's pressure sore) will prevent or delay the healing process (Kiernan 1999), and will therefore need removing to enable healing to progress.

■ Presence of **exudate** (fluid arising from the wound due to increased permeability of capillaries). Is this offensive, coloured, or profuse? Your assessment of presence and extent of exudate will influence your dressing choice. The production of large or increased amounts of exudate or pus could indicate infection, but other signs and symptoms should be taken into account too. A detailed examination of the criteria for identifying a wound infection can be found in Cutting and Harding (1994).

■ Status of the **edge** of the wound: in large and/or deep wounds, the edge of the wound when in the inflammatory and destructive phases, will be oedematous and very red. As this progresses towards the proliferative phase, a white border will appear which is new epidermal tissue, fragile and easily removed.

■ Presence of **foreign bodies**: are there foreign bodies in the wound? This may include cotton wool fibres, pieces of gauze, as well as gravel. All will delay the healing process. The presence of foreign bodies e.g. dirt or grit, can also increase infection risk, and lead to permanent marking (Fletcher 1997). That is why it is necessary for Chloe's wounds to be surgically cleaned of the embedded gravel. It will be important to ensure that she and her father understand why the surgery is required.

■ **Condition of surrounding skin**: is this healthy, dry or moist, flaking or macerated? This is important in considering the type of dressing to be used.

■ **Pain**: is the wound painful? If so, when? During dressing removal, or all the time? Has the pain increased? Is it associated with other signs and symptoms such as malodour, inflammation, increased exudate, and delayed wound healing? The more of these that are present, the greater the likelihood of a wound infection (Miller 1998). However if the pain occurs only on dressing removal, then the type of dressing being used needs reconsideration.

Maceration

Softening and breaking down of skin due to prolonged exposure to moisture. Can occur to surrounding skin when a wound is heavily exudating.

Learning outcome 2:
Be able to record key information in a useful format, which can be used to plan appropriate interventions

Activity

Review the material that you recorded by using the wound assessment tool, and consider the following questions:

• Is it specific and comprehensive enough to help you to plan the wound's management, and to promote continuity of care?
• Has the tool recorded any information about the individual, his/her state of mind, and perception of the wound? If not, is this recorded in your nursing notes?

Now consider the following points in relation to your assessment:

■ The tools employed are generally very wound-specific. They have to be simple to use, yet all encompassing, but not be so inclusive as to waste valuable time and so deter usage.

■ These are legal documents. Have you accurately described the wound environment? Have you avoided the use of colloquialisms, such as 'wound bed appears fine': what does 'fine' mean? Ensure that you use descriptive language that can be interpreted by anyone, not just yourself. This will help to promote continuity of care. A photograph of the wound can be particularly useful for recording wound assessment, and may provide a more objective record of the wound's status, alleviating potential variation in the use of descriptive terms and their interpretation.

■ Can the assessment help you to prepare for the management of the wound? Has it identified, for example, any problems with the existing approach to the dressing, e.g. is the dressing allowing the wound to dry out, or the surrounding skin to become macerated? Was the dressing painful to remove?

Summary
■ Wound assessment requires an holistic approach involving assessment of the whole person and the wound together.
■ Documentation is becoming increasingly important, for management as well as litigation reasons.
■ Accuracy in recording assessment is an important skill to develop and will do much to promote continuity of care.

WOUND MANAGEMENT

You will have noticed by now, from the previous sections, that knowledge required in wound care is extensive, and how the knowledge is used can be subject to the interpretation of the user. Practice will enhance your knowledge and skills; this section will aim to provide some principles to guide your interpretation of good practice in wound management as your experience grows.

In order to achieve a holistic approach it is necessary to manage the wound from a multi-factoral perspective, as well as addressing the specific needs of the wound itself. The characteristics of the individual and the environment and the resources accessible to the client and the wound, must all be considered.

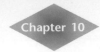
Learning outcomes

By the end of this section you will be able to:

1. Explore the broad aim of wound management.
2. Manage the wound from a multifactoral perspective.
3. Explore approaches to managing the specific need of the wound itself.

Learning outcome 1:
Explore the broad aim of wound management

Activity

In the last section, you carried out a wound assessment. Based on your exploration of this patient and his/her wound explore the broad aim of wound healing for this person, that is, to provide an optimal healing environment. What aspects might this entail?

Discussion points

Environment, in the context of healing, can be interpreted as being the wound environment itself, but also includes the person and the environment in which he is living. To provide an optimal healing environment you will need to address the factors affecting healing identified previously. Social, environmental, spiritual and psychological factors are as important as physical, and a few points relating to these are discussed below.

If the client is unhappy with, for example lack of friendship, and has no one to communicate with, he is unlikely to communicate his feelings regarding the regime of dressings you instigate, and if the client does not understand the regime, he is very unlikely to comply with it. If you are aware of the psycho-social effects of wounds, you can be supportive; this is of relevance to both acute and chronic wounds. Neil and Barrell (1998) point out that the skin is 'a major factor in a person's body image'. The effects on body image of acute wounds can result in a range of psychological reactions including a grief response, anxiety and depression (Magan 1996). A qualitative study conducted by Neil and Barrell (1998) sought to investigate the effects of having a chronic wound, and concluded that people with chronic wounds have to make significant transitions in their lives. Denial, anxiety, pain, immobility and altered body image were experienced. Neil and Barrell (1998) suggest that being aware of this can help health professionals to be understanding, and that effective assessment can promote helpful interventions, referrals, and information provision. Note also that Mr Nixon wants to go home, and being in the hospital environment, contrary to his wishes, may hinder his healing. The risk of cross-infection in the hospital environment remains significant, with wounds being a common site for hospital acquired infection (*see* Chapter 3). Consid-

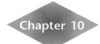

eration of his home environment will be necessary, for when he is discharged.

Learning outcome 2:
Manage the wound from a multifactoral perspective

Your consideration of factors affecting healing will enable you to plan care for the whole person by liaising with the multidisciplinary team and including relatives and the client, to put into practice your plan of action, thus providing an optimal healing environment. Note that involvement of the patient and/or carer are essential in the process of wound healing (Williams and Young 1998) and, as discussed earlier in this chapter, removing or reducing underlying causes of the wound is paramount.

Table 10.5 Promoting wound healing: suggested multidisciplinary team (MDT) involvement for Mr Nixon

MDT member	Role
Ward nurse	Care related to addressing factors affecting wound healing, e.g. blood glucose control, promoting nutrition, relieving stress/anxiety etc. Wound assessment and dressings, education of patient/carer and health promotion, support and information giving, liaison with other nurses, relatives and MDT
Specialist nurses: infection control, diabetes, nutritional support, tissue viability, dermatology, discharge liaison.	Specialist advice and support for patient and family, and ward team, to address the factors affecting wound healing. Equipment provision and resources
Physiotherapist	Promote mobility and correct positioning: education and advice
Occupational therapist	Positioning, mobility and dressing aids, seating, adaptations to home
Social worker	Discharge arrangements and support at home e.g. arranging meals on wheels, day centre, financing of home adaptations
Podiatrist	Foot care
Doctor	Blood glucose control, prescriptions, surgical debridement of pressure sores and ulcer (if required), identifying and treating other health problems which may delay healing, liaison with GP
Pharmacist	Advice on wound care products
Dietician	Assessment and advice re dietary supplements
Primary Health Care Team: district nurse, health visitor, GP, practice nurse	Medical and nursing care in the community after discharge; assessment of health needs in the community
Chaplain	Spiritual needs and support

1. **Possess high thermal insulation**. A study by Lock (1979) (cited in Myers 1983) with pigs found 108% increased cell division at the edge of wounds maintained (through use of a film dressing or a polyurethane foam) at a high temperature (30–35°C), when compared with wounds left open (attaining a temperature of 21°C), or covered with a gauze dressing (attaining a temperature of 25–27°C). It has been demonstrated that 40 minutes is required for a wound to return to room temperature after cleaning, and 3 hours for mitotic cell division and leucocyte activity to restart (Myers 1982).

2. **Maintain a high humidity at the wound/dressing contact**. Winter (1962), in a classic piece of research, dispelled the myth of dry wounds being necessary to prevent bacterial infection. Instead he demonstrated that film dressings increased humidity at the wound surface, doubling the rate of epithelialization. A moist surface enabled the epithelial cells to migrate across the wound more easily, than when the wound was dry.

3. **Remove excess exudate from the wound surface**. The aim here is to prevent the wound becoming macerated by the profuse exudate in certain types of wounds such as pressure sores, burns, fistuli, and drain sites. This remains a difficult task for a dressing to achieve, but there are products aimed specifically at heavily exudating wounds.

4. **Be impervious to micro-organisms**. Thus preventing airborne bacteria from reaching the wound through the dressing, and bacteria on the wound surface from entering the environment causing cross infection (Dealey 1999).

5. **Not shed any fibres or leak out toxic substances**. Dressings which leave particles in wounds prolong the inflammatory response, thus delaying healing (Wood 1976). Gauze, gamgee and cotton wool have no place in contact with a wound bed. They do have a use still in addressing other criteria. e.g. maintaining temperature, as a secondary dressing.

6. **Allow easy removal from the wound without causing damage to the newly formed tissue**.

Handling qualities of an effective wound dressing are that it should: (Dealey 1999):

- Be easy to apply and remove
- Conform well to the wound surface
- Be comfortable
- Not require frequent dressing changes.

Box 10.6 Criteria for an effective wound dressing

Your choice of dressing will relate to your assessment of the individual, whilst taking into account the attributes of an effective wound care product. Particularly important to consider are of course, stage of wound healing, site of wound, pain relief, and amount of exudate, but many other individual factors too. For example, if the wound is malodorous, a charcoal dressing can help to relieve this (Dealey 1999). A detailed review of the advantages and disadvantages of different categories of wound dressings can be found in Feedar (1995). Note that the dressing should keep the wound bed warm (Myers 1982), and that dressing changes can cool the wound and slow down the healing. This should be taken into account when planning dressings, and carrying the dressing out. Also, always consult the manufacturer's instructions when applying dressings.

Dressings for diabetic foot ulcers must be chosen with particular care (Foster 1999), but Gill (1999) identifies that many dressing trials exclude diabetics, making it difficult to make evidence-based decisions on product choice. The use of hydrocolloids for these wounds appears to be particularly controversial but Gill (1999), in a critical review, suggests that this product has often been used in an incorrect manner i.e. left in place for too long a time, without inspecting the wound. The criteria for an ideal dressing for a diabetic foot ulcer, as suggested by Foster *et al.* (1994), can be found in Box 10.7. A trial by Foster *et al.* (1994), compared the use of alginates with polyurethane dressings for non-infected diabetic ulcers, and found that the ulcers healed with either dressing, but the polyurethane dressing handled better. In addition to dressing the ulcer, general foot care (*see* Chapter 5, Box 5.3) is also essential, including aspects such as not soaking the feet and drying the skin carefully (McConnell 1998).

Foster and Moore (1999) note that despite the vast range of dressings that are available, many require more sound evidence for their use than is

---

The ideal dressing for the diabetic foot ulcer should:

- Perform well in the enclosed environment of a shoe, and not take up too much space
- Absorb large quantities of exudate but enable drainage
- Withstand the pressures and shear of walking
- Not be associated with side effects
- Not depend, for its maximum effect, on being left in place for more than 24 hours. As diabetic ulcers can deteriorate very rapidly they must be checked every day
- Be easy to remove/lift for inspection.

Box 10.7 The ideal dressing for a diabetic ulcer (Foster *et al.* 1994)

currently available i.e. although trials have been performed, they have often used insufficient numbers of people. In addition, as noted at the start of this chapter, there are constantly being new products developed. Clinical guidelines for the management of venous leg ulcers, based on a systematic review of available evidence, have been developed by the RCN (1998). There are also currently a number of systematic reviews relating to wound dressings in progress within the Cochrane Institute, results of which will be available 2000–2001. Key groups of dressings, and their uses, are summarized in Table 10.6

The patient/client will need educating about his wound care, and the dressing.

Activity

If you were being discharged home with a dressing *in situ*, or had had a dressing applied by the community nurse, what sort of things would you want to know about it?

You would probably want to know some of the following:

- Can I get the dressing wet? If not, how can I manage activities such as washing?
- When should the dressing be redone, and by whom?
- What should I do if the dressing becomes loose/uncomfortable/ too tight, falls off, or soaks through?
- What should I expect of the wound? e.g. when will it heal?
- Will the wound be painful? If so, how can I deal with this?
- How would I know if the wound was getting infected?
- Are there any special instructions which I should follow?

You might have thought of other things which you would want to know too, and remember that this information is also important to people receiving in-patient care, in order to allay anxiety, build confidence and promote self-care. Parents will wish to know similar things about their child's dressing, but may have special concerns such as how to keep the dressing in place. Certainly, with children there may be particular considerations when choosing a wound dressing. For example, Casey (1999) notes that for children in nappies, it can be difficult to prevent contamination of the wound by faeces or urine if it is in the nappy area, but that occlusive, waterproof dressings can help. It is also important that wounds are kept free of contamination by dirt etc. while playing. Young children may be inquisitive or resent the addition of a dressing to their bodies when they are still developing a clear picture of their own physical self. Therefore dressings will need to be securely applied and 'finger proof'. Note that written information is useful to back up verbal instructions, because it is difficult for people to retain a lot of new information particularly when under stress. Written patient information should be readable, understandable and culturally

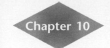

Table 10.6 Wound dressings (based on Foster and Moore 1999; Dealey 1999)

Dressing type	Examples	Description	Uses
Simple	Mepore	Simple wound covering which provides protection from contamination and absorbs mild exudate.	Wounds healing by primary intention e.g. a straightforward surgical wound.
Adhesive film dressings	Opsite, Tegaderm Bioclusive	A transparent, vapour permeable adhesive fim dressing which acts as a barrier to bacteria and water, and therefore allows bathing/showering. Allows observation of wound. Can be left in place for several days.	Primary wound closure e.g. a straightforward surgical wound. To protect skin susceptible to damage from shearing. Shallow granulating and epithelializing wounds, with low to moderate exudate. Abrasions. Can be used as secondary dressings with alginates, or with hydrogels if there is hard necrotic tissue present.
Tulles Medicated and non-medicated	Jelonet (impregnated with soft paraffin), Bactigras (with chlorhexidine), Inadine (with povidine-iodine)	Open weave cotton or rayon dressing impregnated with soft paraffin, antiseptics or antibiotics. Granulation tissue cells can move through the open weave of the dressing, causing damage and pain on removal, and fibres can be left in the wound. Non-absorbent.	Infected wounds healing by secondary intention, with minimal exudate, abrasions, minor burns.
Hydrogels	Intrasite gel, Sterigel	A dressing based on starch polymers, which provides a moist wound environment, and promotes debridement.	Dry, necrotic, and granulating wounds. Light to moderately exudating wounds. Abrasions. Require a secondary dressing.
Foam dressings	Allevyn Tielle	A highly absorbant dressing made from polyurethane or silicone. Available as a flat dressing and a cavity dressing.	Heavily exudating wounds, full thickness cavity wounds healing by secondary intention. Granulating and epithelializing wounds.

Continued

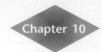

Table 10.6 Wound dressings (based on Foster and Moore 1999; Dealey 1999)

Dressing type	Examples	Description	Uses
Hydrocolloids	Granuflex, Comfeel plus, Tegasorb	A polyurethane foam sheet fixed onto a semi-permeable film. Provides a moist environment, promotes debridement, granulation and epithelialization. A protective barrier against micro-organisms. Can cause maceration of surrounding skin. Also available as a paste or powder, for cavity wounds.	Has wide application, for both chronic wounds, and acute wounds such as abrasions. Moderately but not heavily exudating wounds. Necrotic, infected, sloughy, granulating or epithelializing wounds. Can be left in place for several days and bathing/showering can take place with the dressing *in situ*.
Alginates	Kaltostat, Sorbsan	Made from the sodium and calcium salts of alginic acid – a seaweed derived polymer. Reacts with wound exudate to form a gel which, it is believed, promotes wound healing. This can be irrigated off leading to a less painful dressing change. Highly conforming and encourages clotting. Available as a flat dressing, rope and ribbon.	Used for moderately to heavily exudating wounds, including infected wounds. Can be used to pack puncture and cavity wounds. For sloughy and granulating wounds. May require secondary dressing.
Hydrofibre dressings	Aquacel	An absorbant dressing which provides a moist wound healing environment.	Infected wounds, and acute surgical wounds healing by secondary intention. Can be left in place for up to 3 days.

relevant however, if it is to be effective in promoting self-care and relieving anxiety (Wilson and McLemore (1997).

Leg ulcer bandaging
A systematic review by Cullum *et al.* (1999) concluded that compression increases venous ulcer healing rates when compared with no compression, that multi-layered systems are more effective than single layered systems, and that high compression is more effective than low compression. However

compression should **only** be used in the absence of significant arterial disease, and therefore, as discussed earlier in this chapter, arterial blood supply to the feet must first be assessed. Treatment will need to be continued after healing, as without compression, the underlying problem – venous hypertension – will return, and a leg ulcer will form once more (Williams and Young 1998). Therefore patient education and involvement is essential to try to improve compliance with this regime.

Before selecting a compression bandage each patient is assessed individually and lifestyle considered (Williams and Young 1998). Bandaging should extend from the base of the toes to the knee (Scully 1999). RCN guidelines (1998) state that leg ulcer bandaging should be applied by a trained practitioner, have adequate padding and be capable of sustaining compression for at least a week. You should get the opportunity to observe leg ulcer bandaging in practice, possibly at a clinic, or with the district nurse. Try to find out about a local leg ulcer clinic, and arrange a visit.

How can I minimize pain and discomfort?

Unfortunately patients may often associate their wounds with pain. A study of 694 patients with a variety of chronic wounds found that almost half experienced pain (Lindham *et al.* 1999). Any care in relation to wounds can cause fear and distress, be this removal of a surgical drain, a dressing change or removal of skin closing devices such as staples, clips or stitches. A person with a traumatic wound, such as Chloe, will have already experienced pain when the injury occurred, and the thought of having a wound dressing could be very distressing. A summary of factors contributing to pain associated with wounds, and possible solutions, can be found in Table 10.7.

It is important that pain is assessed and that the source of pain is identified, so that steps can be taken to alleviate this. Clear links have been found between anxiety and pain, and providing information can reduce this (Hayward 1975). Analgesia prior to dressing change may be required, particularly with children (MacQueen 2000), opiates being necessary if pain is severe, but otherwise non-steroidal anti-inflammatory drugs or simple analgesics. Sufficient time for them to take effect before the dressing, should be ensured (Emflorgo 1999). Nitrous oxide (entonox) can also help some people, and can be effective even for young children (Casey 1999). Other pain reduction strategies include use of relaxation and distraction, and involving patients by removing their own dressings. MacQueen (2000) suggests that a child can remove his own dressing while bathing/showering, which can make the experience less frightening. The Hospital Play Therapist may be able to accompany the child during the dressing procedure, providing

Table 10.7 Factors causing pain associated with wounds, and possible solutions (adapted from Hollinworth 1997)

Factors	Solution(s)
Use of cold fluids for cleansing/irrigation	Use fluid at body temperature
High-pressure irrigation	Consider reducing pressure, and use of analgesia and other pain relieving strategies
Use of forceps on sensitive tissue	Use gloves instead
Use of plastic spray which stings	Consider benefits of use versus discomfort. If used, warn patient, and be supportive
Pain on removal of dressings	• Careful choice of product. • Information giving and explanations about the procedure. • Correct dressing removal technique. Refer to manufacturer's instructions. • Use of analgesia, and other pain relieving strategies such as relaxation, distraction.

support and employing distraction strategies to help the child cope with the experience.

Casey (1999) notes the importance of giving the child opportunity to express concerns about dressing changes. An infant or small child can sit on the parent's lap while the dressing takes place, while an older child such as Chloe, can have her father sitting with her. However, whilst parental presence during dressings is beneficial to the child, parents can find observing painful procedures being performed on their children emotionally distressing (Callery 1997). Nurses should, therefore, be sensitive to the parents' needs for support. MacQueen (2000) also suggests the use of play, and that dressing times for children should be kept to a minimum, thus reducing discomfort. Therefore, planning carefully and preparing everything in advance is essential, as well as choosing an uncomplicated dressing which takes minimal time to apply. Casey (1999) emphasizes that pain management must be effective from the start, as the child would otherwise quickly start to associate wound dressings with pain. This statement could equally apply to adults, particularly where there is a chronic wound which will require ongoing wound dressings.

Careful choice of dressing will also minimize wound pain. Adherent dressings e.g. gauze, paraffin gauze, cause pain on removal, as they dry out, and tissue can grow through the fabric. Therefore never use gauze as a primary dressing, and if using paraffin gauze, redress daily. Some products are much less painful to remove (e.g. hydrocolloids, alginates, foam, hydrogels), so give preference to these. Occlusive dressings, such as hydrocolloids, have been found to relieve pain at the wound site (Feedar 1995). Some products e.g. hydrocolloids and film dressings, lose adhesiveness as days go by, so leaving them *in situ* for the maximum time possible will promote easy removal. Irrigation can ease removal with some dressings. To remove film dressings, lift the edge, and stretch the dressing up and away rather than peeling it back which is more painful (Jones and Milton 2000).

Activity   Identify possible strategies for wound care for Mr Nixon, Christopher, Alison and Chloe, based on the information within this chapter. Some aspects may be difficult as you would need a more detailed assessment of these individuals, but try to suggest options. Remember to consider: use of clean or sterile technique, debridement, cleansing, wound dressing, and pain management.

Points which you might have identified can be found in Table 10.8.

Table 10.8 A possible wound care strategy for Christopher, Mr Nixon, Alison and Chloe

	Christopher	*Mr Nixon*	*Alison*	*Chloe*
Wound type	Dirty surgical wound on buttock	1. Necrotic sacral pressure sore 2. Infected diabetic neuropathic ulcer on toe	Clean surgical wound on forearm	Contaminated lacerations/abrasions on face
Use of sterile or clean technique?	Sterile	Clean	Sterile	Clean prior to surgery, sterile post surgery
Debridement needed?	Was performed surgically	Yes. Identify an appropriate option for this individual	Not required	Is being performed surgically
Cleansing?	Yes, bathing, showering or irrigation with warm saline	Could bath or shower, or the wounds could be irrigated with warm saline when the dressings are renewed. Feet should not, however, be soaked. Consider use of antiseptic for infected toe ulcer (Miller 1998).	Not required Can bath or shower as she wishes	Cleansing prior to surgery would be minimal as the superficial nature of these wounds causes extreme pain. Post-surgery, cleansing would depend on condition of wounds, e.g. irrigate with warm saline if excess exudate.

Continued

Table 10.8 *Continued*

	Christopher	Mr Nixon	Alison	Chloe
Which dressing?	Pack wound with alginate, then apply secondary dressing	1. Hydrogel or hydrocolloid to sacrum 2. Toe could be dressed with an alginate or foam dressing, which could be removed daily for toe inspection.	Not necessary after first 24 hours (Weiss 1983) but Alison may find it to be more comfortable if her wound is covered with a film dressing until her clips are removed.	If required post-surgery, film dressings would be appropriate, or a thin hydrocolloid can reduce pain of abrasions by preventing nerve endings from drying out (Dealey 1999). In practice, facial wounds are rarely dressed.
Pain management	Assess client. Information giving and explanations. Regular analgesia e.g. non-steroidal anti-inflammatory drugs. The alginate dressing should be comfortable to wear and painless to remove.	Assess client. Information giving and explanations. Hydrogel, hydrocolloid, foam and alginate dressings are all comfortable to wear and their removal should be painless. Regular analgesia if needed. Neuropathic ulcers are usually painless.	Assess pain. Information giving and explanations. Regular analgesia may be needed. Removal of film dressing with care. Removal of skin closures will need careful preparation, reassurance and support.	Assess pain. Information giving and explanations. If dressings are present, remove with care. Regular analgesia may be needed. Removal of skin closures will need careful preparation, reassurance and support.

Summary

- A structured and multifactoral approach to the management of the person with a complex wound, including multidisciplinary team involvement, is proven to produce the best results.
- Wound assessment must precede effective wound management, which then requires the application of suitable cleansing methods, the most appropriate dressing to cover the wound, and pain relieving strategies. Application of these skills in the care of each individual, is the product of knowledge and experience.

CHAPTER SUMMARY

This chapter has aimed to introduce an understanding of how wounds heal, with an emphasis on the systemic nature of wound healing, and the range of factors which may this process. An awareness of how wounds can be assessed and managed, taking into account their underlying causes, has been promoted. An individualistic and holistic approach to wound care has been emphasized, and different options available for managing wounds have been discussed.

The reader has been encouraged to take every opportunity to apply knowledge to practice, and to start to gain experience in observing wounds and identifying their stage of healing. There has been an emphasis on involving patients/clients and their families, on working with the multidisciplinary team, on accessing expert knowledge, and being aware of the need to continually update. This chapter did not attempt to include specialist knowledge and it is intended that further in-depth reading in relation to individual topics such as leg ulcers and burns, would be undertaken by the reader.

To conclude, an understanding of wound care is important for all nurses; this chapter has aimed to introduce key principles to act as a foundation for future learning.

REFERENCES

Angeras, M.H., Brandberg, A., Falk,A. and Seeman, T. 1992. Comparison between sterile saline and tap water for the cleaning of acute traumatic soft tissue wounds. *European Journal of Surgery* **158**, 347-50.

Bergstrom, N., Demuth, P.J. and Braden B.J. 1987 A clinical trial of the Braden Scale for predicting pressure sore risk. *Nursing Clinics of North America* **22** (2), 417–28.

Boore J. 1978, *Prescription for Recovery*. London: RCN.

Bremmelgaard, A., Raahave, D. and Beier- Holgersen *et al.* 1989. Computer aided surveillance of surgical infections and identification of risk factors. *Journal of Hospital Infection* **13**, 1-18.

Briggs, M. 1996. Surgical wound pain: a trial of two treatments. *Journal of Wound Care* **5**, 456-460.

Bryant, R. 1992. Preface. In: Bryant, R. (ed.) *Acute and Chronic Wounds: Nursing Management*. St Louis: CV Mosby, xi-xii.

Callery, P. 1997. Paying to participate: financial, social and personal costs to parents of involvement in their childrens care in hospital. *Journal of Advanced Nursing* **25**, 746-52.

Casey, G. 1999. Wound management in children. *Paediatric Nursing* **11** (5), 39-44.

Clancy, J. and McVicar, A. 1997. Wound healing: a series of homeostatic responses. *British Journal of Theatre Nursing* **7** (4), 25-34.

Cooper, D. 1992. Wound assessment and evaluation of healing. In: Bryant, R.(ed.) *Acute and Chronic Wounds: Nursing Management*. St Louis: CV Mosby, 69-90.

Cooper, R. and Molan, P. 1999. The use of honey as an antiseptic in managing pseudomonas infection. *Journal of Wound Care* **8**, 161-64.

Cruse, P. and Foord, R.1980. The epidemiology of wound infection, a ten year prospective study of 62,939 wounds. *Surgical Clinics of North America* **60**, 27-40.

Cullum, N. and Roe, B. 1995. *Leg Ulcers: Nursing Management, a Research Based Guide*. Harrow: Scutari Press.

Price, B. 1993. Diseases and altered body image in children. *Paediatric Nursing* **5** (6), 18-21.

Reid, J. and Morison, M.1994. Towards a consensus: classification of pressure sores. *Journal of Wound Care* **3**, 157-160.

Royal College of Nursing 1998. *Clinical Practice Guidelines: the Management of Patients with Venous Leg Ulcers.* London: RCN.

Scully, C. 1999. In on a limb. *Nursing Times* **95** (27), 59-60, 62, 65.

Siana, J. and Gottrup, F. 1992. The effects of smoking on tissue function. *Journal of Wound Care* **1** (2), 37-41.

Silhi, N. 1998. Diabetes and wound healing. *Journal of Wound Care* **7**, 47-51.

Thomas, S. 1990. *Wound Management and Dressings.* London: Pharmaceutical Press.

Thomas, S., Jones, M., Shutler, S. and Jones, S. 1996. Using larvae in modern management . . . maggot therapy. *Journal of Wound Care* **5** (2), 60-69.

Thomas, S., Andrews, A. and Jones, M. 1998. The use of larvae therapy in wound management. *Journal of Wound Care* **7**, 521-524.

Thomas, S. 1997. *A Prescribers Guide to Dressings and Wound Management Materials.* Cardiff: Value for Money Unit.

Thomlinson, D. 1987. To clean or not to clean. *Nursing Times* **83** (9), 71, 73, 75.

Waterlow, J. 1988. The Waterlow card for the prevention and management of pressure sores: toward a pocket policy. *Care – Science and Practice* **6** (1), 8-12.

Weiss, E.L. 1995. Connective tissue in wound healing. In: McCulloch, J.M., Luther, C., Kloth, L.C. and Feedar, J.A. (eds.) *Wound Healing Alternatives in Management*, 2nd edn. Philadelphia: F.A. Davis, 16-31.

Weiss, Y. 1983. Simplified management of operative wounds by early exposure. *International Surgery* **68**, 237-240

Wiedenbach, E. 1964. *Clinical Nursing: A Helping Art.* New York: Springer Publications.

Williams, C. and Young, T. 1998. *Myth and Reality in Wound Care.* Dinton: Mark Allen Publishing.

Wilson, F.L. and McLeomore, R. 1997. Patient literacy levels: a consideration when designing patient education programs. *Rehabilitation Nursing* **22**, 311-17.

Winter, G. 1962. Formation of the scab and the rate of epithelialisation of superficial wounds in the skin of the young domestic pig. *Nature* **193**, 293-94.

Wood, R.A.B. 1976. Disintegration of cellulose dressings in open granulating wounds. *British Medical Journal* **1**, 1444-45.

Wysocki, A.B. and Bryant, R.A. 1992. Skin. In: Bryant, R. (ed.) *Acute and Chronic Wounds: Nursing Management.* St Louis: CV Mosby, 1-30.

Young, T. 1997. Wound care in the accident and emergency department. *British Journal of Nursing* **6**, 395-6, 398, 400-1.

Young, T. 2000. Managing MRSA wound infection and colonisation. *NTPlus* **96** (14), 14-16.

Zink, M., Rousseau, P. and Holloway, G.A. 1992. Lower extremity ulcers. In: Bryant, R.(ed.) *Acute and Chronic Wounds: Nursing Management.* St Louis: CV Mosby, 164-212.

FURTHER READING

Cohen I.K., Diegelmann, R.F. and Lindblad, W.J.1992. *Wound Healing: Biochemical and Clinical Aspects.* Philadelphia: W.B. Saunders.

Flanagan, M. 1997. *Wound Management.* Edinburgh: Churchill Livingstone.

Chapter

11

Drug administration

Veronica Corben

In almost every practice setting, nurses administer drugs, or supervise their administration. In order to do this safely nurses require a breadth of knowledge including pharmacology, legal and policy issues, calculations and how to administer drugs via a variety of routes. Only a registered nurse can administer drugs unsupervised, but to develop competence requires considerable experience and practice and therefore students need to take every opportunity to build up their knowledge and skills during the pre-registration course.

Included in this chapter are:
- Safety and storage of medicines
- Administering oral medication
- Application of topical medication
- Administering medication by injection routes
- Calculating drug doses

Note that administration of inhaled and nebulized medication is included in Chapter 8 (Respiratory assessment and care) and administration of rectal medication (via suppositories or enemas) is included in Chapter 6 (Meeting elimination needs).

Recommended biology reading

It is important that you have an understanding of how drugs are absorbed, and how they reach the site where their action is required. Thus the following questions will help you to focus on the biology underpinning this chapter's skills. Use your recommended text book to find out:

- What are drugs? What do they do? How do they know where to act? How do they achieve their effects?
- Define the terms bioavailability, agonist and antagonist.
- In order to be delivered to individual cells, drugs must be absorbed into the bloodstream. Few methods of drug administration involve direct injection into a blood vessel. Which routes of administration would be described as enteral and which as parenteral?
- What factors will affect the absorption rate of orally administered drugs?
- What is the first pass effect?
- Drugs often have unwanted side effects. Understand terms such as nephrotoxic, hepatotoxic.
- In order to be effective, levels of the drugs must be within the therapeutic range. What could happen following the administration of a wrong dose?
- Drugs must be metabolized in order to be eliminated from the body. Where does metabolism occur?
- How are drugs excreted from the body?
- What factors will affect the absorption, distribution, metabolism and elimination of drugs?

It will also be useful to revise the layers of the skin.

Note that the introductory chapters in the following books are helpful:

Hopkins, S.J. 1999. *Drugs and Pharmacology for Nurses*, 13th edn. Edinburgh: Churchill Livingstone.
Trounce, J. 1997. *Clinical Pharmacology for Nurses*, 15th edn. New York: Churchill Livingstone.

PRACTICE SCENARIOS

The following practice scenarios illustrate situations where nurses will be administering medication via several different routes, and will require knowledge of these drugs' actions and side effects, as well as how to store and administer them safely. They will be referred back to throughout the text.

■ **Adult**

Miss Ivy Prior is 82, and is a diabetic controlled on insulin. She has been unwell for some time and has been admitted to a medical ward with a chest infection. She lives alone and is normally self-caring. She is prescribed a number of medications, including glycerol trinitrate patches and diuretics for a heart condition, and she is now prescribed antibiotics too.

■ **Child**

Shabana is 5 years old, has tonsillitis and is finding it difficult to swallow. She is currently receiving antibiotics in suspension form and is feverish and lethargic. She also has conjunctivitis for which antibiotic eyedrops are being administered. Her mother is caring for her at home, and she has two other children aged 1 and 3.

■ **Learning disability**

Charles is 18 years old and has cerebral palsy and is an unstable epileptic. He lives at home with his parents, and attends a day centre daily. He is prescribed once daily anti-convulsants, but requires help and supervision in taking them. He also has acne, for which he is now prescribed Fucidin cream three times daily.

■ **Mental health**

Mary Tompkins was first diagnosed as having a schizophrenia type illness 20 years ago, and has had several subsequent relapses. Now in her 40s, she is a cleaner in a local school, and lives alone. Her mental state is variable, but the school staff are used to supporting her when necessary. She attends the health centre for a once monthly depot injection of fluphenazine for her schizophrenia.

SAFETY AND STORAGE OF MEDICINES

There are a number of legal and policy issues relating to storage and safety of drugs which must be adhered to by nurses.

Learning outcomes

By the end of this section you will be able to:

1. Identify key aspects of legislation and policies governing drug administration.
2. Discuss issues concerning safety and storage of medicines.

Learning outcome 1:

Identify key aspects of legislation and policies governing drug administration

You are probably aware that there is government legislation which covers abuse of drugs, sale of medicines over the counter, labelling of medicines, and pharmacies in supermarkets. There are two important acts of parliament which provide this public protection, and infringement of these is a criminal offence.

These are:

■ **The Misuse of Drugs Act, 1971,** which controls the storage, sale and administration of controlled (addictive) drugs (*see below*).

■ **The Medicines Act, 1968,** which controls the labelling, sale and distribution of all medicines, and established a licensing system.

Useful categories of medicines defined in the Medicines Act (Hopkins 1999) are:

1. **Prescription only medicines (POM):** These can only be obtained on a prescription. In hospitals, almost all medicines are POM, (Duthie 1988), and therefore each patient will have a prescription chart.

2. **General Sale List (GSL):** This is a restricted list of simple medicines that can be freely sold through almost any outlet, e.g. garages and supermarkets.

3. **Pharmacy only medicines (P):** These can only be sold in the presence of a pharmacist, but do not require a prescription.

Appropriate examples would be:

1. Antibiotics;
2. Aspirin;
3. Cough mixtures.

There are many other examples of course.

Controlled drugs

Answer: A controlled drug is addictive, because of the probable dependency that could result from it. These drugs may not be as toxic to the body as others that are more easily available. For example, 10 paracetamol tablets could kill you, but these are not controlled. However, access to pethidine, morphine etc., or any other drugs of this family that we call 'opiates' (because they are derived from opium), can cause addiction, with all its consequences, very quickly, if taken for non-therapeutic reasons. Remember, these drugs are therefore dangerous and their sales need controlling because of their addiction, not their toxicity. They are controlled under the Misuse of Drugs Act, 1971, already mentioned.

Since 1985, controlled drugs have been subject to different levels of restriction, (Henry 1998), and are therefore divided into 'schedules', e.g. temazepam, a form of night sedation, is a schedule 4 drug, whereas pethidine is a schedule 2 drug. Scheduled drugs need to be kept in even more safe conditions than others. In in-patient settings, schedule 2 drugs have to be kept within two locked cupboards, and very securely in people's homes. However, the detail of this level of safety has to be negotiated with the people concerned, because it is within their property (Hopkins 1999).

Controlled drugs can only be ordered by a registered nurse, and must be administered by a registered nurse with a second checker, who fits the criteria for a checker for the local drug policy. This may vary in community settings, and where people may be self-medicating. You will need to check these details in each placement, and try to access the appropriate drug policy.

Checking administration of controlled drugs requires an understanding of the gravity of the issue, as detailed above. For this reason, student nurses may be able to check these drugs, but in some areas this may not be permitted. Again, your local drug policy will inform you. Checking during administration involves the whole procedure from preparing the drug with each checker individually calculating the dose, administration of the drug and disposal of any remaining drug and equipment. As a student nurse, you need to feel confident to check and give such drugs. You may decide that you need more observational practice and knowledge before being prepared to take on such a role.

Registers of controlled drugs must include details of stock and drugs administered, and must be signed by both persons providing such detail. They should be kept for at least 2 years (Hopkins 1999).

| **Activity** | Think back to a recent placement experience and try to identify who else needs to be involved in drug administration. Can you think of other organizations which may be involved in drug regulation too? |

You should have included professional bodies and employers.

■ **Professional bodies**, e.g. doctors through their professional body, the British Medical Association, pharmacists through their professional body, and nurses through the UKCC. Pharmacists provide very expert knowledge about drugs, and often have an information adviser who can provide instant and accurate advice. Initiatives to expand the role of the community pharmacist, and to improve General Practitioner collaboration are being developed (Pilling *et al.* 1998). The UKCC issues guidance via statements of principles on many issues including drug administration to all its registered nurses in all branches. It is vital that nurses read these and abide by them, to protect patients/clients, and themselves professionally. The booklet is called 'Principles of safe drug adminstration' (UKCC 1992).

Activity
You may have been provided with a copy of the above booklet but otherwise look at a copy in the library, or ask a registered nurse to show you her copy of the UKCC booklet.

■ **Employers** produce similar drug policies for their individual organizations. This includes private health-care settings as well as NHS Trusts. These contain much useful information in a usually easily read form, and they refer to the student role and other issues too. They should always be accessible in placements, even if you do not have your own copy. It is one of the most important documents in all areas of practice!

Activity
Have a look and see where the drug policy is kept in your current, or next, practice placement.

Learning outcome 2:
Discuss issues concerning the safety and storage of medicines

The Duthie report (1988) recommended new safe procedures for storing and handling drugs.

Activity
When you are next in practice, ask a practitioner what these safety procedures are and check them with the points below.

You should have found out about the following:
■ **A safe place.** This will be different depending on the setting, for example in hospital, this will be in a locked cupboard or immobilized medicine trolley, but in a person's home it could be the kitchen table, if she lives alone as in Miss Prior's case. **Remember**: even lotions and cleaning agents need to be stored like medicines, in a locked or safe place, especially where there are children around, as in Shabana's family. Controlled (addictive) drugs, e.g. morphine, should be kept within two locked cupboards.

■ **A cool place**. Medicines are often quite unstable chemically, and may even be manufactured with a stabilizer included in the chemical compound. They generally become more unstable if warm, hence a cool dark place, away from direct sunlight is most suitable. This is why medicines are generally stored in dark bottles. Some drugs actually need to be stored in a refrigerator e.g. insulin, and some antibiotics and sedatives. In residential settings of any kind, a separate locked drugs fridge should be used which has a visible temperature gauge on the outside, and the temperature is regulated to 8°C (Hopkins 1999).

■ **Stock rotation**. Like your larder, medicines need to be kept in chronological order, with new ones put to the back, and the older ones used first. Charles and Miss Prior might need help to remember this. Remember: where there is an expiry date with a month and year, it is the last day of the month when it expires, and it can therefore be used until then.

■ **Labelling of medicines**. All medicines have an approved (generic) and a brand (proprietary) name. The approved name is the chemical name and is used by all drugs companies. The brand name may be different depending on the company who has produced it. For example, cold remedies may contain the same constituents, but be marketed under different names. This could cause confusion, so all prescriptions should display the approved name, especially in hospital settings (Sexton and Braidwood 1999) and this is strictly controlled under the Medicines Act (1968). Medicines are also labelled with a batch number on the container. This is specific to the batch of medicines produced at the same time. For this reason too, medicines should never be transferred from one container to another. There is also the danger of labels being misread and different medicines being mixed in the same container.

■ **Holding drugs keys**. These should always be held by a registered nurse, preferably the nurse in charge. As a student therefore, you should never hold keys. In areas where there is no registered nurse, e.g. some learning disability settings, you may be advised not to get involved in drug administration, because staff will be unable to comply with professional regulations (UKCC 1992) although they will have a different policy in place. Talk to your lecturers about this.

Summary

■ It is crucial that drugs are stored safely, whether in hospital or in the community, and in appropriate conditions, thus maintaining their effectiveness.

■ Nurses need to be familiar with legislation and local policies concerning storage of drugs and be aware of issues that could affect their safety.

ADMINISTERING ORAL MEDICATION

By the end of this section you will be able to:

1. Identify the different types of available oral medication.
2. Identify issues about nurse and patient/client preparation for safe oral drug administration.
3. Understand how to administer oral medication safely.

Learning outcome 1:
Identify the different types of available oral medication

Activity	What types of oral medication have you seen? Devise a list with a colleague.

You may have considered:

■ **Tablets.** These are convenient, are accurately dosed and relatively cheap. They often contain additives to prevent disintegration in the gastrointestinal tract.

■ **Capsules.** These are oval-shaped, with a coat of hard gelatin. They are useful for bitter drugs, and for unpleasant liquid, e.g. Chlormethiazole. Miss Prior's antibiotics may be capsules. Remember: never open capsules as they are made to be swallowed whole (Trounce 1997).

■ **Elixirs and syrups.** These flavoured and sweetened liquids are particularly useful for children, as in Shabana's case. Many are sugar-free, especially those for children.

■ **Emulsions.** These are a mixture of oil and water, e.g. liquid paraffin. They need to be shaken well to mix the contents.

■ **Linctus.** This is a sweet syrupy preparation, e.g. cough linctus.

Sublingual and buccal medication

Note that there are two other forms of medications which although taken into the mouth, are not swallowed:

*   **Sublingual medication:** These are produced as sprays or as tablets, and are absorbed through the mucosa under the tongue. As the sublingual area is very vascular, absorption and effect of the drug occur rapidly.
*   **Buccal:** These medications are usually produced as tablets, and are put onto the gum under the lip. Again, effect of the drug is rapid.

When this route is used very careful instructions should be given, so that the patient/client fully understand that sublingual and buccal tablets should not be swallowed.

Learning outcome 2:
Identify issues about nurse and patient/client preparation for safe oral
drug administration

Remember that the administration of drugs must be under direct supervision
of a registered nurse until you qualify.

■ **Activity**   What precautions and preparations would you need to consider before giving
medication to a patient or client by any route? A prescription chart may help you
with your answer.

*Box 11.1 outlines the points you should have considered and these are
discussed in more detail below.*

- Patient/client identity
- Allergies
- Consent
- Timing of the drug
- Route of the drug
- Prescription
- Dose.

Box 11.1 Drug administration: checks which should be made

■ **Identity**. How do you know that this is the correct person for the drug?
The use of identity bands in residential settings may provide the answer.
However, the client may not have a name band, e.g. in out-patient
settings, a new patient, or long-term residents, e.g. in learning disability
settings. Neither Shabana, Mary nor Charles will have identibands. You
will need to ask the person, or a friend or relative to tell you his name
and date of birth, where possible. If you merely ask the person to
acknowledge what you think his name is, he may agree regardless,
because of his developmental level of functioning or if he is too unwell
to think clearly.

■ **Allergies**. Does the person have any allergies, e.g. antibiotics? If so, he
could have an allergic reaction to the drug which could produce a serious
local or systemic reaction – anaphylaxis. Anaphylaxis is a potentially life-
threatening condition, and is discussed in detail by Henderson (1998).

■ **Consent**. Does the person or the next of kin understand what the drug
is for, and agree to it being given? Only in rare circumstances does this
not apply. Can you think what these might be? A situation where it
might be acceptable to administer drugs without consent, would be if the
medication is considered essential (e.g. life saving) and the person is

unconscious, very unwell, or unable to understand for developmental reasons. Clients who are detained under section 3 of the Mental Health Act (1983) (Department of Health and Welsh Office 1993) may be administered drugs to treat their mental health condition without consent, even if they have declined this treatment. Which people in the scenarios may find compliance with treatment hard? Your answer could include any of them. Appropriate presentation of the drug, e.g. in user-friendly containers, will increase compliance (Ling 1999), as well a clear explanation about the drug and rationale for its prescription. The explanation should take into account level of understanding and developmental stage, as in Shabana's case.

■ **Timing of the drug.** Is the drug due now; or is it prescribed only if required by the person? Some drugs need to be taken with food if they need an acid medium in which to be metabolized, whereas others, e.g. flucloxacillin, should be taken on an empty stomach because an acid medium would break the drug down before it can be absorbed in its useful form (Caldwell 1999). Miss Prior is taking diuretics, which are usually prescribed in the morning, to prevent a diuresis late in the day or at night.

■ **Route.** How is the drug to be given, and is this the most appropriate route? Consider whether the oral route would be appropriate if, for example, the person is vomiting.

■ **Prescription.** Is this written clearly throughout, including the drug itself (using the approved name), the date and signature of the doctor, and the route and time of administration? Is the person's name, and any special instructions, such as 30 minutes before food, clearly written? If any of this information is unclear or missing, the registered nurse must not give the drug (Henry 1998). Any alteration must be signed and dated by the doctor. In an emergency, verbal messages may be taken over the phone by a registered nurse, and the prescription chart signed by the prescribing doctor within 24 hours. Many employers request that the drug is repeated to two nurses over the phone. Student nurses should not become involved in verbal messages. You may find that abbreviations are used on prescription charts.

■ **Activity** Discuss with a colleague whether abbreviations would be acceptable on a prescription chart.

Your discussion should have included that internationally recognized abbreviations are acceptable, but that these must be clearly written. Many of these are translations from Latin! Locally developed abbreviations should not be used. What abbreviations have you seen?

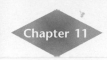
Developing Practical Nursing Skills

■ **Activity**

Try to interpret the abbreviations below, which are all widely recognized. (Answers are at the end of the chapter.)

nocte, prn, mane, po, qds, bd, stat, tds, ml, pv, inh, neb, od, inst, caps, elix, kg, mg, mcg.

■ **Dose**. Does the dose appear correct for the person? Oral doses will often be larger than intravenous doses. This is because oral drugs have to pass through the gut and liver before entering the circulation, and some of the drug may be lost here, rather than entering the circulation directly. This is called the first pass effect. (Check up on your reading if necessary.) This is also why enteral drugs take longer to work than parenteral, which do not have to pass via the liver first. You will also need to consider whether the dose involves a complex calculation, or is it to be given to a child? In both these cases, two nurses will be needed (Sexton and Braidwood 1999), of which one may be a student. At home, however, Shabana's mother will administer her medicines unsupervised.

■ **Activity**

Check with your local drugs policy about your role as a student in being a checker for drug calculations and for administering drugs to children.

Remember, if a calculation has to be done, both nurses need to work it out separately and then compare the answer. Otherwise it is really only one calculation.

Learning outcome 3:
Understand how to administer oral medication safely

What should you always do before any patient interaction? You should of course hand wash thoroughly (*see* Chapter 3).

Before administering any drug, you should:

• Know what the drug is
• How it works
• The normal dosage
• Any side effects
• Any extra precautions you may need to tell the person.

There is a compendium called the British National Formulary (updated twice yearly) which is there to provide such information. All clinical areas should have one. The compendium may help in Miss Prior's case, where she is taking a variety of medicines together, and you may want to know about their interactions. Remember that for some prescriptions, as already discussed, it is necessary to have two people to check and administer them. The local drug policy will always help you to identify these circumstances.

Having made the checks discussed in Learning outcome 2, you should now identify the appropriate bottle or packet of medicine that corresponds with the prescription. Check all the prescription details with the bottle label, and also the expiry date and any special instructions. If the tablets are in a bottle, tip the correct amount into the lid, and then tip into a medicine glass or spoon. Remember the lid is as clean as the inside of the medicine bottle. Many tablets are now supplied in blister packs, so that they can be individually sealed, and then pushed out through a foil backing into a medicine pot so that no touching is necessary (Hopkins 1999).

For children and some clients with swallowing difficulties, most oral medicines will be in liquid form. Many paediatric suspensions are sold with a double-ended spoon, which can measure 2.5 and 5 ml volumes. If administering liquids, firstly shake the bottle for even distribution, then hold the bottle with the label uppermost, so that the medicine cannot flow over the label and deface it, and pour gently into a measuring glass, at eye level for accuracy. If the dose is one millilitre or less, use a one ml syringe and aspirate it directly from the bottle or via a quill, and then put the lid back on the bottle. It may also be useful to use a syringe for withdrawing larger quantities e.g. 5 ml, as they are more accurate than medicine pots. Note that there are special oral syringes available which have a different appearance from usual syringes. They should always be used if available to reduce risk of mistakes, e.g. by giving an oral medication intravenously in error, which would have serious or even fatal, consequences. Many parents now choose to buy 5 ml syringes from chemists.

Activity

For this exercise you need a tube of Smarties, a small cup, a bottle of water and a syringe. You should be able to access a syringe in the skills laboratory, but you may need permission – do check. Practise tipping a Smartie out into the lid and then into the cup without touching the Smartie. Then try drawing water up from the bottle with a syringe.

You will next need to decide how to administer the drug. Can the person self-administer or do you need to administer it on a spoon? Do tablets need crushing and would they be more acceptable to a child if put in jam or ice cream etc? Parents will usually be the best people to advise, and to administer medication to their child. Is the medicine best put into the mouth from a syringe? In Shabana's case, how well can she swallow today? There are some tablets which should not be crushed, such as long-acting or enteric-coated tablets, e.g. prednisolone, where their action is damaged by the crushing action (Sexton and Braidwood 1999). For obvious reasons (prevention of cross-infection), never touch the medication with your hand. If the person cannot self-administer, put it into the person's mouth using some form of utensil.

> **■ Activity**
>
> Now try feeding Smarties on a spoon from a cup to a willing volunteer, taking care not to touch the Smarties.

You may have to consider the preparation of the medicine. Liquids are much more quickly absorbed than tablets, because the gastrointestinal transit time is reduced (Caldwell 1999). They are also more convenient for children, and may be better for learning disability clients too, where dysphagia, (difficulty in swallowing) may be present. If these are unavailable, it may be necessary to crush tablets in food to ease swallowing. Gentle downward stroking motions over the larynx may help with swallowing (Wong 1993). Always provide adequate fluids, (about 50 ml for an adult) to ensure medication has been swallowed, and allow a choice of fluid, particularly with children.

Think also about the positioning of the person before swallowing. A baby or child may need holding, and an adult will also require effective support. Sitting up well (if not contraindicated) will make swallowing much easier. Ensure that the person has swallowed all the medication before documenting. A patient may pocket tablets, spit them out when you have gone, or be unable to totally clear them from the mouth. Reward a child, at least verbally, if the medication is taken well, but avoid negative behaviour if the reverse occurs.

When documenting drug administration, ensure that the registered nurse's signature is used, as it is she who is accountable for the administration, not the student. However, if you were the second checker for a controlled drug you should sign the register, along with the registered nurse. After drug administration, clear away all equipment, and wash your hands again if indicated.

> **■ Activity**
>
> Consider how you would dispose of unwanted medication. Tick below those methods you think should be used.

1. Return to chemist or pharmacy.
2. Put into a waste bin.
3. Put down a sink.
4. Flush down the lavatory or sluice.
5. Kept safe for another time.

You should have ticked numbers 1, 3 and 4, and 5 in some circumstances (Duthie 1988). Medicines can always be returned to chemists or the hospital pharmacy for disposal. Small quantities of medicine that have either been dropped, or taken out of the container and then not required, can be disposed of via the domestic waste, a sink or toilet, providing it is not contraindicated as being harmful even in small quantities, e.g. cytotoxic drugs. Medicines should never be put as they are into a waste bin, where someone else could have access to them. Unused medicines can be kept safe for another time, provided they have been kept in the original container, and are not part of a previous course, e.g. antibiotics, when the course should always be completed.

> **Activity**   Have a look at your local drug policy and see what it says about disposal of drugs.

Summary

- Drug administration by a student must be under direct supervision by the registered nurse.
- Both preparation and administration should be performed systematically ensuring that drug policy is adhered to, promoting safety and prevention of cross-infection.
- Careful assessment should ensure that the administration of an oral medication is performed in an acceptable and appropriate manner for the individual, taking into account factors such as age and swallowing ability.

APPLICATION OF TOPICAL MEDICATION

The topical route consists of drug administration via the epidermis (outer layer of the skin) and external mucous membranes. It therefore includes administration into eyes and ears.

Learning outcomes

By the end of this section you will be able to:

1. Understand indications, and preparations used, for the topical route.
2. Show awareness of how topical medication is administered, and the particular precautions that are necessary.

Learning outcome 1:
Understand indications, and preparations used, for the topical route

> **Activity**   Identify reasons for using the topical route in the practice scenarios.

Your discussion should have included Shabana and Charles, for whom this method would be less uncomfortable than swallowing or injection. It also permits local rather than systemic absorption of the drug, which reduces its side effects on the body generally, and this would be important for Shabana and Charles also. The epidermis is fully developed in the young child after one year, and this is therefore a good route for effective drug administration (Choonera 1994).

Not many medications are available in topical form, but this route is becoming increasingly used, particularly in the patch form, such as for pain relief (fentanyl), angina (glyceryl trinitrate), and for children, particularly local anaesthesia (emla cream). Many topical medications are designed to give a 24-hour slow release of the drug and therefore continuous action. This would be very helpful to Miss Prior for her heart condition. Topical preparations also include drops e.g. into eyes and ears, where absorption occurs through the mucous membranes. Shabana's antibiotic eye drops will be locally absorbed this way.

Topical preparations come in several forms:

■ **Pastes**: These contain little water in their composition, and are therefore fairly stiff, and may be difficult to spread (Hopkins 1999). Lids need to be carefully secured to prevent drying when exposed to the air, which would make them even drier in texture.

■ **Creams**: These are made of an oil-based preparation, and are therefore easier to spread and less prone to solidification.

■ **Ointments**: These may be water or oil-based, are semisolid, and are usually available in a tube. It may be advisable to discard the first centimetre (Jamieson *et al.* 1997), as this may have been contaminated by previous exposure to air, especially when using eye preparations. Eye ointment should always be applied to the inside of the lower lid (*see* Fig. 11.1), and the eye held closed afterwards for a short time, where possible. This will enable the ointment to settle. Applications of ointment to the eye are therefore usually applied at night. Vision may be blurred afterwards for a while.

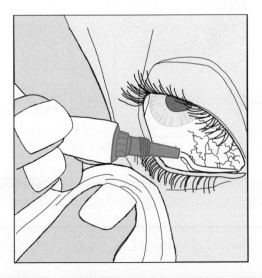

Figure 11.1 Administration of eye ointment

425

■ **Patches**: Medication in this form comes sealed in a small patch, with a peel-off sheet, which exposes the adherent part to be placed on the skin. You need to follow the instructions for where it should be placed, but most are attached to the abdomen or chest, in a relatively hairless region if possible, and the site is alternated each time the patch is changed, usually every 24 hours.

■ **Activity**   Read the manufacturer's instructions enclosed in the packet next time you see a patch used. Are you following them exactly? You need to check the skin for local irritation at the site of the patch each time it is changed.

■ **Drops**: Drops are presented in solution in either single use containers called minims, or in a larger bottle with a pipette type end or dropper. Care must be taken to ensure that they are used for one person only, that the expiry time once opened is observed (usually 28 days) and that they are refrigerated if indicated. Slowly squeeze the bulb, and drop vertically (Jamieson *et al.* 1997), from as near to the patient as possible, but without actually touching the eye with the dropper which would contaminate it. When putting into eyes, put inside the lower lid (*see* Fig. 11.2). Children need extra support to keep the eye still whilst instilling drops. Shabana's mother will need to know to keep the drops refrigerated, and to use one minim for each eye each time, unless a bottle has been provided.

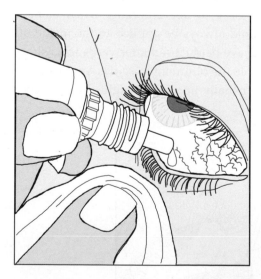

Figure 11.2 Administration of eye drops

■ **Activity**   If you have access to a dropper, you may want to practise this skill onto a target on a piece of paper.

■ **Sprays**: These are produced in containers under pressure, and enable a fine spray to be directed onto the area requiring it, e.g. nasally.

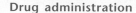

Learning outcome 2:
Show awareness of how topical medication is administered, and the particular precautions that are necessary

Activity

Many of the principles which we have already discussed, e.g. explanation and consent, infection control and safety issues etc., apply to topical medication as well. Can you think of any extra precautions that might be necessary when administering topical medications?

You should have included:

The position of the person is important to ensure that all the topical medication is applied. For application of eye drops/ointment, this should be with the face horizontal, the person preferably lying flat. For application into ears, lying with the ear to be treated uppermost is most effective, and for nasal sprays, the person should be upright.

Careful hand washing is essential. Eyes in particular are highly susceptible to infection, which can have a devastating effect on sight. For application of pastes, lotions etc. to the skin, gloves should be worn if someone other than the patient is applying the medication. This is partly for infection control issues, both from you to the patient and vice versa, and also as some absorption may occur into your skin. Steroid creams should be applied sparingly (Sexton and Braidwood 1999). Where possible, encourage people to do this for themselves. Charles, for example, may be able to apply his cream, although he is likely to need guidance and supervision at first. A young child, like Shabana, may need coaxing from her mother to co-operate. Eye drops can sting, and leave an aftertaste at the back of the throat. If eye medication is being applied to both eyes, apply it to the least affected one first, to prevent potential spread of infection. Following application of topical medication, consideration must be given to remaining in the position for several minutes, or for the type of covering, if any, to be applied. With creams etc. to the skin, this may include advice about clothing, and instructions about any possible staining or soiling. Nasal medication should be administered 20 minutes before food so that the nasal passages are clear for eating.

Remember: always evaluate the effectiveness of the treatment and report and document progress or deterioration to the doctor, or nurse in charge.

Summary
- Topical drugs are prepared in many different formats, and have a number of advantages, such as direct action on the affected area, and slow absorption through the skin.
- Specific instructions should be followed carefully.
- Measures to prevent cross-infection when administering topical medication are particularly important.

ADMINISTERING MEDICATION BY INJECTION ROUTES

Nurses in most settings will give injections on occasions, and it is a practical skill, therefore, that you will want to acquire during your pre-registration course. Note that parenteral means the administration of medication by a route other than via the gastrointestinal tract. This route includes all drug administration by injection and topical routes also. Enteral means absorption via the gastrointestinal tract only. This then includes all forms of oral administration. It will help you to review again the first pass effect and parenteral routes.

By the end of this section you will be able to:

1. Appreciate the rationale for this choice of route.
2. Understand the principles of, and issues relating to administering a drug by injection.
3. Discuss health and safety issues, especially for nurses, when giving injections.
4. Understand the key points in administering intramuscular and subcutaneous injections.

Learning outcome 1:
Appreciate the rationale for this choice of route

Activity   What injection routes have you seen used and where do you think the point of the needle rested on administration? Why do you think these routes were chosen?

Injection routes

You may have seen injections into muscle (intramuscular), into the fat layer under the skin (subcutaneous), into veins through a cannula (intravenous) or under the skin (intradermal). Injections can also be given into joints, into the epidural space or directly into the heart. **Note that as a student nurse you can only give intramuscular (IM) and subcutaneous (SC) injections, and this must be under constant supervision**. It is therefore only the IM and SC routes which will be discussed.

Note that to use the intravenous route you will require further training, and supervised practice as a registered nurse. The intradermal route is used mainly for local anaesthetic prior to invasive procedures. Registered nurses in some specialities may undergo preparation to give intradermal injections. The other injection routes mentioned are mainly used by medical staff.

Rationale for injections

Below are some of the reasons for use of the injection route:

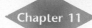
- Rapidity of effect. The drug is more rapidly absorbed into the circulation when it avoids the gastrointestinal tract completely (Campbell 1995).
- When patients are nil by mouth.
- When drugs are destroyed by digestive enzymes in the gut, e.g. insulin.
- When long-term release of a drug is required, e.g. depot injections in mental health clients, especially if non-compliance is a problem.

Key features about the intramuscular (IM) route:

- Skeletal muscle is well perfused with blood vessels, and has relatively few pain receptors (Campbell 1995), so it should be fairly painless. However, not everyone would agree with this!
- The effects are more rapid than the subcutaneous route, because of the good blood supply, so it takes approximately 10 minutes for the effect to begin (Newton et al.1992).
- Absorption can last for 2–3 weeks if desired, using oil-based, slow release preparations, e.g. fluphenazine, as in Mary's scenario.
- In adults, up to 5 ml maximum can be given into one site, but only 1–2 ml in deltoid muscle. In children, a much smaller amount would be acceptable.

Key features about the subcutaneous (SC) route

- A large variety of sites are available as any subcutaneous tissue can be used (Campbell 1995).
- It is usually less painful than the intramuscular route as it has even less pain receptors.
- The speed of action is slower because of the poorer blood supply but medication administered has, therefore, a longer duration, which may be useful, e.g. for continuous 24-hour pain control.
- The person's ability to absorb needs to be checked. If peripheral circulation is poor, the drug may stay in the subcutaneous region. This could be a problem for Miss Prior as she has a heart condition.

Learning outcome 2:

Understand the principles of, and issues relating to, administering a drug by injection

Remember, all safety procedures for the oral route apply to injections too.

Activity

Consider the following issues in relation to IM and SC injections. What have you seen in practice?

- Skin cleaning.
- Injection sites.
- Syringe and needle selection.

Compare what you have observed with the points below:

Skin cleaning

Views vary considerably about this. The study of Lawrence *et al.* (1994) indicated that a 5-second disinfection time using alcohol based swabs, results in a 97% reduction in all bacteria except spore-forming bacteria. Other studies have suggested that social cleanliness is sufficient (Dann 1969; Koivisto and Felig 1978). What appears to be clear is that if alcohol swabs are used, the skin needs to be cleansed for 5 seconds and allowed to dry for 30 seconds (Simmonds 1983). In practice, alcohol swabs are now rarely used prior to injections, with apparently no adverse effects. Alcohol swabs are always contraindicated when subcutaneous insulin and heparin are administered, as alcohol interferes with the drug action and hardens the skin (Workman 1999).

Injection sites

Intramuscular sites

These are indicated in Fig. 11.3. If the gluteus maximus muscle in the buttock is used, it is important to quarter the buttock first and then to administer in the upper outer quarter, to ensure that the sciatic nerve is avoided totally. Any other quarter could cause nerve injury. Note that this site is not recommended for infants and children, because the muscle mass is relatively small. Research has indicated that when injecting IM, it is beneficial to spread the skin (as indicated in Fig. 11.4) to provide a Z-track, which reduces the chance of leakage and pain (Beyea and Nicholl 1995). Once the needle has entered the skin, it need not be stretched, as the exit point is now Z-shaped. This method will be advantageous when giving Mary her injection.

Subcutaneous sites

These are very numerous, but the main ones are shown in Fig. 11.5. When administering by this route, ensure a skin fold is gently pinched to free the adipose tissue from the underlying muscle (Workman 1999). Miss Prior should be encouraged to continue to give her own injections whilst in hospital, to maintain her independence.

Syringe and needle selection

Syringes are selected according to the volume to be given. Volumes of 1 ml and under must be given in a 1 ml syringe, because of the smaller units of graduation, usually 0.1 ml (Beyea and Nicholl 1995). Remember some drugs require a special syringe e.g. insulin, as this is marked off in units, which is how insulin is prescribed. Insulin syringes incorporate a needle as well.

Dorso-gluteal site
(upper outer quadrant of buttock)

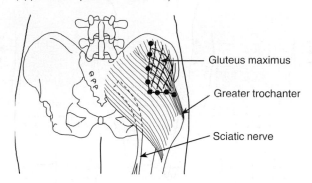

Gluteus maximus

Greater trochanter

Sciatic nerve

Deltoid muscle site
(upper outer third of upper arm)

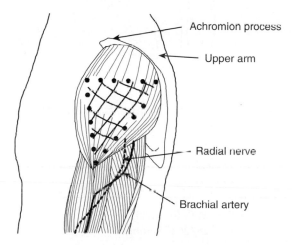

Achromion process

Upper arm

Radial nerve

Brachial artery

Quadriceps site
Vastus lateralis – anterior middle third of thigh
Rectus femoris – outer middle third of thigh

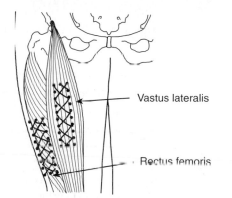

Vastus lateralis

Rectus femoris

Figure 11.3 Intramuscular injection sites

(a)

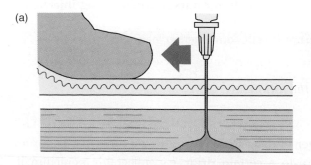

(b)

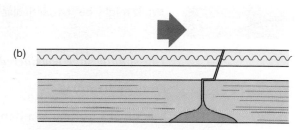

Figure 11.4 The Z-track technique. (a) Skin spread to the left on administration of intramuscular medication, (b) Skin released afterwards, showing formation of Z-track as a result

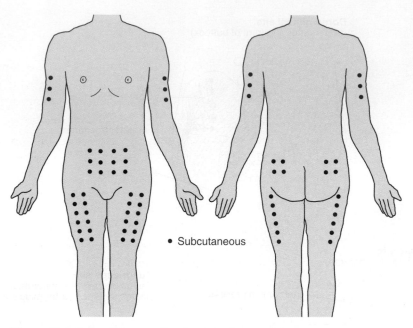

Figure 11.5 Subcutaneous sites for injection

Needles are selected according to the route and sometimes according to the body adipose of the person.

The following is a guide:

Intramuscular:	*Subcutaneous:*
Adult: 1½ × 21 G, (green)	5/8 × 21 G (orange)
Child: 1¼ × 23 G (blue)	5/8 × 25/26 G (orange)

Needles are colour coded for easy identification.

Learning outcome 3:
Discuss health and safety issues, especially for nurses, when giving injections

Activity

What might be the particular hazards with administering injections?

You should have considered the following:

Drug contamination

Use gloves if there is a danger of drug toxicity producing a dermatitis, or as a result of frequent exposure to a certain drug, e.g. injectable penicillin if touching the skin repeatedly, will be absorbed in enough quantity to possibly provoke a resistance.

Needlestick injury

Never re-sheath used needles because these are now contaminated. Leave them uncovered on the injection tray and dispose of immediately into a designated sharps container. A study by De Laune (1990) revealed that 50% of needlestick injuries occurred when needles were re-capped. Also put all syringes, needles and glass ampoules into the sharps container. Never overfill these and separate the needle and syringe using the tapered slot on the top of the box (Campbell 1995). Despite these precautions, needlestick injuries can still occur (particularly when sharps boxes are overloaded), so what should you do?

- Remove the needle quickly.
- Encourage the wound to bleed by applying indirect pressure.
- Then place the injured area under cold running water.
- Cover with a dressing or plaster if required.
- Complete an incident form.
- The Occupational Health Department policy will advise you as to whether further action is necessary.
- Try to ensure that it does not happen again!

Note: if there is any chance of contact with the person's blood, always wear gloves. *See* Chapter 3 (preventing cross infection) and check your local Infection Control Policy for further guidance.

Note also that, unless the injection is prepared beside the person, you will need to re-sheath the **unused** needle carefully after drawing up the drug, to prevent the needle becoming contaminated on exposure to air.

Learning outcome 4:

Understand the key points in administering intramuscular and subcutaneous injections

Activity	Discuss with a colleague or lecturer any anxieties you may have about giving injections, and how this could affect your ability to administer safely. Remember, although injections can be uncomfortable, they have been prescribed to enhance recovery or relieve symptoms.

The steps when giving an IM or SC injection are discussed in points 1–17 below:

1. Ensure that the drug is due to be given, written up correctly, and that the patient or next of kin has given consent. Look back to an earlier part of this chapter for information re consent if necessary.
2. Wash your hands properly.
3. Assemble equipment: Injection tray or equivalent, appropriate syringe and needle, cotton wool swab, (or alcohol swab if local policy), medication and diluent if required.

4. Check details of the medication, then draw up medication either directly from the vial, or if a powder, by mixing according to the manufacturer's instructions.

  – Always use the exact volume and diluent recommended to provide the most therapeutic concentration, and hold the syringe at eye level to achieve this.

  – Remember to check the vial for cracks, precipitation or cloudiness.

  – With multi-dose vials which have already been used, clean with an alcohol swab and allow to dry before piercing.

  – One dose vials which have been newly opened do not need to be cleaned.

    Note: there is no need to change needles after drawing up the liquid as the needles are made of steel and cannot be blunted easily. Also, the more you tamper with the equipment, the more the risk of contamination. However, it is better to use a small gauge needle when drawing up fluids from a glass vial in case there are any glass particles in the fluid (Jamieson *et al.* 1997). You may then need to change the needle to the correct size.

5. Recheck the person's details and medication, consent and name band if appropriate. The approach you take to the person is very important in developing rapport and reducing anxiety about the injection. It is better not to state, nervously, that this is your first injection!

6. Position the person comfortably, supporting limbs if necessary. Babies and children are better held firmly. It is however rare now to see the intramuscular route used for children of any age, except when administering immunizations.

7. Identify the site. With **IM sites** look again at Fig. 11.3. The upper, outer aspect of the leg must be divided into three to identify the correct third, or divide the buttock into four to ensure that the upper outer quadrant is used. As can be seen, the deltoid muscle is in the outer aspect of the top of the arm. Take into account the volume of drug to be administered and convenience to the person, when choosing the site. You should also rotate sites, if repeated injections are being given.

Activity

What would be the IM site of choice for:

(a) A fully dressed woman who needs an IM tetanus injection (0.5 ml).
(b) A patient lying on his back in bed, who has abdominal pain which is worse on movement, and requires an IM injection of 100 mg of pethidine (2 ml), and 10 mg of metochlopramide (2 ml).

The obvious sites would seem to be:

(a) The deltoid muscle, as this can take an injection of up to 1 ml, and is less intrusive for this woman, who need only roll her sleeve up.

(b) This volume injection must go into the thigh or the buttock. As this man has pain on movement, it would be better to inject into his thigh so that he does not have to move.

8. Clean the skin if required to do so.

9. Intramuscular injections: spread the skin. Subcutaneous injections: bunch the skin.

10. Hold the needle at 90 degrees for all IM or SC injections, except where the SC needle is not pre-packed with the syringe and you are attaching an orange needle which is therefore more than 8 mm in length, in which case hold at 45 degrees (Workman 1999) (*see* Fig. 11.6)

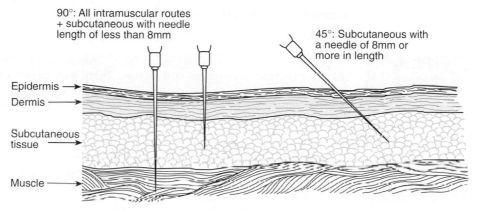

90°: All intramuscular routes + subcutaneous with needle length of less than 8mm

45°: Subcutaneous with a needle of 8mm or more in length

Epidermis
Dermis
Subcutaneous tissue
Muscle

Figure 11.6 Subcutaneous and intramuscular injections: diagram to show skin, subcutaneous and muscle layers, and needle insertion

11. Gently insert two-thirds of the needle into the skin, leaving a third free in case the needle should break and need removing from beneath the skin (Jamieson *et al.* 1997).

12. With IM injections, pull back on the plunger. If blood appears in the syringe, support the skin, withdraw the needle and recommence. This is because the needle must have entered a capillary, and therefore the route would then be intravenous rather than IM. If no blood appears, administer the drug slowly at the recommended rate (if one is prescribed). Note that drawing back on the plunger is unnecessary with SC injections which are entering much less deeply and so are very unlikely to enter a capillary.

13. Observe the person carefully throughout the procedure, providing reassurance as necessary.

14. Quickly withdraw the needle, supporting the skin with the cotton wool swab and apply gentle pressure over the site. Do not rub the skin. Can you think why this might be? You will cause local irritation and may alter

the drug absorption rate by doing so. This would be an issue for both Miss Prior and Mary.

15. Ensure the person is comfortable. Check that there is no untoward form of reaction, either systemic or local. All nurses should be aware of signs of anaphylaxis (a severe allergic reaction). *See* Henderson (1998) for further reading.

16. Dispose of equipment according to local policy (*see* Chapter 3, Sharps disposal; Waste disposal).

17. Document on prescription chart, in the person's notes or wherever is required.

Remember: the signature should be that of the registered nurse taking accountability for the administration, not the student, unless both are required.

> **Activity**
>
> You may have the opportunity to access equipment in the skills laboratory so that you can practise drawing up an injection. There may be an artificial skin pad available which you can practise injecting into. This can help you to become familiar with the equipment and technical aspects of the skill, and thus increase your confidence.

Injections are an invasive procedure and there can be untoward effects.

> **Activity**
>
> You will yourself have experienced injections. What do you think are the main untoward effects?

You may have identified:

■ **Pain**

This may be unavoidable, but can be reduced by distraction techniques, especially when administering to children – think about what form this could take. However, injections, especially IM, are avoided with children whenever possible as they can be traumatic, and might lead to needle phobia. Other routes will be used whenever possible. If an injection must be given, applying the local anaesthetic cream (emla) an hour in advance, will reduce the pain. Emla cream can only be given to children of over one year, because the epidermis is too thin before this. Keeping the skin taut also helps to reduce pain as it stretches the small nerves, and reduces sensitivity (Stilwell 1995). With an IM injection, try to encourage the person to relax, as injecting into a tense muscle will be more painful.

■ **Tissue damage**

Again a degree of this is probably unavoidable. However, damage due to the needle may be reduced by good technique and using the most appropriate needle. For example, if the adult is very thin, it may be more appropriate to use a blue rather than a green needle. Damage may be due to the drug being administered. This can be avoided by ensuring correct dilution according to manufacturer's instructions, and by using the appropriate technique, e.g. always use the Z-track technique (Beyea and Nicholl 1995) for depot injections. Bruising may sometimes be unavoidable, e.g. when giving subcutaneous anticoagulants, such as fragmin, because of the anticoagulant nature of the drug. Rotating sites, as in Miss Prior's case, will prevent local damage.

■ Infection

Using non-touch technique (*see* Chapter 3) in the preparation and administration of an injection should render this very rare. Occasionally a local abcess may develop in a very vulnerable patient. This could become more generalized if untreated. It may be necessary to consider using alternative sites where the risks are less.

■ Hypersensitivity

Obtain a clear allergic history from the person before giving a drug for the first time. Ensure that you observe the patient/client carefully during administration and after, especially during the first few doses. Because of the first pass effect, the action and therefore reaction of the person will be faster than using the oral route.

■ Staining of the skin

This may occur with pigmented drugs like iron. Using the Z-track method should leave intact tissue above the injected material in an indirect line, therefore preventing leakage to the surface tissue (Campbell 1995).

Summary
- Student nurses can give intramuscular and subcutaneous injections under supervision. It is advantageous to take opportunities during the course to observe and then practice, so that skill and confidence develops.
- It is important to understand the sites, equipment and hazards involved in IM and SC injections, and to be aware of how complications can be avoided.

CALCULATING DRUG DOSES

Nurses often worry about their ability to calculate drug doses (Woodrow 1998). However, if you follow the simple rules and standard formulae you cannot go wrong! One of the commonest issues concerns the ability of nurses to do basic maths like understanding decimals, rather than using the

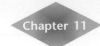

formulae. Therefore if you think you have a problem with basic maths, talk to a friend or family member, and ask them to help you solve it. The application of the formulae is for most people the easy part.

This section will cover key areas in drug calculations, and include some exercises and answers. For further study you are referred to:

Lapham, R. and Agar, H. 1995. *Drug Calculations for Nurses: A Step by Step Approach.* London: Arnold.

Learning outcomes:

By the end of this section you will be able to:

1. Understand the need for effective numeracy skills in practice.
2. Handle fractions and decimals in calculations.
3. Understand conversion of units within drug calculations.
4. Use a drugs formula to calculate medication.

Learning outcome 1:
Understand the need for effective numeracy skills in practice

Activity Consider what the outcome of occasionally getting a calculation slightly wrong would be. Can you ever be justified in giving a person an inaccurate dose?

The answer must always be no. You have to be 100% accurate all the time. Even a small discrepancy will mean that the patient will not receive the prescribed dose, and this could be very harmful. Also, not understanding the full implications of decimals could mean that a patient receives ten times more or less than the prescribed dose if the point is one place wrong.

Activity Discuss with your colleagues the advantages and disadvantages of using calculators to calculate drug doses. Should these be allowed? They are now commonplace in schools and are freely available to all.

There is great debate about this. They can increase accuracy and are certainly useful for complex calculations (Shockley *et al.* 1989). However, there may be occasions when a calculator is unavailable or not working. It is also only as good as its operator, hence if the wrong numbers are put in by mistake, the answer will be wrong. Also, if you are totally unable to work without a calculator, you cannot estimate easily what the right answer will be, and therefore have no way of checking that the calculator answer is about right.

It would seem sensible, therefore, to be able to calculate drug doses manually and by calculator, to prevent any chance of error.

Learning outcome 2:
Handle fractions and decimals in calculations

Fractions, e.g. ⅜

■ In the above fraction (sometimes written as 3/8) the lower figure tells you how many times the whole has been divided, e.g. into eighths. If the lower figure was 4, this would tell you that the whole had been divided in quarters. The top number tells us how many of that division there are e.g. this fraction tell us that there are three eighths. If the fraction was ½, it would tell us that there is one half.

■ Try to think of the line between the two numbers as a dividing line. To convert the fraction into a decimal, you need to divide the bottom number into the top: Thus: ⅜ = 3 divided by 8. This obviously will not go into whole numbers, so the answer is going to be 0. something.

■ The figures after the decimal point indicate a different type of fraction, this time expressed in tenths or decimals. These are the units we use in fractions of drug doses. Most calculations will divide into relatively easy numbers, because the nurse has to be able to give that proportion of the drug without dividing into complicated amounts, e.g. a dose of ⅛ tablet or 0.0065 ml etc. would, of course, be unrealistic and unsafe. 3 divided by 8 = 2.66.

Calculation exercise 1: Try the following conversions into decimals: (answers at the end)

(a)   ⅙ =
(b)   ⁶⁄₁₂ =
(c)   ²⁵⁄₇₅ =
(d)   ½₀ =
(e)   ⁷⁄₁₀ =
(f)   ⁶⁄₃₀ =

To divide and multiply decimals

Your calculations will always involve multiplying and dividing by units of 10 (see next section). Because decimals represent fractions in tenths, this makes these processes very easy:

■ To multiply by 10, move the decimal point one place to the right:

e.g. $0.05 \times 10 = 0.5$; $5.8 \times 10 = 58$

■ If you want to multiply by another unit of ten, e.g. 1000, move the decimal point to the right by the number of 0s. In the case of 1000, three places, in the case of 100, two places. e.g.

$0.06 \times 1000 = 60$; $5.0 \times 1000 = 5000$; $0.67 \times 100 = 67$.

■ If there are no more figures to move the point over, add 0 to fill the spaces:

e.g. $5.8 \times 100 = 580$.

■ To divide by 10, or multiples of, do the reverse:

e.g. $\frac{500}{10} = 50$; $\frac{6.3}{100} = 0.063$; $\frac{25}{1000} = 0.025$.

Calculation exercise 2: (answers at the end)

(a) $2.5 \times 100 =$

(b) $0.3 \times 1000 =$

(c) $54 \times 10 =$

(d) $\frac{36}{100} =$

(e) $\frac{125}{1000} =$

(f) $\frac{5.5}{1000} =$

Learning outcome 3:

Understand conversion of units within drug calculations

It is essential to use the same units throughout a drug calculation – you cannot work with both micrograms and milligrams, or millilitres and litres. Therefore you need to convert the drug doses in the calculation into the same units. It does not matter which unit you change them into. There is a simple rule for conversion which is the rule of thousands.

Everything that needs converting is achieved by either dividing or multiplying by a thousand. This is because:

1000 micrograms = 1 milligram
1000 milligrams = 1 gram
1000 grams = 1 kilogram
1000 millilitres = 1 litre.

With a few exceptions, these are the units used in drug prescriptions. So:

■ To convert 5 milligrams (mg) into micrograms (mcg), you need to multiply by 1000 = 5000 micrograms.

■ To convert the other way, you need to divide by 1000, e.g. 50 micrograms to milligrams = 0.05 mg.

In essence, to convert to a larger unit, you need to divide the figure, because there will be less of them.

To convert to a smaller unit you need to multiply because there will be more of them.

Calculation exercise 3 (answers at the end)

(a)   2000 mcg =   mg

(b)   2 litres =   ml

(c)   50 mg =   grams

(d)   3 mg =   mcg

(e)   3500 ml =   litres

(f)   125 mcg =   mg

Learning outcome 4:
Use a drugs formula to calculate medication

Remember: there is one magic formula for all calculations! There are no exceptions and it can be used for tablets, and liquids for oral doses or injections. The formula is:

■
$$\frac{Dose\ prescribed}{stock\ dose\ \times\ stock\ volume\ (if\ a\ fluid)} = dose\ to\ be\ given.$$

For example:

■ 500 mg of amoxycillin is needed for Miss Prior, and the stock dose is 250 mg capsules.

Thus, to follow the formula:

Dose prescribed = 500 mg
Stock dose = 250 mg
$^{500}/_{250}$ = 2 capsules

If Shabana was prescribed amoxycillin, her dose might be (depending on her weight) 250 mg. She would require the medicine as a liquid, a suspension, and the stock bottle may be 125 mg per 5 ml. Thus the calculation would be:

$^{250}/_{125} \times 5 = 10$ ml.

Now try Exercise 4. Remember that in each calculation you must ensure that the drugs are in the same units before you apply the formula.

Calculation exercise 4 (answers at the end)

(a)   200 mg trimethoprin required. Stock dose = 100 mg tablets

(b)   100 mg chlorpromazine required. Stock dose = 25 mg tablets

(c)   10 mg diazepam elixir required. Stock dose = 5 mg/5 ml

(d)   0.25 mg digoxin required. Stock dose = 250 mcg tablets

(e)   240 mg paracetamol elixir required. Stock dose = 120 mg/5 ml

(f)   50 mg morphine elixir required. Stock dose = 10 mg/5 ml

(g)   40 mg pethidine required. Stock ampoule = 50 mg/ml

(h)   6 mg morphine is required. Stock ampoule = 10 mg/ml

(i)   Heparin 2000 units required. Stock ampoule = 5000 units/ml

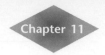

Most paediatric drugs are calculated on the child's weight. It is very important therefore that their weight is measured and recorded accurately, and that this is monitored constantly in a sick child. This may result in the drug dosage changing rapidly.

Summary

- All nurses must be able to calculate drug doses accurately, and for this a basic understanding of fractions and decimals is needed.
- There are formulae which can be used when a calculation is required, and it is important to develop skill in their application.
- Students will not carry out drug calculations unsupervised, but it is advisable to start working on this skill at an early stage, in preparation for registration, and as students may be asked to be second checkers for a calculation at some stage during the pre-registration course.

CHAPTER SUMMARY

This chapter has demonstrated the importance of having a basic understanding of the laws concerning drug administration, and of the use of local drugs policies to ensure these are adhered to in practice.

You should also now be able to understand the need for a working knowledge of the drugs you are giving, and be able to calculate doses accurately.

The chapter has stressed the importance of safe practice with regard to drug administration and the student role, and should help you to understand the reasons for different routes of administration. It should enable you to confidently manage to administer drugs safely in a variety of clinical settings.

Remember: the golden rule in drug administration is to be honest to yourself. If you do not understand or agree with what is being given for any reason, you must challenge the situation you find yourself in.

ANSWERS TO 'ABBREVIATIONS EXERCISE', AND DRUG CALCULATION EXERCISES 1–4

Abbreviations

Nocte = at night; prn = when necessary; mane = in the morning; po = orally; qds = four times daily; bd = twice daily; stat = immediately; tds = three times daily; ml = millilitre; pv = vaginally; inh = inhaled; neb = nebulized; od = once daily; inst = instilled; caps = capsules; elix = elixir; kg = kilograms; mg = milligrams; mcg = micrograms.

Exercise 1

(a) $\frac{2}{6} = 0.33$

(b) $\frac{6}{12} = 0.5$

(c) $\frac{25}{75} = 0.33$

(d) $\frac{4}{20} = 0.2$

(e) $\frac{7}{10} = 0.7$

(f) $\frac{6}{30} = 0.2$

Exercise 2

(a) $2.5 \times 100 = 250$

(b) $0.3 \times 1000 = 300$

(c) $54 \times 10 = 540$

(d) $\frac{36}{100} = 0.36$

(e) $\frac{125}{1000} = 0.125$

(f) $\frac{5.5}{1000} = 0.0055$

Exercise 3

(a) 2000 mcg = 2 mg

(b) 2 litres = 2 000ml

(c) 50 mg = 0.05 grams

(d) 3 mg = 3000 mcg

(e) 3500 ml = 3.5 litres

(f) 125 mcg = 0.125 mg

Exercise 4

(a) 2 tablets

(b) 4 tablets

(c) 10 ml

(d) 1 tablet

(e) 10 ml

(f) 25 ml

(g) 0.8 ml

(h) 0.6 ml

(i) 0.4 ml

REFERENCES

Beyea, S.C. and Nicholl, L.H. 1995. Administration of medication via the intramuscular route: an integrative review of the literature and research based protocol for the procedure. *Applied Nursing Research* **5** (1), 23–33.

Caldwell, N.A. 1999. Drug absorption, distribution, metabolism and elimination. In: Luker, K.A and Wolfson D.J. (eds.) *Medicines Management for Clinical Nurses.* Oxford: Blackwell Science, 31–50.

Campbell, J. 1995. Injections. *Professional Nurse* **10**, 455–58.

Choonera, I. 1994. Percutaneous drug absorption and administration. *Archives of Diseases of Childhood* **71**, 73–4.

Dann, T.C. 1969. An argument that routine skin preparation before injection is not necessary. *Lancet* **2**, 96–98.

Department of Health and Welsh Office. 1993. *Code of Practice: Mental Health Act 1983.* HMSO.

De Laune S, 1990. Risk reduction through testing, screening and infection control precautions. *Infection Control Hospital Epidemiology* **11**, 563–65.

Duthie, R.B. 1988. *Guidelines for the Safe and Secure Handling of Medicines: A Report to the Secretary of State for Social Services by the Joint Committee of the Standing Medical Nursing and Midwifery and Pharmaceutical Advisory Committees.* London: HMSO.

Henderson, N. 1998. Anaphylaxis. *Nursing Standard* **12** (47), 49–55.

Henry J.N. 1998. *BMA New Guide to Medicines and Drugs.* London: Dorling Kindersley.

Hopkins, S.J. 1999. *Drugs and Pharmacology for Nurses*, 13th edn. Edinburgh: Churchill Livingstone.

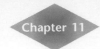

Jamieson, E.M., McCall, J.M., Blythe, R. and Whyte, L.A. 1997. *Clinical Nursing Practices*, 3rd edn. New York: Churchill Livingstone.

Koivisto, V.A. and Felig, P. 1978. Is skin preparation necessary before insulin injection? *Lancet* **1**, 1072–73.

Lapham, R. and Agar, H. 1995. *Drugs Calculations for Nurses: A Step by Step Approach*. London: Arnold.

Lawrence, J.C., Lilly, H.A. and Kidson, A. 1994. The use of alcohol wipes for disinfection of injection sites. *Journal of Wound Care* **3** (1), 11–14.

Ling, M. 1999. The patient's role in optimising treatment. In: Luker K.A. and Wolfson D.J. (eds.) *Medicines Management for Clinical Nurses*. Oxford: Blackwell Science, 104–29.

Medicines Act 1968. London: HMSO.

Misuse of Drugs Act 1971. London: HMSO.

Newton, M., Newton, D. and Fudin, J. 1992. Reviewing the three big injection routes. *Nursing* **2** (9), 34–42.

Pilling, M., Geoghegan, M., Wolfson, D.J. and Holden, J.D. 1998. The St Helens and Knowsley Prescribing Initiative: a model for pharmacists-led meetings with GPs. *Pharmacy Journal* **260**, 100–2.

Sexton, J.A. and Braidwood, C.C. 1999. The nurse's role in medicines administration - operational and practical consideration. In: Luker K. A. and Wolfson D.J. (eds.) *Medicines Management for Clinical Nurses*. Oxford: Blackwell Science, 237–57.

Shockley, J., McGurn, W., Gunning, C. *et al*. 1989. Effect of calculator use on arithmetic and conceptual skills of nursing students *Journal of Nursing Education* **28** (9), 402–5.

Simmonds B.P. 1983. CDC guidelines for the prevention and control of nosocomial infections: guidelines for the prevention of intravascular infections. *American Journal of Infection Control* **11** (5), 183–9.

Stilwell, B. 1995. Injections. *Community Outlook* **1** (1), 21–2.

Trounce, J. 1997. *Clinical Pharmacology for Nurses*, 15th edn. New York: Churchill Livingstone.

United Central Council for Nursing, Midwifery and Health Visiting. 1992. *Standards for the Administration of Medicines*. London: UKCC.

Wong D.L. 1993. *Whaley and Wong's Essentials of Paediatric Nursing*, 4th edn. St Louis: Mosby.

Woodrow, P. 1998. Numeracy skills. *Nursing Standard* **12** (30), 48–55.

Workman, B. 1999. Safe injection technique. *Nursing Standard* **13** (39), 47–53.

Applying and prioritizing practical nursing skills

Lesley Baillie

This book has covered a range of assessment skills and interventions, which you could require in your nursing practice, as a foundation for developing the specialist branch practical skills, which you will need. You should also now have a firm grasp of how you can learn practical skills and the importance of a caring attitude and a sound underlying knowledge, as well as being able to carry out the skill. It is expected that in the care setting, practical nursing skills will be carried out within the philosophy of care for that environment, which in some instances, will require the use of a structured framework of care. In some settings, this may be in the form of an integrated care pathway: a multidisciplinary plan relating to a specific diagnostic group.

This chapter is divided into two sections.
- ■ In Section 1, we will focus on four new scenarios, and you will be asked to identify what assessment skills and interventions might be required, and how they might be carried out, in the situations described.
- ■ In Section 2, a detailed account of the actual care carried out by the nurse will then be given, illustrating how in some instances, care had to be re-prioritized because of unexpected events.

The importance of the relationship between the nurse carrying out the practical skills, and the person and family, is clearly indicated. Throughout the text you will be referred back to previous chapters in the book so that you can re look at details about how these skills are carried out. The emphasis is on

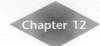
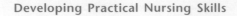

consolidation but some additional, more branch-specific information is included with references for further reading.

The scenarios were developed in collaboration with practitioners. Identifying features have been changed, and some details omitted in order to preserve anonymity.

SECTION 1: THE PRACTICE SCENARIOS

■ Adult setting: Graham and his situation

Graham is 29 years old and was transferred to your ward for rehabilitation 3 days ago. He had sustained a **spinal cord injury** after a recent accident, and the affected vertebra has been surgically fixed.

The wound was closed with staples, which will be removed next week. Graham has no movement or sensation in his legs. He has normal sensation and movement in his upper body and arms. The referring hospital had carried out an MRSA (*Methicillin-resistant Staphylococcus aureus: see* Chapter 3) screen, as is routine, and had found it to be negative, so Graham is in a bay with five other patients. Currently Graham is on bed rest but he should be able to start getting up soon. Since admission Graham has been withdrawn, and he has barely communicated with either staff or other patients. He has had no visitors yet as his family live some distance away. However his mother and sister are due to visit this afternoon.

You know that he is being nursed on a pressure relieving mattress, and has an in-dwelling urethral catheter. His appetite has been poor since admission and he is receiving **intravenous fluids**.

Nasogastric feeding is being considered. Graham's movement is hampered by his intravenous infusion in his left arm, and he is also complaining of pain in his right shoulder.

This morning the night staff hand over that he has been pyrexial overnight, and has had some diarrhoea. A stool specimen was collected this morning. He has been verbally abusive to them on a number of occasions. He has complained of nausea this morning and vomited a small amount.

Action

Now identify what assessment/monitoring skills and care are likely to be required by Graham this morning, and how you could organize and prioritize his care. In Section 2 you can find out what actually happened during the morning.

■ Child setting: Harry and his family

Harry is a 14-month-old infant who has sustained 17% scalds to face, right arm and middle chest from freshly made black tea.

Spinal cord injury

Is a major change in an individual's life, which is sudden and devastating in its effects (Davis 1997). Nolan and Nolan (1998) note that its sudden and traumatic onset enables no preparation, and is followed by a long hospital stay.

Intravenous (IV) fluid administration

IV therapy can cause phlebitis (inflammation of the vein wall) and sepsis, and thus care of IV sites, giving sets and IV lines is an important nursing role (Willis 1999). Campbell (1998a; 1998b) looks at prevention of phlebitis in detail.

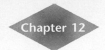

Burns in children
Children under two years who have sustained a burn of over 10% of their total body surface area will be considered to have a severe thermal injury, and the immediate priority will be to initiate resuscitative procedures, if needed, and minimize hypovolaemic shock (Colson 1995). Colson identifies other immediate priorities as prevention of respiratory problems, and pain relief, while intermediate aims will be to prevent wound infection and promote healing. It is recognized that this injury is highly traumatic to both child and parents, and psycho social support is essential (Colson 1995).

Parents' anxiety
About dressings and treatments is discussed by Francis (1990), who suggests that the possible discomfort caused to the child by these procedures further increases guilt feelings of parents.

Status epilepticus
A series of fits where consciousness is not regained between each one. This is a serious condition and needs urgent treatment.

He was admitted to the Burns Unit 2 days ago until his condition had stabilized, and he is now fit for transfer to the children's ward. Harry and his parents are brought down to the ward by a staff nurse from the Burns Unit during the afternoon.

You show them into the side room (consisting of one parent's bed and a cot) where Harry is to be nursed, and you then get a hand-over from the staff nurse, at the nurse's station. The staff nurse informs you that Harry's mum is heavily pregnant and due to deliver in 4 weeks. Harry's intravenous fluids were discontinued 4 hours ago, and he therefore still needs to have a strict record of his input and output kept. Harry is obviously not yet potty-trained, and so is wearing nappies. His face is being irrigated regularly with normal saline and he has dressings over his chest and arm. Regular analgesia is keeping his pain under control. The dressings will need to be removed tomorrow morning so that Harry's burns can be reviewed by the consultant to assess whether skin grafts will be necessary. Harry's parents are very anxious about this and would like Harry to be asleep during this procedure.

After the staff nurse returned to her own ward, Harry's father comes up to the staff and says that the room is too small, and asks if they can return to the high-dependency area in the Burns Unit where there is much more space.

Now identify what assessment/monitoring skills and care are likely to be required by Harry during the late shift, and how these might be carried out and prioritized. Remember to take into account the whole needs of the family, and the anxiety of Harry's parents. In Section 2, you can find out what actually happened.

■ Learning disability setting: Jenny and her situation

You are working on a small staffed unit for people with severe learning disabilities. Jenny is one of the residents, and you will be looking after her this morning. Jenny is 46 years old, has severe learning disabilities and has been in residential care all her life. She cannot communicate verbally, but she does make eye contact, she points, and appears to recognize her name. She can indicate her dislikes non-verbally, but generally has difficulty making her wishes known. She does not respond well to being touched. Her parents visit about once per month. Jenny walks unaided, and likes to wander around the unit. She seems to enjoy outings from the unit, and has a befriender who takes her swimming on a regular basis. Staff are working actively with this befriender to explore other areas of common interest such as music in a community setting.

Jenny is an epileptic who, despite medication, has a major fit about once a week. If she has a fit, her balance is affected afterwards for a while. She has a history of going into **status epilepticus**, and her prescription chart advises that, if she fits, diazepam 10 mg should be administered rectally.

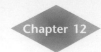

Individual
Programme Plan
An individual
programme plan seeks
to comprehensively
address the needs of
an individual with
learning disabilities
through a systematic
and structured
process. This process is
sometimes referred to
as life-planning.

Key worker
The role of the key
worker necessitates a
close and regular
involvement with the
client. Major aspects
of the role involve
identifying those
people that have a
major involvement in
the life of the client
and gathering relevant
information that
relates to their care
and lifestyle, for the
purpose of an
Individual Programme
Plan. Individual
Programme Plans and
the role of the key
worker are discussed
in detail by Gilbert
(1993).

Depressive illness
Fennell (1989) states
that at any given time,
15–20% of adults are
suffering significant
levels of depressive
symptoms. It seems
that depression is
caused by no single
factor, but an
interaction between a
variety of biological,
historical,
environmental, and
psycho-social variables
(Fennell 1989).

Jenny's medications are listed with their main uses and side effects in Table 12.1. As the prescription chart implies, Jenny does have a tendency towards constipation. Jenny usually takes her medication well, although verbal encouragement is sometimes required. Jenny's self-help skills are very limited despite efforts to develop these in the past. In keeping with Jenny's **Individual Programme Plan**, her **key worker** is aiming to develop her skills for independent living to their optimum level. However, due to her developmental level it is unlikely that there would be much success in the developing of further self-help skills. Consequently the emphasis is on maintaining existing skills and working towards goals that relate to increased community presence.

Jenny has a poor appetite. She feeds herself but needs constant verbal encouragement. If she appears fatigued by the process of feeding herself some physical help is offered. Her favourite meal is breakfast, but she is reluctant to eat or drink during the rest of the day, pushing the food away. Particular care is taken to ensure that breakfast is to her liking, substantial and that adequate time is allowed. Jenny is weighed monthly, and has recently been assessed by the dietician, who suggested that high-protein drinks should be encouraged. These are accepted by Jenny with variable success. There are two snacks which she particularly enjoys, and the unit is able to provide these.

Jenny is unable to wash or dress but co-operates during these routines by moving her limbs appropriately and pushing her arms through sleeves in response to physical prompts. Jenny is incontinent of urine and faeces. However she is taken to the toilet at regular intervals e.g. after meals, and then sometimes uses the toilet. She wears a pad and pants during the day and an all-in-one pad at night. The unit has contact with the continence advisor for advice on maintaining the integrity of the skin and ensuring maximum comfort for the client.

Towards the end of the handover from the night staff, you hear a loud noise and immediately investigate its source. You find Jenny lying on the floor by her bed. It is assumed that she has had a fit and fallen out of bed.

Action
Now identify what assessment/monitoring skills and care are likely to be required by Jenny this morning, and how you could organize and prioritize her care. In section 2 you will find an overview of what actually happened during the morning.

■ Mental health setting: Edith and her situation
Mrs Samuels, an 86-year-old widow, usually lives in a local residential home. She has asked to be called Edith. She is currently staying in the admission unit for the elderly mentally ill, due to a **depressive illness**, the cause of which is still being explored. Box 12.1 lists common symptomatology associated with depression.

Table 12.1 Jenny's medication: its main uses and side effects (Trounce 1997)

Drug prescribed	Main uses	Main side effects
Carbamazepine 500 mg b.d. orally	Tonic-clonic seizures, trigeminal neuralgia, bipolar depression	Rashes, dizziness, drowsiness, depression of the white blood cells, occasionally jaundice and excessive salivary secretion
Sodium valporate 700 mg b.d. orally	Tonic-clonic and absence seizures	Fall in platelet count, drowsiness, hair thinning and weight gain
Lamotrigine 125 mg b.d. orally	Partial and tonic-clonic seizures	Ataxia, nausea, headaches, rashes
Senna 7.5 mg o.n. orally	A stimulant purge given to prevent or treat constipation	Griping
Latulose 10 ml o.n. orally	An osmotic purge given to prevent or treat constipation	Flatulence and distention
Paracetamol 1 g orally p.r.n. for pain/fever	A minor analgesic, and antipyretic	Uncommon at normal dosage. Causes severe liver damage in over-dosage
Diazepam 10 mg rectally p.r.n.	A benzodiazepine given as a minor tranquillizer, but also used in status epilepticus	Few side effects but continued use can cause fatigue and memory problems.
Phosphate enema p.r.n. for constipation	Constipation, or prior to bowel investigations	Trauma to ano-rectal mucosa, localized tissue reaction

Sadness and tearfulness
Guilt
Irritability
Anxiety and tenseness
Inability to react emotionally
Inability to enjoy or be interested in normal activities
Low energy
Withdrawal
Difficulty in concentrating
Preoccupation with feelings of badness and insoluble difficulties
A feeling that basic bodily functions are disturbed
Difficulty in sleeping
Decline in appetite
Loss of sexual desire
Feelings of hopelessness
Suicidal thoughts.

Box 12.1 Symptoms of clinical depression (Fennell 1989)

The staff in the home and her GP were concerned that her low mood was affecting her nutritional intake, and her ability to carry out everyday activities. Edith also has osteoarthritis, and usually walks with a zimmer frame. However her mobility has deteriorated due to her low mood, and her anxiety about falling. Her mobility assessment (which is repeated weekly) has found that Edith is able to stand and transfer with one nurse but is unable to walk at present. Her manual dexterity is poor and she has a tendency to drop things. An anti-depressant has been prescribed, and staff aim to try to encourage her independence. A nutritional assessment identified her as at high risk of malnutrition, and a dietician referral was made. A supplementary high-protein drink is prescribed twice daily, and Edith's weight is monitored weekly. A food intake chart is also maintained. The Waterlow pressure sore risk assessment tool found her not to be at risk of pressure sores currently. She is continent, and will ask to use the toilet.

Edith has her own room, which has an en-suite bathroom. During the week occupational therapists organize activities for the clients, but not at the weekend. Whilst in the unit Edith's niece has visited each week, and the home staff have been in several times. Edith usually likes watching television and reading, although she currently shows little interest in either. Her niece describes her as being a naturally quiet person. Edith's medication, with its actions and main side effects, can be seen in Table 12.2.

It is Saturday morning, and the night staff hand over that Edith has had a comfortable night.

Action

Now identify what assessment/monitoring skills and care are likely to be required by Edith this morning, and how you might organize and prioritize her care. In section 2 you will find an overview of what actually happened during the morning.

See **Chapter 2**
The nurse's approach.

Spinal cord injury and changes to body image
These are covered in depth by Davis (1997), who indicates that the change in body image resulting from spinal cord injury, is an important psycho-social factor, of an increasing priority once the acute post-injury phase is over, and rehabilitation is in place.

SECTION 2: IMPLEMENTATION OF PRACTICAL SKILLS

■ Adult setting: Graham's morning

Box 12.2 lists assessment skills and interventions which you might have included, and these are discussed in more detail below.

The nurse (Clare) caring for Graham first greeted him, and explained that she would be carrying out his care this morning. She recognized that it was important to gain Graham's trust (UKCC 1996), and to try to build up a rapport with him.

Clare was aware that Graham was isolated from his family and friends, and was having to come to terms with **altered body image**, and a major change to his expectations for the future.

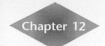

Table 12.2 Edith's medication: its uses, and side effects (Trounce 1997)

Drug prescribed	Main uses	Main side effects
Digoxin 62.5 micrograms o.d.	Heart failure. Atrial fibrillation.	Heart rhythm/rate disturbance (too slow, coupled beats, complete heart block), nausea and vomiting, confusion in the elderly.
Co-amilofruse 2.5/20 mg o.d.	Mainly used in heart failure. Consists of frusemide (a loop diuretic) combined with amiloride (a potassium-sparing diuretic). Prevents the potassium loss which would occur if frusemide was given alone.	Uric acid retention causing gout. Decreased glucose tolerance. Sodium depletion.
Lofepramine 100 mg o.d.	A tricyclic antidepressant, used in depressive illness.	Anticholinergic effects, dry mouth, constipation, fall in blood pressure, increased appetite and weight gain. Note lofepramine has the least side effects of this group of drugs, and causes minimal sedation.
Lansoprazole 30 mg o.d.	Inhibits gastric acid secretion. Used to treat peptic ulcers.	Headache, nausea, diarrhoea and rashes.
Docusate 2 tablets nocte	A stool softener, used to prevent or treat constipation.	None listed.
Co-proximal 2 tablets qds	Comprised of two analgesics: paracetamol and dextropropoxyphene (a codeine). Used for pain that does not respond to paracetamol alone.	Vomiting. Slightly addictive. Constipation as the codeine decreases intestinal peristalsis.
Temazepam 10 mg nocte prn	A benzodiazepine given as a hypnotic to induce sleep.	Continued use can cause fatigue and memory problems. Main problem is dependence causing difficulty in sleeping when the drug is withdrawn.

Psychological distress
A number of studies have suggested that psychological distress associated with physical illness affects physical recovery, rate and extent of rehabilitation, and causes psychological pain and anguish (Nicholls 1993).

See **Chapter 8**
Measuring and recording temperature.

He has also been through surgery with the accompanying discomfort entailed, and has only recently transferred to the ward, which is another upheaval for him. While Graham's physical needs were of a high priority, Clare was aware that care relating to his **psychological distress** was very important too.

From the night report it was obvious that Graham was unwell, and Clare knew that it would be important to monitor his temperature regularly.

Graham refused any breakfast as he did not feel well enough but agreed to drink a small amount of fluids. Graham was prescribed a number of drugs by a variety of routes. It was essential that Clare administered these with adherence to the drug policy and with a knowledge of the drugs' actions and side effects. Due to Graham's immobility and recent surgery, he was a high-risk patient for developing thromboembolic complications, so his morning

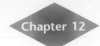

- Build a rapport and give psychological support
- Explain all procedures
- Maintain correct positioning
- Monitor observations
- Drug administration
- Source isolation
- Turns
- Maintain/encourage fluids and diet
- Prevention of thromboembolic complications
- Hygiene needs and skin care
- Catheter care
- Wound care
- Nursing documentation.

Box 12.2 Assesment skills and interventions for Graham

See **Chapter 11**
Drug administration.

Heparin
Is an anticoagulant which is not absorbed by mouth, so is given intravenously or subcutaneously (Trounce 1997).

See **Chapter 9**
Pressure sore risk assessment; pressure sore prevention.

See **Chapter 3**
Source isolation.

medication included subcutaneous heparin. Clare also gave Graham para-cetamol 1 g to reduce his pyrexia.

Graham was obviously at high-risk of pressure sores. On the particular mattress on which he is being nursed it is usually sufficient to turn patients from side to side every 6 hours. However Clare decided that as Graham was pyrexial he needed to be turned 3-hourly at present, being aware that his pyrexia increased his pressure sore risk. Clare needed help from another nurse with each turn, and the move, using a sliding sheet, had to be carefully co-ordinated due to Graham's spinal surgery. Skin care is very important for the person who has no sensation, but especially for Graham due to his diarrhoea. Clare planned to bed bath Graham and turn him soon after breakfast. This time with Graham would also give Clare further opportunity to try to build a relationship with him.

However, shortly after breakfast, a phone call from microbiology informed Clare that Graham's blood cultures had grown MRSA. Whilst it is not neces-sary for every patient with an infection to be nursed in a side room (Parker 1999), the Trust policy advised that in these circumstances it was necessary, particularly as Graham had diarrhoea and vomiting. Clare spent sometime explaining to Graham about this, and also arranged for the doctor to see him. The doctor spent time with Graham, reviewing his condition and explaining the treatment that he would need. Antibiotics were prescribed. Clare explained that Graham had vomited this morning so both were written up intravenously, to be given by the registered nurse.

Clare was aware that being nursed in isolation can cause depression, anxiety and a lack of control (Parker 1999), but she found an immediate

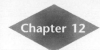

See **Chapter 6**
Effects of incontinence.

See **Chapter 6**
Administration of suppositories and enemas.

See **Chapter 3**
Hand washing, use of gloves and aprons, waste disposal, source isolation.

See **Chapter 5**
Meeting hygiene needs.

See **Chapter 6**
Management of incontinence.

See **Chapter 6**
Caring for the person with a urinary catheter.

See **Chapter 10**
Principles of wound care.

See **Chapter 2**
The nurse's approach: communication.

See **Chapter 5**
Oral hygiene; facial shaving

See **Chapter 9**
Pressure sore prevention; prevention of other complications of immobility.

Foot drop
Plantar flexion of the foot due to weakness or paralysis of the anterior muscles of the lower leg.

See **Chapter 3**
Source isolation

positive change in Graham's mental state as she and another nurse, Tom, moved Graham into the side room. Graham said that he was pleased to have a room on his own, as the six-bedded bay was noisy and so he couldn't sleep, and he had been very embarrassed when he had had diarrhoea.

Clare acknowledged how he was feeling, but explained that it wasn't his fault, that the care needed was part of her and Tom's everyday work, and that they were investigating the underlying cause so that it could be treated. Once his diarrhoea has been resolved, Graham's neurological impairment will mean that a bowel regime, to prevent constipation and/or incontinence, will be necessary, and this is likely to involve the use of oral aperients, and suppositories.

Graham's room was set up for source isolation, and so all entering the room would wear gloves and aprons, and follow the policy for disposal of infected waste. Graham was currently very dependent in meeting his hygiene and elimination needs due to his restricted arm movements and general poor condition. A high standard of hygiene was essential to prevent further complications, and to promote well-being. Graham agreed that he would like a wash now, and Clare and Tom gave him a bed bath. Whilst doing this, they observed his skin carefully. They found that his skin was dry so aqueous cream was applied. On cleaning his skin, they found that his buttocks were becoming excoriated. After careful drying, cream was applied. Whilst bathing, Clare washed around Graham's catheter, and observed Graham's wound for any signs of infection.

Clare needed to try to maintain Graham's dignity and her communication with him helped to make the bed bath an opportunity to build a rapport. Throughout this care, they found Graham to be very communicative and he talked about his family, obviously looking forward to their visit. Graham cleaned his teeth, and Clare observed that his mouth was in good condition. Clare combed Graham's hair for him. Due to his anticoagulant therapy Clare did not want to risk shaving Graham, as he could bleed. Graham thought that his mother would bring him an electric razor, which would be safer. All Graham's bed linen was changed, and he was turned and carefully positioned, using pillows to support his limbs, prevent **foot drop** and reduce pressure, especially between his knees. Clare and Tom knew that the physiotherapist would be visiting shortly to carry out passive exercises.

Before leaving Graham, Clare checked that he could reach his drink, his TV control, and his call bell, being aware that Graham could be very isolated being immobile and in a side room. Graham was much more cheerful than he had been previously, but Clare was aware that being in isolation could become increasingly lonely as time went by. Psychological consequences of source isolation are reviewed in depth by Gammon (1999).

Clare ensured that Graham's nursing documentation was maintained and updated throughout the morning. She remained concerned about Graham's lack of nutrition, and decided that a dietician referral was necessary. Particular strategies used by Clare during the morning were her calm and empathetic approach and her listening skills. She also carefully explained everything to Graham and negotiated how his care would be carried out.

■ Child setting: Harry and his family's day

Box 12.3 lists assessment skills and interventions which you might have included. These are discussed in detail below.

- Build a trusting relationship with Harry and his family, and listen to their concerns
- Negotiate involvement in care
- Fluid intake, and accurate measurement of input/output
- Pain assessment and management
- Prevention of cross-infection
- Monitor vital signs
- Wound management
- Nutritional intake for Harry and family
- Provision of appropriate environment and stimulation for Harry.

Box 12.3 Assessment skills and interventions for Harry

Rose, the nurse in charge, offered Harry's father the opportunity to stay in a flat within the hospital but this was not acceptable to him. He said that both he and his wife must be in the same room, as Harry's mum needed him to help care for Harry, and therefore they needed three beds – one each for the parents and the cot for Harry. The nurse in charge, Rose, recognized their anxiety, and the need to listen to their underlying concerns. However, returning to the Burns Unit was not a reasonable option, as the Burns Unit needed that room for any new major burns patient, and now that Harry was over his acute episode, a children's ward was a more appropriate environment for the family. It was important to explain this to the family in a friendly and non-defensive manner, and begin to build a trusting relationship with Harry and his parents. Trust is fundamental to a successful, and effective health-care relationship (Ham 1997), and in an acute environment must be developed from the start. There was admission documentation to complete, and there were important priorities of care to be carried out, but Rose was aware that in order to care for Harry, her first priority was to reach a compromise about the sleeping arrangements. Rose understood that beneath Harry's parents' demands, they were feeling anxious and fearful, and appreciated that Harry's serious injury would have had a major impact on them (Noyes 1999). Rose's approach reflected the practice of family-centred care, recognized as an important philosophy in child health-care and incorporated into health-care policy (Department of Health 1991).

See **Chapter 2**
The nurse's approach.

However, the cubicle could not safely hold three beds, because if Harry had become suddenly unwell, access to him would have been hazardous. The cubicle next door was larger, and was also unoccupied, and it had a more comfortable bed for Harry's mother, so this was a better option. Rose was also able to access a reclining chair which would fit into this cubicle, which could be used for Harry's mum to sit in if it was more comfortable, or for his father if he wished to be in the same room to sleep. The cubicle next door was now empty, so Rose felt that this could be offered to Harry's father, on the understanding that if it was needed for an admission, he would have to move out. Rose therefore explained these options to Harry's parents, and they agreed that he could stay on the children's ward.

With Harry's parents now more accepting of their new environment, Rose needed to identify the important elements of care. These included: ensuring adequate fluid intake and output, ensuring Harry was free from pain and discomfort, promoting adequate dietary intake for Harry and his parents – particularly his pregnant mother, protecting Harry from infection, monitoring Harry's vital signs, and caring for Harry's wounds.

Harry appeared to be comfortable and free from pain, but Rose would continue to administer Harry's prescribed regular analgesia, and involve his parents in monitoring his pain. Harry was at risk of dehydration due to the fluid loss from his burns, so Rose explained the need for an adequate fluid intake to his parents. Rose discussed with Harry's parents what sort fluids he liked to drink, and explained that they needed to encourage him to take plenty of drinks from his bottle which would need to be recorded on a fluid chart. Rose also explained the need to monitor Harry's fluid output, which would be done by weighing his wet nappies. Harry's parents would call a nurse to take the nappies for weighing, who would then record the amount on the fluid chart. Thus the nurse and Harry's parents negotiated the contribution each would make to his care. This is recognized as an important element of children's nursing (Fradd 1996).

See **Chapter 4**
Bottle feeding the infant.

See **Chapter 6**
Assisting with elimination.

A young child with a burn has an increased susceptibility to infection (Parker 1999), and therefore protective isolation was a necessity, with Harry's parents, other visitors and all staff entering his cubicle, needing to wash hands. Again it was important for Rose to explain the rationale for this to Harry's parents. Harry was also to lay on his cot on a sterile green towel, as an additional protection against infection.

See **Chapter 3**
Hand washing.

See **Chapter 7**
Measuring and recording temperature and pulse.

See **Chapter 8**
Measuring and recording respirations.

See **Chapter 11**
Administering oral medication.

See **Chapter 4**
Recognizing the contribution of nutrition to health.

See **Chapter 4**
Promoting healthy eating.

See **Chapter 8**
Monitoring respirations.

See **Chapter 11**
Principles of wound care.

Harry's vital signs needed to be monitored and Rose assessed that initially Harry's temperature and pulse should be measured 2-hourly, as it was likely that he might become pyrexial due to his recent burns, and the risk of developing an infection. Rose measured his temperature with the tympanic thermometer, as this was tolerated well, and he allowed her to count his pulse and respirations.

On finding that Harry was pyrexial, Rose administered the prescribed paracetamol orally, with the help of Harry's parents, via an oral syringe.

Harry's burns caused an increased nutritional demand due to the requirements for additional nutrients for wound healing. Rose also recognized the need for Harry's mother to eat a healthy diet because of her pregnancy.

The children's ward has a special menu for children, and Harry's parents were able to choose suitable food for him, and feed him. Rose monitored Harry's food intake to ensure that it was sufficient. He initially ate only small amounts and so Rose encouraged his parents to feed him nutritious drinks, particularly milk, thus illustrating how nurses and parents work together in partnership (Casey 1988). Parents are usually given meal vouchers to eat in the staff canteen, but as this was some distance away, Harry's mother was provided with a meal on the ward.

Due to Harry's burns to his face and chest, and the swelling that can result, the best position for Harry was to be propped up in a sitting position, to minimize swelling to his airway. He also needed to be observed for any respiratory distress. Care for the burns at this stage was to irrigate Harry's face with saline. Rose's approach to Harry was important, to try to reduce apprehension and fear about this procedure. Dressings were *in situ* on his arm and chest which were to remain undisturbed overnight, but observed for exudate. Had they leaked through, Rose would have applied further padding over the dressings. Harry's parents continued to express concern about the procedure of removing his dressings in the morning. Rose explained that actually giving him a general anaesthetic (as they were suggesting) was best avoided, as he may need a general anaesthetic if skin grafts are required, and it is preferable not to have more anaesthetics than necessary. However, Rose suggested that oral sedation could be given, that any stuck areas could be soaked with saline and removed slowly and gently, and that they could stay with Harry throughout, if that was what they wanted. Harry's parents accepted this compromise. Again this demonstrates negotiation skills, and the need for nurses to be flexible and sensitive to parents' needs (Darbyshire 1995).

By the time Rose finished her shift she had been able to build a trusting relationship with Harry and his parents, whilst also attending to the essential care which Harry required.

■ Learning disability setting: Jenny's morning

Box 12.4 lists assessment skills and interventions which you might have included. These are discussed in detail below.

See **Chapter 7**
Assessing neurological status.

Rachel took considerable time in making the environment safe, and ensuring that Jenny was fully conscious and secure. Because of Jenny's level of disability, her level of consciousness was difficult to assess. When she called Jenny's name, she turned her head and established eye contact. Jenny lay quietly for a moment while Rachel checked visually for any signs of injury. When touched Jenny pushed away, and used the bed to attempt to push

---

- Maintenance of airway
- Assessment and monitoring of neurological status
- Maintaining a safe environment
- Assistance with mobility
- Reassurance and explanations
- Administration of medication
- Promoting nutrition
- Assistance with hygiene and elimination
- Providing a stimulating environment
- Involvement in community activities
- Maintaining documentation.

Box 12.4 Assessment skills and interventions for Jenny

---

herself into a standing position. Unusually Jenny did accept some physical help from Rachel and another member of staff to get up off the floor, which required careful risk assessment by Rachel, as the floor is a dangerous place to move and handle clients. Once on her feet, she was able to walk to the dining room and sit down at the table. Rachel discreetly observed her whilst assisting other clients to the breakfast table until she was satisfied that Jenny had made a good recovery.

See chapter 11
Administering oral medication.

Probably because of her recent fit, Jenny refused to eat breakfast, and kept pushing her plate away. She also refused her medication, even when verbal encouragement was offered. Rachel was aware that Jenny's medication (particularly her anti-convulsants) was important, and so she planned to try to encourage her to accept her medication at different intervals later. She also encouraged Jenny to take a nourishing drink to ensure that her blood sugar levels were at an adequate level.

See **Chapter 4**
Recognizing the contribution of nutrition to health.

After breakfast, Rachel took Jenny to her bedroom to offer her the opportunity to choose her clothing, but she showed no interest in doing so. Rachel carefully observed Jenny's motor function throughout. She then collected the

See **Chapter 3**

Hand washing; Waste disposal.

See **Chapter 6**

Assisting with elimination.

See **Chapter 5**

Assisting with bathing.

See **Chapter 9**

Assessment of pressure sore risk.

See **Chapter 5**

Oral hygiene.

See **Chapter 11**

Administering of oral medication.

necessary toiletry items and clean clothes for Jenny's toilet routine. She removed her pad, disposing of it as per unit policy. Throughout Jenny's personal care Rachel ensured that she washed her hands as necessary to prevent cross-infection between residents. Rachel was careful to respect Jenny's privacy during her toilet routine but needed to remain close by to offer assistance. Jenny's bowel motions are monitored, due to her constipation. Rachel was aware that Jenny had had a bowel action the previous day, and would not therefore need an enema this morning. Rachel is aware that Jenny has an increased risk of a urinary tract infection, due to her poor fluid intake, so Jenny is observed for signs of urinary tract infection.

After using the toilet, Jenny was encouraged to wash her hands at the sink, but Rachel needed to do most of this activity for her. Jenny enjoys having a bath, so Jenny ran a bath for her, carefully checking the temperature of the water. Rachel attempted to carry out Jenny's plan, by asking her to undress herself, assisting as necessary, and giving verbal reinforcement according to Jenny's level of co-operation. Jenny did raise her limbs where appropriate to assist with clothing removal, and Rachel praised her, saying 'Well done Jenny'. In the bath, Jenny was encouraged to wash her face but did not respond to this request. While assisting with Jenny's bath, Rachel observed her skin condition, being aware that her incontinence could put her skin at risk of pressure sores. After her bath, Rachel dressed her. With each item of clothing, she named the item (e.g. 'here's your blue cardigan'), before dressing her. Again Jenny would help by stretching out an arm for example, and Rachel praised her. Rachel asked Jenny to clean her teeth but Jenny did not respond to this so Rachel assisted her with this task, and also brushed her hair. Throughout Jenny's washing and dressing routine Rachel ensured that her privacy was maintained within the bathroom.

With Jenny's personal care complete, Rachel took Jenny to the lounge to sit down. At this point she tried to encourage her to take her medication, and this time Jenny accepted it. Rachel observed carefully to ensure that she swallowed the tablets. Rachel then tried to encourage her to have a drink but Jenny pushed the cup away. At this point Rachel noticed that Jenny did have a bruise developing on her forehead which must have been sustained when she fell out of bed. Rachel talked to Jenny about this, and observed for any signs of discomfort. It did not appear to be too painful for her. Rachel would continue to observe for signs of discomfort or drowsiness.

Usually Jenny would go for a walk outside during the morning, but due to her fit and fall, she seemed to prefer to be quiet this morning, but she did get up and walk around the unit on a few occasions. Jenny does not like to watch television. She does enjoy classical music and Rachel put on her favourite tape for a short period before lunch. At lunch, Rachel found that unusually, Jenny was hungry and ate quite well. She was due to go swimming in the afternoon so Rachel intended to reassess her condition and discuss any possible needs for increased observation with the person taking her swimming. Rachel ensured that she documented Jenny's care, and an accident form was completed relating to Jenny's fall and her bruise.

Overall Rachel feels that it is important to find other meaningful community based activities for Jenny to enjoy. As the named nurse responsible for Jenny's care, she is actively working with her Key Worker and befriender to do this. She will be reporting back on this need at Jenny's next Individual Programme Plan meeting in a month's time. She is concerned that Jenny's medication makes her drowsy. Her medication is reviewed regularly, but her present medication appears to be the best combination of tablets to control her epilepsy. Rachel is concerned about Jenny's nutrition. Her food and fluid intake is observed, but Rachel thinks this should be documented more systematically. She intends to discuss this also at the next Individual Programme Plan meeting.

Rachel's priorities for Jenny this morning were to ensure a full recovery from her fall and to provide reassurance and encouragement while meeting Jenny's daily needs.

See **Chapter 4**

Assessing nutritional status and developing a plan of action.

■ Mental health setting: Edith's morning

Box 12.5 lists assessment skills and interventions which you might have included, and these are discussed in more detail below.

- Explanation and negotiation of interventions
- Provision of support and encouragement
- Promote self-confidence and esteem
- Observation of motivation and mood
- Drug administration
- Assistance with mobility
- Promote nutrition
- Assistance with hygiene and elimination
- Encourage interaction and activity
- Maintain documentation.

Box 12.5 Assessment skills and interventions required for Edith

See **Chapter 5**
Oral hygiene.

Robert, the nurse looking after Edith this morning, checked on his group of clients after handover. Edith woke up at around eight o'clock and as Robert knows that to have her dentures in is important for her dignity and her speech, he rinsed them for her and she was able to put them in place. The use of therapeutic communication skills are essential to maximise the nurse-client relationship (Cutting and Hardy 1997). Thus Robert's approach to Edith

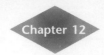

See **Chapter 2**
Self-awareness;
Communication skills.

included the use of effective communication skills and self awareness, being sensitive to her non-verbal cues, which would indicate her mood and motivation. Robert discussed with Edith how she would spend the morning. She requested to use the toilet first, and then wanted to wash and dress, and go to the dining room for her breakfast. Robert therefore fetched her wheelchair, so that he could assist her to the toilet. Edith was very anxious about falling, lacking confidence about her ability to stand, and therefore Robert needed to use verbal prompting and encouragement. A trusting relationship can take time to build up, but as Robert has been looking after Edith since her admission, he has been able to build a therapeutic relationship, which is central to the process of helping (Peplau 1988; Cutting and Hardy 1997).

See **Chapter 9**
Assisting with
mobilization.

After Edith had been transferred onto the toilet Robert left her alone, with the call bell, thus giving her privacy. Afterwards, Robert transferred her back to the wheelchair and took her to the sink. With verbal prompting, Edith removed her nightdress. Robert ensured that she was kept covered to preserve her dignity. She was prompted verbally to wash and dry herself, to maintain her independence. When this was completed praise and encouragement was given, e.g. 'That's really good Edith'. With verbal prompting from Robert, Edith dressed herself. Robert needed to hand her each item of clothing individually. He attempted to engage her in conversation during her washing and dressing, and was able to gain some response from her, which enabled him to identify areas of interest to encourage Edith's motivation.

See **Chapter 6**
Assisting with
elimination.

See **Chapter 5**
Meeting hygiene
needs.

Once her personal care was completed, Robert washed his hands, and then pushed Edith to the dining room for her breakfast. Edith was given choice about her breakfast and decided on cereal and a cup of tea. Robert was aware that being given choice and small portions would make food more acceptable to Edith. He made himself a cup of tea too, and sat down with her at the table, as he has found previously that this is a helpful strategy to encourage clients with poor appetites to eat and drink. Many older people will refuse to eat/drink due to depressive illness and dietary changes can affect older people dramatically, so it is essential to maintain nutrition (Burleigh 1997). Robert was able to offer verbal encouragement and reinforcement, whilst chatting with Edith. After Edith had consumed her breakfast with verbal encouragement, Robert dispensed her prescribed medication orally. Her medication does have various side effects of which Robert is aware (*see* Table 12.2) and is able to observe for. Because of her difficulty with fine finger movements, he administered the tablets on a spoon, and observed Edith closely to ensure that they were swallowed effectively.

See **Chapter 3**
Hand washing.

See **Chapter 4**
Assessing nutritional
status and developing
a plan of action.

After breakfast Robert took Edith to the toilet at her request. Edith has a history of being constipated, which has been exacerbated by her antidepressant medication, and she has needed an enema on several occasions since admission. Robert is aware that attending to Edith's elimination needs

See **Chapter 11**
Administering oral
medication.

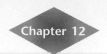

See **Chapter 6**
Assisting with elimination.

See **Chapter 9**
Preventing other complications of immobility.

See **Chapter 4**
Promoting healthy eating.

See **Chapter 4**
Assessing clients' nutritional status and developing a plan of action.

See **Chapter 8**
Measuring and recording temperature.

promptly will help to maintain urinary continence, and prevent constipation, by enabling her to take advantage of the gastrocolic reflex. Robert made sure that Edith had the opportunity to wash her hands at the sink, and then took her to the dayroom, and, again with verbal encouragement, transferred her into an armchair. He asked her if she would like her book from her room, being aware that with her limited mobility she could become isolated and bored, which would be compounded by her low mood. At this point he assisted Edith with her menu choice, discussing with her, her likes and dislikes. He also explained that snacks, such as sandwiches, could be made for her on the unit, if that would be preferable to her. During the morning Robert and other staff organized some activities in the dayroom, such as word games. They also spent time in conversation with the clients. At mid morning, Edith was encouraged to have her high protein drink. Robert gave her choice over the flavour, and again sat down with her and had a cup of coffee himself, giving Edith verbal encouragement e.g. 'You're doing well'.

At lunchtime, Robert offered Edith a choice from the menu. He ensured that a small portion of her liking was prepared and presented attractively, and Edith ate a small amount of food.

Throughout the morning Robert ensured that Edith's documentation was maintained and updated, and this included recording her food intake. He also noted her mood level during the morning, observing both her verbal and non-verbal communication and motivation. He was aware that her mental state could affect her ability to respond to temperature and that he should therefore observe for any signs that she was too hot or too cold. Throughout Robert's care of Edith, he had been trying to achieve a balance between encouraging her to do things for herself thus promoting her confidence and self-esteem, without pressurizing her, which would be counterproductive.

CONCLUSION

This book started by highlighting that being able to perform a range of practical nursing skills in a competent manner is a necessary accomplishment for a registered nurse. The scenarios within this chapter have illustrated how these skills might be prioritized within the care of one person on one day, highlighting the dynamic nature of the practice setting. In every scenario, competency by the nurse in carrying out these practical skills was essential for the well-being of the recipient of care. However, these scenarios also demonstrated the therapeutic use of self, to develop rapport, build a trusting relationship, promote self-esteem and confidence, and engender a feeling of security and being cared for. The scenarios also illustrated the use of effective communication, particularly listening, and negotiation skills. An empathetic approach enabled the nurses to understand underlying emotions and needs in order to

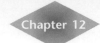

make an effective response to the individual. Respect for individual choice in relation to care was also apparent in the scenarios explored.

It has been the intention of this book to enable you to develop a foundation in practical nursing skills. There will be many more skills which you will need to develop, but you should now have a good insight into how to learn practical skills, the components of a practical skill and the importance of an appropriate attitude and an informed knowledge base, as well as being able to carry out the psychomotor element. I will conclude by emphasizing once more, the importance of carrying out practical skills within the context of caring, and ensuring that their effect on each individual is beneficial and healing.

REFERENCES

Burleigh, S. 1997. Care of the elderly. In: Thomas, B., Hardy, S. and Cutting, P. (eds.) *Stuart and Sundeen's Mental Health Nursing: Principles and Practice*. 357–75.

Campbell, L. 1998a. IV-related phlebitis, complications and length of hospital stay: 1. *British Journal of Nursing* **7**, 1304–12.

Campbell, L. 1998b. IV-related phlebitis, complications and length of hospital stay: 2. *British Journal of Nursing* **7**, 1364–73.

Casey, A. 1988. A partnership with child and family. *Senior Nurse* **8** (4), 8–9.

Colson, J. 1995. Nursing support and care: meeting the needs of the child and family with altered integumentary function. In: Carter, B. and Dearmun, A.K. (eds.) *Child Health Care Nursing* Oxford: Blackwell Science, 469–99.

Cutting, P. and Hardy, S. 1997. Therapeutic nurse-patient relationship. In: Thomas, B.; Hardy, S. and Cutting, P. (eds.) *Stuart and Sundeen's Mental Health Nursing: Principles and Practice*, 33–44

Darbyshire, P. 1995. Parents in paediatrics. *Paediatric Nursing* **7** (1), 8–9.

Davis, P.S. 1997. Spinal cord injury and changes to body image. In: Salter, M. (ed.) *Altered Body Image*. London: Ballière Tindall, 267–85.

Department of Health 1991. *The Welfare of Children and Young People in Hospital*. London: HMSO.

Fennell, M.J.V. 1989. Depression. In: Hawton, K., Salkovskis, P.M., Kirk, J. and Clark, D.M. (eds.) *Cognitive Behaviour Therapy for Psychiatric Problems*. Oxford: Oxford University Press, 169–234.

Fradd, E. 1996. The importance of negotiating a care plan. *Paediatric Nursing* **8** (6), 6–9.

Francis, A.L. 1990. Support for parents of burned children. *Nursing*, **4** (7), 7–10.

Gammon, J. 1999. The psychological consequences of source isolation: a review of the literature. *Journal of Clinical Nursing* **8**, 13–21.

Gilbert T. 1993. A systematic approach to care. In: Brigden P. and Todd M. (eds.) *Concepts in Community Care for People with a Learning Difficulty*. Basingstoke: Macmillan Press.

Ham, S.P. 1997. Concept analysis of trust: a coronary care perspective. *Intensive and Critical Care Nursing* **13**, 351–6.

Nicholls, K.A. 1993. *Psychological Care in Physical Illness*, 2nd edn. London: Chapman and Hall.

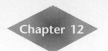

Nolan, M. and Nolan, J. 1998. Rehabilitation following spinal injury: the nursing response. *British Journal of Nursing* **7**, 97–104.

Noyes, J. 1999. The impact of knowing your child is critically ill: a qualitative study of mothers' experiences. *Journal of Advanced Nursing* **29** (2), 427–35.

Parker, L.J. 1999. Current recommendations for isolation practices in nursing. *British Journal of Nursing* **8**, 881–7.

Peplau, H.E. 1988. *Interpersonal Relations in Nursing: A Conceptual Frame of Reference for Psychodynamic Nursing.* London: Macmillan.

Trounce, J. 1997. *Clinical Pharmacology for Nurses*, 15th edn. London: Churchill Livingstone.

United Kingdom Central Council 1992. *Guidelines for Professional Practice.* London: UKCC.

Willlis, J. 1999. IV therapy: an expanding role with implications for education. *Nursing Times* **95** (25), 48–9.

Index

Page numbers in **bold** refer to figures and page numbers in *italic* refer to tables

Index

Index

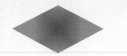

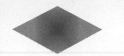

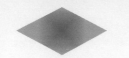

Index